8th International Symposium on
THERAPEUTIC ULTRASOUND

To learn more about AIP Conference Proceedings, including the Conference Proceedings Series, please visit the webpage **http://proceedings.aip.org/proceedings**

8th International Symposium on
THERAPEUTIC ULTRASOUND

Minneapolis, Minnesota   *10 – 13 September 2008*

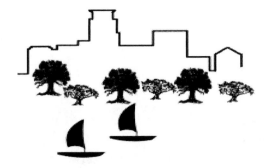

EDITOR

Emad S. Ebbini
University of Minnesota
Minneapolis, Minnesota

All papers have been peer reviewed

SPONSORING ORGANIZATIONS
International Society for Therapeutic Ultrasound
Imasonic
SuperSonic Imagine
Onda Corporation
EDAP
JJA-Instruments
Phillips
Focused Ultrasound Surgery Foundation
China Medical Technologies

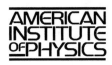

Melville, New York, 2009
AIP CONFERENCE PROCEEDINGS ■ VOLUME 1113

Sep/ue
PHYS

Editor:

Emad S. Ebbini
Department of Electrical and Computer Engineering
University of Minnesota
EECS Building - Room 4-174
200 Union Street S.E.
Minneapolis, MN 55455-0167

E-mail: emad@umn.edu

L.C. Catalog Card No. 2009923705
ISBN 978-0-7354-0650-6
ISSN 0094-243X
Printed in the United States of America

CONTENTS

1 - ADAPTIVE FOCUSING IN THE PRESENCE OF STRONGLY SCATTERING OBJECTS

2 - BIOLOGICAL EFFECTS

3 - CAVITATION AND BUBBLES

4 - CLINICAL AND PRE-CLINICAL STUDIES

7 - TREATMENT MONITORING AND GUIDANCE

8 - QUALITY ASSURANCE

9 - THERAPEUTIC DEVICES

Preface

The International Society for Therapeutic Ultrasound held its 8th annual symposium in Minneapolis in 2008. Since their inception in 2001, ISTU meetings have provided a much needed forum that brought together scientists, engineers, and medical practitioners interested the advancement of the basic science, system and device technology, and clinical application of therapeutic ultrasound. While certain aspects of therapeutic ultrasound research have been prominently featured in a number of international meetings over the last two decades, the ISTU meetings play a unique role in showcasing the depth and breadth of therapeutic ultrasound research worldwide. The ISTU 2008 meeting in Minneapolis fulfilled its role of providing researchers from Asia, Europe and North America to present their latest results and share ideas on the latest developments in the field. The meeting featured 12 invited talks from leading researchers covering topics from the basic science of therapeutic ultrasound to the latest advances in system and device technology and clinical applications. In addition, 167 contributed abstracts were defended in oral and poster formats during the three-day meeting. These included 51 abstracts with a student as a lead author, an encouraging sign of the health and vitality of ISTU and the field of therapeutic ultrasound.

Several ISTU meetings have recognized some of the early pioneers who have contributed to the basic science of the therapeutic ultrasound. The ISTU 2008 meeting recognized Professor Floyd Dunn for his outstanding contributions on the bioeffects and biophysics of ultrasound. This award was named the William and Francis Fry Award and was presented to Professor Dunn by Professor William D. O'Brien, Jr. from the University of Illinois at Urbana-Champaign. On behalf of the ISTU Board, I would like to thank Professor Dunn for coming to Minneapolis to receive this recognition and Professor O'Brien for presenting him with the award. We were honored by the presence of the second and third generation scientists following the tradition of the first generation scientists whose names grace this award.

For the first time the ISTU 2008 Organizing Committee instituted the ISTU Early Career Award, which was approved by the ISTU Board in its meeting on September 11, 2008. Professor Lawrence Crum chaired a committee that included Dr. Katsuro Tachibana and Dr. Gail ter Haar selected Dr. Michael Bailey as the recipient of the 2008 ISTU Early Career Award from a list of 12 candidates who applied or were nominated for this award. Having observed the selection process, I am proud of the quality of our young members and their potential for great achievements in the future. I can also attest to the difficulty of the committee's task in making the final selection as the quality of the top candidates was quite high. I would like to express my deepest gratitude for Professor Crum and the committee for accepting this hard task under less-than-favorable circumstances to make the selection. Congratulations to Dr. Bailey on being the first recipient of the ISTU Early Career Award.

Following the tradition of previous ISTU meetings, a student paper competition was held at ISTU 2008, which was organized by a committee co-chaired by Professor Nadine Barrie-Smith (Penn State) and Dr. Ralf Seip (Philips Research). In addition to the co-chairs, Dr. Jessica Foley (Insightec), Professor Jahan Tavakkoli (Bryson University), and Dr. Balasundar Raju (Philips Research) participated as judges. Fifteen finalists were selected before the meeting and were asked to prepare poster presentations of their papers. These posters were judged on September 11 and 12 and the winners were announced at the Symposium Banquet on September 12. The winners were Lisa Treat (Harvard), Caroline Maleke (Columbia, 2nd), Charles Caskey (University of California Davis, 3rd). Congratulations to the winners and many thanks for the selection committee on a job well done.

The lasting legacy of any scientific meeting is in its proceedings that will make the research findings available to the larger scientific community. We have received nearly 98 manuscripts for inclusion in the proceedings of ISTU 2008, of which we have accepted 86. These papers were organized in the following categories:

- Bioeffects
- Cavitation and Bubbles
- Drug and Gene Delivery
- Therapeutic Systems and Device Technology
- Treatment Planning and Modeling
- Treatment Monitoring and Guidance
- Adaptive Focusing
- Quality Assurance
- *In Vivo* Animal Studies
- Clinical and Pre-clinical Studies

It is hoped that you will find these papers useful, both in terms of providing a good view of the state-of-the-art for therapeutic ultrasound and special relevance to your research and/or application interests. I would like to thank all the authors who have contributed their manuscripts for publication consideration in the proceedings. I also would like to take this opportunity to thank the Technical Program Committee (Dr. Katsuro Tachibana and Professor Chris Diederich, Co-Chairs) on their efforts in reviewing the abstracts and their suggestions regarding session organization.

ISTU 2008 and these proceedings would not have been possible without the tireless efforts of a number of colleagues at the University of Minnesota. I would like to especially thank my students Yayun Wan, John Ballard, Dalong Liu and Andrew Casper. They have exceeded every expectation and made vital contribution to this effort at every juncture. We have also received generous staff support from the Department of Electrical and Computer Engineering and the Institute of Engineering in Medicine at the University. I would like to especially thank Ms. Jeanine Maiden for her extraordinary efforts with budget issue during the University transition to a new electronic fund management system which presented us with significant challenges. I also would like to acknowledge Ms. Jessica Schynoll for her efforts on maintaining e-mail list for ISTU 2008. On behalf of these and other dedicated individuals who helped with this effort, it has been our pleasure seeing you in Minneapolis and bringing you the proceedings of the meeting.

Finally, I would like to thank the members of the ISTU Board for giving us the opportunity to organize ISTU 2008 in Minneapolis. We are also grateful to all of our sponsors who made it possible to cover the costs of the proceedings and subsidize the registration of students and invited speakers. This support was absolutely critical for this meeting and we hope they will continue to support future ISTU meetings. Speaking of future ISTU meetings, ISTU 2009 will be held in Aix en Provence September 23 - 26, 2009 (http://www.istu2009.org) . We hope to see you there.

Sincerely,

Proceedings Editor
ISTU 2008 General Chair

ISTU 2008 Committee Membership

ISTU Board

ISTU 2008 Scientific Advisory Committee

- Kullervo Hynynen, PhD President
- Emmanuel Blanc
- Jean-Yves Chapelon, PhD
- Constantin Coussios, PhD
- Emad Ebbini, PhD
- Vera Khokhlova, PhD
- Narendra Sanghvi, MSEE
- Jacques Souquet, PhD
- Katsuro Tachibana, MD, PhD
- Gail ter Haar, PhD
- Z. Wan, PhD
- David Wild
- Bradford Wood, MD
- Feng Wu. MD, PhD

New Members

- Chris Diederich, PhD
- Katherine Ferrara, PhD
- Gerald Harris, PhD
- Joo Ha Hwang, MD, PhD
- Ralf Seip, PhD
- Toyoaki Uchida, MD

Early Career Award

- Lawrence Crum, Chair
- Gail ter Haar
- Katsuro Tachibana

Student Competition Award

- Nadine Barrie-Smith, co-Chair
- Ralf Seip, co-Chair
- Jessica Foley
- alasundar Raju
- Jahan Takkavoli

Technical Program Committee

- Chris Diederich, PhD Technical Chair
- Katsuro Tachibana, MD, PhD, Clinical Chair
- Michael Bailey, PhD
- Timothy Bigelow, PhD
- Gregory Clement, PhD
- Constantin Coussios, PhD
- Lawrence Crum, PhD
- Emad Ebbini, PhD
- Gerard Fleury, PhD
- Jessica Foley, PhD
- Brian Fowlkes, PhD
- Victor Frenkel, PhD
- Kullervo Hynynen, PhD
- Vera Khokhlova, PhD
- Elisa Konofagou, PhD
- Cyril Lafon, PhD
- Robert McGough, PhD
- David Melodelima, PhD
- Robert Muratore, PhD
- Narendra Sanghvi, MSEE
- Ralf Seip, PhD
- Nadine Smith, PhD
- Sham Sokka, PhD
- Jacques Souquet, PhD
- Mickael Tanter, PhD
- Gail ter Haar, PhD
- Vesna Zderic, PhD

Local Organizing Committee

- Emad Ebbini, Chair
- John Ballard
- Andrew Casper
- Dalong Liu
- Jeanine Maiden
- Jessica Schynoll
- Yayun Wan

AWARDS

The William J. and Francis J. Fry Award

Presented to Professor Floyd Dunn in recognition of outstanding contributions in the area of bioeffects and biophysics of ultrasound. Professor Dunn received his PhD in 1956 from the University of Illinois. His PhD dissertation entitled "Determination of Ultrasonic Dosage Relations for the Mammalian Central Nervous System," was obtained under the guidance of Professor W.J. Fry. Professor Dunn joined the faculty of the University of Illinois be-

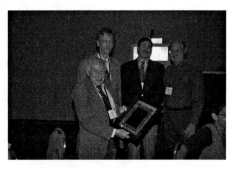

tween 1956 and 1996 and he is currently Professor Emeritus. His research interests are in the investigation of the ultrasonic propagation properties of living systems, viz., velocity, attenuation, absorption, scattering, impedance; study of the physical mechanisms of interaction of ultrasound and biological media, viz., thermal, cavitation, other mechanical mechanisms; ultrasonic toxicology; ultrasonic dosimetry; measurement of ultrasonic fields in liquid and liquid-like media and development of measurement and sound field production instrumentation; and ultrasonic microscopy.

Professor Dunn has collaborated internationally with researchers in Japan, United Kindom and China and held visiting professorships at several international institutions. He has also received major awards from the Acoustical Society of America, the institute of Electrical and Electronic Engineering, the American Institute of Ultrasound in Medicine, and American Cancer Society. He is a fellow of the Acoustical Society of America, the American Institute of Ultrasound and Medicine, the Institute of Electrical and Electronic Engineering, American Association for the Advancement of Science, the Institute of Acoustics (UK), and the American Institute For Medical and Biological Engineering. He is a member of both the National Academy of Engineering and the National Academy of Sciences.

The ISTU 2008 Early Career Award

Presented to Dr. Michael Bailey, Center of Industrial and Medical Ultrasound (CIMU), University of Washington. Dr. Bailey's strong publication record and numerous contributions to the biophysics of lithotripsy were cited by the letter writers and the selection committee. The award was presented by Dr. Kullervo Hynynen, the President of the Board, on September 12, 2008.

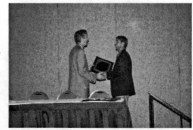

The ISTU 2008 Student Competition Winners

First Prize Lisa Treat (Harvard-MIT Health Sciences and Technology, US): Impact of Focused Ultrasound-Enhanced Drug Delivery on Survival in Rats with Glioma.

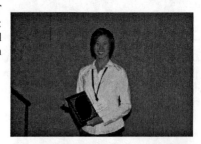

Second Prize Caroline Maleke (Columbia University, US): Real-time HIFU Monitoring Using Harmonic Motion Imaging (HMI).

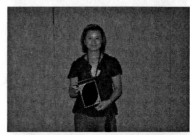

Third Prize Charles Caskey (University of California at Davis, US): Observation of Microbubbles in Gel Phantom Helps Identify Important Factors in Developing Safe Contrast-based Delivery Techniques.

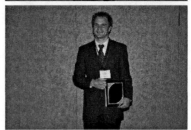

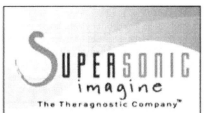
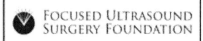
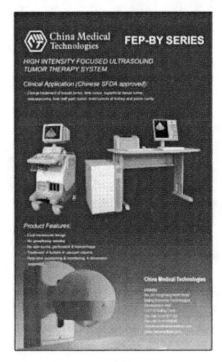

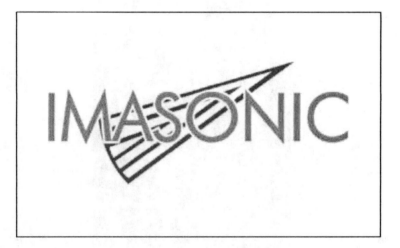

ADAPTIVE FOCUSING IN THE PRESENCE OF STRONGLY SCATTERING OBJECTS

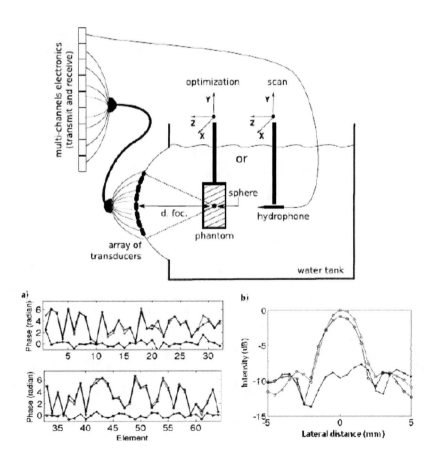

Standing wave suppression for transcranial ultrasound by random-modulation

Sai Chun Tang and Gregory T. Clement

Focused Ultrasound Laboratory, Department of Radiology,
Brigham and Women's Hospital, Harvard Medical School,
221 Longwood Avenue, Boston, MA 02115.

Low frequency transcranial ultrasound (<1MHz) is being investigated for a number of brain therapies, including stroke, tumor ablation, and localized opening of the blood brain barrier. However, lower frequencies have been associated with the production of undesired standing waves in the brain. Presently, we examine an approach to suppress standing waves during continuous wave transcranial application. This investigation uses a small randomization in the frequency content of the signal for suppressing standing waves. The approach is compared to single-frequency continuous wave operation as well as to a sweep-frequency input. Acoustic field scans within an *ex-vivo* human skull demonstrate the near-elimination of standing waves using the randomized input signal. It is expected that the process may play a critical role in providing a safer application of the ultrasound field in the brain and may have application in other areas where standing waves may be created.

Keywords: Standing wave suppression, transcranial ultrasound, random frequency modulation.
PACS: 87.50.yt

I. INTRODUCTION

Transcranial ultrasound has demonstrated the potential to serve as a therapeutic tool in the treatment of a range of disorders [1]. High-intensity focused ultrasound (HIFU) therapies include ablation for the treatment of tumors [2], [3], with the additional potential to treat Parkinson's disease [4], and other conditions [5]. Substantial clinical promise has further been shown in the enhancement of tissue plasminogen activator (tPA) for thrombolysis in stroke treatment [6]-[8]. Moreover, the ability for ultrasound to locally open the blood brain barrier (BBB) presents the prospect of using ultrasound to assist in delivering drugs to targeted regions in the brain [9].

Each of these therapies requires ultrasound penetration through the skull, which distorts and attenuates the beam. These deleterious effects caused by the skull become successively more severe with increasing frequency due to increased attenuation. Conversely, submegahertz frequencies - particularly frequencies below ~500 kHz [10], [11] - have been shown to pass through the skull with relatively small aberration. This property of submegahertz ultrasound has led to low-frequency studies for ablative treatments [12], sonothrombolysis, and opening of the BBB [13].

Low frequency ultrasound, however, can be associated with certain risks for adverse bioeffects. There is also an increased potential of inducing standing waves [14] as a result of longer wavelengths and reduced absorption in the brain tissue. The

CP1113, *8th International Symposium on Therapeutic Ultrasound,* edited by E. S. Ebbini
© 2009 American Institute of Physics 978-0-7354-0650-6/09/$25.00

occurrence of such standing waves at and away from the therapeutic target locations has been suggested as a source of hemorrhaging during low frequency transcranial thrombolysis [15]-[17]. Motivated by these observations, as well as the use of similar frequencies for opening the BBB [13] and ablating tumors [12], we examine an approach for eliminating standing waves in the skull during continuous wave (CW), or near-CW application of ultrasound. We hypothesize that small randomization in the frequency content of the application signal is sufficient to significantly reduce or eliminate standing waves. In this manner, the randomization will cause a break in the ultrasound symmetry between forward and reflected waves that does not allow standing waves to establish. It is further predicted that, given a sufficient spread in bandwidth, intensity fluctuations in the nearfield will be homogenized as a result of the frequency dependence on the spatial locations of nulls in the field. Frequency sweeps have long been understood to reduce the effects of standing waves, and have been implemented in various ultrasound products, such as ultrasonic cleaners [18]. Recently, suppression of standing waves has been investigated using a frequency chirp. Mitri et al. [19] used this approach to suppress standing waves in vibro-acoustography. Erpelding et al. [20] used a similar approach to inhibit standing waves in bubble-based radiation force measurements. Building on these previous studies, we compare the present randomized approach to the frequency sweep with similar frequency content.

II. MATERIALS AND METHODS

A. Signal generation

A 250 kHz piezoelectric transducer with 50mm diameter and 10cm radius of curvature was used to generate all acoustic fields. Two different signal types were generated in order to compare the efficacy of the acoustic standing wave suppression. In the first signal, the frequency was swept linearly with time by modulating a carrier signal with a lower frequency triangular wave. This sweep signal was created by feeding a triangular wave with a frequency of 3.9 kHz from a function generator to another function generator that modulated the 250 kHz carrier frequency with the input triangular signal. The second signal was created by modulating a carrier signal with a random noise signal so that the instantaneous frequency deviated from the center frequency in a random manner. This random-signal-modulated signal was generated by a circuit built in-house. This circuit consisted of a voltage-controlled-oscillator with a center frequency of 250 kHz and a bandwidth of 50k Hz (±10% of the center frequency) fed by a random noise modulation signal. Likewise, the center frequency and bandwidth of the swept signals were 250 kHz and 50 kHz. Both signals were amplified by an RF power amplifier. Control experiments with single-frequency CW excitation at 250 kHz without modulation were also performed. Voltages across the transducer excited by the spread-spectrum (sweep and random) and the single-frequency signals were set to 10V RMS and measured by an oscilloscope. As explained in the next section, the number of waveforms acquired for averaging for the sweep and the random frequency are 10 and 100 respectively.

B. Acoustic field scan experiments

The experiments were carried out inside a tank filled with degassed de-ionized water. The tank was lined with rubber sheets to reduce reflections from the walls. A 1mm diameter PVDF needle hydrophone was used to sense the acoustic pressure within an *ex-vivo* human skull. The needle hydrophone was mounted on a three-axis positioning system controlled by a PC and was aligned 45° with respect to the ultrasound propagation direction. The transducer axis of symmetry was chosen as the Cartesian z-axis, with the origin at the center of the transducer. The transducer was respectively excited by the spread-spectrum signals and the single-frequency signal then amplified by an RF power amplifier. The transducer excitation voltage was set to 10Vrms. Acoustic field patterns were scanned over the x-z plane (y=0) for the swept, random, and single-frequency CW signals. The hydrophone was scanned from (x,z) = (-30mm,20mm) to (30mm,70mm) with a spatial resolution of 0.5mm in both dimensions for the sweep and single-frequency CW signals. The length of the waveform data at each hydrophone position for the single and sweep-frequency signals were 2ms and 10ms respectively. The spatial resolution and the length of the waveform data for the random-signal-modulation were 1mm and 100ms respectively. The number of sample points per each waveform frame was set to 10^4 and the oscilloscope sample rate was 10 Mega Samples/second so that the time length of each waveform frame was 1ms. The acquired waveforms were transferred to the PC through a GPIB cable.

III. RESULTS

The averaged acoustic field on the x-z plane (y=0) inside an *ex-vivo* human cranium are shown in Fig. 1. The plots show the relative pressure field represented by the hydrophone voltage in linear scale. Ten and a hundred data frames were used for averaging the rms values of the sweep and the random-frequency signal, respectively, at each hydrophone position. The field patterns shown in the figure illustrate that the sweep-frequency method provided an improvement on the reduction of the standing wave effect compared to the single-frequency excitation. However, the standing wave effect with the sweep excitation was still clearly visible. The acoustic field scan on the x-z plane inside the cranium with the random-modulation excitation, as shown in Fig. 1c, reveals that applying the random-modulation scheme substantially suppresses the standing wave effect in the ultrasound main beam (|x|<5mm). An inconspicuous standing wave effect was observed outside the main beam, but the intensity was significantly lower than that inside the main ultrasound beam. Both the average and the peak intensity at x=-15mm (outside the main beam) were more than 3 times less than that at x=0mm (inside the main ultrasound beam) from z = 40m to 60mm.

IV. DISCUSSION

Random modulation of the driving frequency was found to be highly effective in eliminating standing waves. One metric of this success is a comparison of the

5

amplitude peak, p_{max}, to minimum, p_{min}, over a region with the average amplitude of p_{avg}. We examined the value

$$R = \frac{p_{max} - p_{min}}{p_{avg}} \qquad (1)$$

along the axis of propagation between 40 mm and 60 mm from the transducer face after propagating through both the plate and the skull. In the plastic plates, with the 250 kHz single-frequency CW signal the ratio was R= 0.354, for the sweep-frequency the ratio was R= 0.102, and for the random-signal modulation it was R=0.063. A similar trend was recorded in the skull where the single-frequency ratio was R= 0.276, for the sweep-frequency the ratio was R= 0.174, and for the random-signal the ratio was R=0.135. Care was taken to assure accurate comparison between the sweep and the random spread-spectrum techniques. Signal content was directly monitored from the voltage input to the transducer so that the signals of the sweep and random-frequency inputs were verified to match in spectra as closely as possible. The aim of the study was to test the ability of random-frequency modulations introduced into the input signal of an ultrasound emitter to inhibit standing waves in the human skull. The approach was examined at 250 kHz, due to the frequency's direct implications from recent studies in transcranial tumor ablation, sonothrombolysis and targeted opening of the blood brain barrier. The method, however, is expected to readily generalize to any application where it would be advantageous to eliminate standing waves.

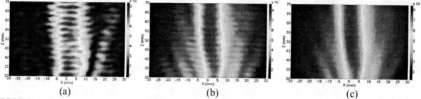

(a)   (b)   (c)

FIGURE 1. Measured hydrophone rms voltage on the x-z plane in an *ex-vivo* human cranium when the transducer was excited by the signal with (a) single frequency, (b) sweep frequency, and (c) random-signal modulation.

V. CONCLUSION

Experiments have indicated the effect of inducing random-frequency modulations on ultrasound standing waves. Results indicate the approach's ability to inhibit standing waves both within a human skull, as well as within a plastic cavity of parallel walls. The random approach was found to be superior to the established swept-frequency method. The method may have application in stroke treatment, transcranial ablative therapies and in studies using ultrasound to open the blood brain barrier. Application is further expected to translate to an assortment of situations where suppression of standing waves is desired.

ACKNOWLEDGMENTS

This work was supported by NIH grants U41 RR019703 and R01 EB003268.

REFERENCES

1. K. Hynynen and G. Clement, "Clinical applications of focused ultrasound - The brain," Int J Hyperthermia, vol. 23, no. 2, pp. 193-202, 2007.
2. G. T. Clement, P. J. White, R. L. King, N. McDannold, and K. Hynynen, "A magnetic resonance imaging-compatible, large-scale array for trans-skull ultrasound surgery and therapy," J Ultrasound in Med, vol. 24, no. 8, pp. 1117-1125, 2005.
3. K. Hynynen, N. McDannold, G. Clement, F. A. Jolesz, E. Zadicario, R. Killiany, T. Moore, and D. Rosen, "Pre-clinical testing of a phased array ultrasound system for MRI-guided noninvasive surgery of the brain - A primate study," Eur J Radiology, vol. 59, no. 2, pp. 149-156, 2006.
4. W. J. Fry and F. J. Fry, "Fundamental neurological research and human neurosurgery using intense ultrasound," IRE Trans Med Electron, ME-7, pp. 166-181, 1960.
5. W. J. Fry, "Ultrasound in neurology," Neurology, vol. 6, no. 10, pp. 693-704, 1956.
6. M. Daffertshofer and M. Fatar, "Therapeutic ultrasound in ischemic stroke treatment: experimental evidence," Eur J Ultrasound, vol. 16, no. 1-2, pp. 121-130, 2002.
7. R. Mikulik and A. V. Alexandrov, "Acute stroke: therapeutic transcranial Doppler sonography," Front Neurol Neurosci, vol. 21, pp. 150-161, 2006.
8. H. Kawata, N. Naya, Y. Takemoto, S. Uemura, T. Nakajima, M. Horii, Y. Takeda, S. Fujimoto, A. Yamashita, Y. Asada, and Y. Saito, "Ultrasound accelerates thrombolysis of acutely induced platelet-rich thrombi similar to those in acute myocardial infarction," Circ J, vol. 71, no. 10, pp. 1643-1648, 2007.
9. K. Hynynen, N. McDannold, N. Vykhodtseva, and F. A. Jolesz, "Noninvasive MR imaging-guided focal opening of the blood-brain barrier in rabbits," Radiology, vol. 220, no. 3, pp. 640-646, 2001.
10. A. Y. Ammi, T. D. Mast, I. H. Huang, T. A. Abruzzo, C. C. Coussios, G. J. Shaw, and C. K. Holland, "Characterization of ultrasound propagation through ex vivo human temporal bone," Ultrasound Med Biol, vol. 34, no. 10, pp. 1578-1589, 2008.
11. F. J. Fry, S. A. Goss, and J. T. Patrick, "Transkull focal lesions in cat brain produced by ultrasound," J Neurosurg, vol. 54, no. 5, pp. 659-663, 1981.
12. N. McDannold, E. Zadicario, M. C. Pilatou, and F. A. Jolesz, "Preclinical testing of a second-generation MRI-guided focused ultrasound system for transcranial brain tumor ablation," Proc 16th Scientific Meeting, International Society for Magnetic Resonance in Medicine, 2008.
13. K. Hynynen, N. McDannold, N. Vykhodtseva, S. Raymond, R. Weissleder, F. A. Jolesz, and N. Sheikov, "Focal disruption of the blood-brain barrier due to 260-kHz ultrasound bursts: a method for molecular imaging and targeted drug delivery," J Neurosurg, vol. 105, no. 3, pp. 445-454, 2006.
14. T. Azuma, K. Kawabata, S. Umemura, M. Ogihara, J. Kubota, A. Sasaki, and H. Furuhata, "Schlieren observation of therapeutic field in water surrounded by cranium radiated from 500 kHz ultrasonic sector transducer," Proc IEEE Ultrason Symp, vol. 2, pp. 1001-1004, 2004.
15. M. Daffertshofer, A. Gass, P. Ringleb, M. Sitzer, U. Sliwka, T. Els, O. Sedlaczek, W. J. Koroshetz, and M. G. Hennerici, "Transcranial low-frequency ultrasound-mediated thrombolysis in brain ischemia: increased risk of hemorrhage with combined ultrasound and tissue plasminogen activator: results of a phase II clinical trial," Stroke, vol. 36, no. 7, pp. 1441-1446, 2005.
16. W. C. Culp and T. C. McCowan, "Ultrasound Augmented Thrombolysis," Current Med Imaging Reviews, vol. 1, no. 1, pp. 5-12, 2005.
17. J. F. Aubry and M. Fink, "Transcranial Ultrasound-Mediated Thrombolysis: Safety Issue," Proc 7th Int Symp on Therapeutic Ultrasound, 2007.
18. B. Louis and G. B. Long, "Sonic washer," US Patent 2985003, 1961.
19. F. G. Mitri, J. F, Greenleaf, and M. Fatemi, "Chirp imaging vibro-acoustography for removing the ultrasound standing wave artifact," IEEE Trans Med Imaging, vol. 24, no. 10, pp. 1249-1255, 2005.
20. T. N. Erpelding, K. W. Hollman, and M. O'Donnell, "Bubble-based acoustic radiation force using chirp insonation to reduce standing wave effects," Ultrasound Med Biol, vol. 33, no. 2, pp. 263-269, 2007.

Energy-Based Adaptive Focusing of waves: Application to Ultrasonic Transcranial Therapy

E. Herbert, M. Pernot, G. Montaldo, M. Tanter and M. Fink

Laboratoire Ondes et Acoustique ESPCI, CNRS UMR 7587, INSERM
10, rue vauquelin 75005 Paris, FRANCE

Abstract. We propose a general concept of adaptive focusing through complex media based on the estimation or measurement of the wave energy density at the desired focal spot. As it does not require the knowledge of phase information, this technique has many potential applications in acoustics and optics for light focusing through diffusive media. We present here the application of this technique to the problem of ultrasonic aberration correction for HIFU treatments. The estimation of wave energy density is based on the maximization of the ultrasound radiation force, using a multi-elements (64) array. A spatial coded excitation method is developed by using *ad-hoc* virtual transducers that include all the elements for each emission. The radiation force is maximized by optimizing the displacement of a small target at the focus. We measured the target displacement using ultrasound pulse echo on the same elements. A method using spatial coded excitation is developed in order to estimate the phase and amplitude aberration based on the target displacement. We validated this method using phase aberration up to 2π. The phase correction is achieved and the pressure field is measured using a needle hydrophone. The acoustic intensity at the focus is restored through very large aberrations. Basic experiments for brain HIFU treatment are presented. Optimal transcranial adaptive focusing is performed using a limited number of short ultrasonic radiation force pushes.

Keywords: Adaptive focusing, aberrations, focused ultrasound, transcranial therapy, HIFU
PACS: 42.15, 43.80

INTRODUCTION

High Intensity Focused Ultrasound (HIFU) brain therapy has been highly limited by the distortions of the ultrasonic wavefront induced by the skull bone [1]. Large phase aberrations induced by a strong discrepancy of the speed of sound between brain tissues and the skull bone lead to a drastic decrease of the acoustic intensity at the focus and a potential shift of the focus location. In the past decade, several techniques based on time reversal or phase conjugation have been developed in order to restore a sharp focus through the skull [2]. These techniques rely on the use of the wave propagation simulation through the skull guided by a prior CT-scan of the skull bone. These techniques allow restoring a good focus in the brain, but are time consuming and are not fully optimal due to modeling and positioning errors.

In this paper, we propose a new aberration correction approach that is practicable *in-vivo* and fully optimal. Contrary to the previous techniques, our method does not require the measurement of Green's function through the skull bone. The principle

CP1113, *8th International Symposium on Therapeutic Ultrasound*, edited by E. S. Ebbini
© 2009 American Institute of Physics 978-0-7354-0650-6/09/$25.00

relies on the non-invasive estimation of the wave energy at a desired location through the radiation force effect. Urban et al. [2] proposed recently the use of the radiation force as a method for improving the focusing of a phased array through heterogeneous medium. The basic principle relies on the idea that the optimization of the focusing at a target location can be achieved through the maximization of the mechanical excitation induced by the radiation force. They developed an iterative technique that worked successfully with a few elements (16).

Based on a different approach, we have developed a novel aberration correction technique based on the estimation of the wave energy. This general method estimates the phase corrections that maximize the energy deposition using a limited number of spatial coded excitations. Here, this technique is applied to the problem of transcranial focusing. Experiments are first performed through an ex vivo human skull in order to demonstrate the potential of this technique to restore the focusing. Secondly, the aberration correction technique is performed based on local motion induced by the radiation force in order to estimate the wave energy. As shown in this paper, this technique is fully optimal to restore non-invasively a sharp focus, can be applied to a large number of elements with a good accuracy and allows a strong reduction of the acquisition time.

THEORY

In this technique, the optimization of the intensity at the target is achieved through maximization of the acoustic radiation force at the same point. The local force per unit of volume generated by an ultrasound beam in tissues can be written as:

$$\mathbf{f} = 2\alpha I \mathbf{e}_z / c \tag{1}$$

where I is the acoustic intensity, α is the absorption coefficient of the tissue and c is the speed of sound and ez is the direction of the wave propagation. Let's assume that two transducers are transmitting a continuous wave at the same frequency ω towards the focus though an aberrator. If the respective waves received at the focal point are expressed as $s_1(t) = ae^{i(\omega t)}$ and $s_2(t) = be^{i(\omega t + \varphi)}$, the total intensity at the focus is given by:

$$I = a^2 + b^2 + 2ab\cos\varphi = A + B\cos\varphi \tag{2}$$

In order to determine the phase aberration φ, an additional phase shift x is introduced between the two transducers on the emission signals. When x is varied, the intensity becomes modulated as a cosine function:

$$I(x) = A + B\cos(\varphi + x) \tag{3}$$

Thus, by measuring I(x) for at least three different x in the range $[0;2\pi]$, the three unknowns A, B and φ can be retrieved by solving the equation system.

However, this method cannot be applied directly to the problem of large phased arrays, due to the fact that two small elements cannot generate enough radiation force at the focal point. In order to use this technique with a large number of small elements, it is necessary to combine all the small individual elements into large "virtual elements".

9

Linear combinations of the elements are performed using the Hadamard matrix H_{ij}. The "virtual elements" T_i are composed of all the individual elements S_j and can be expressed as:

$$T_i = H_{ij}S_j = \begin{bmatrix} 1 & 1 & 1 & 1 & ... \\ 1 & -1 & 1 & -1 & ... \\ 1 & 1 & -1 & -1 & ... \\ 1 & -1 & -1 & 1 & ... \\ : & : & : & : & ... \end{bmatrix} S_j \qquad (4)$$

It is then possible to use the technique described before using couples of elements T_i, to determine the phase aberration between the elements T_i. A reference element T_{ref} is arbitrary chosen, and the phase shifts between all the elements and T_{ref} are determined by estimating the intensity for at least three additional phase shifts. Once the aberrations have been determined for the virtual elements, the phase aberration of the "real elements" S_i is computed by inverting H_{ij}.

$$S_j = H_{ij}^{-1}T_i \qquad (5)$$

This method requires estimating the intensity for a number of emission equals to 3 times the number of elements N. For each emission the intensity is estimated by the measurement of the displacement induced by radiation force.

CORRECTION OF SKULL BONE ABERRATIONS

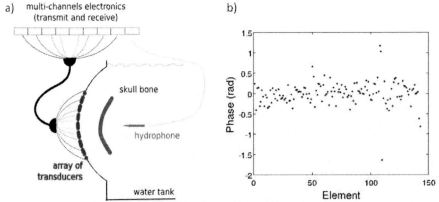

FIGURE 1. a) Experimental setup b) Phase estimation error

In this part, the feasibility of using this technique for correcting aberrations induced by a skull bone is shown. 145 elements of a large 300 element high power array were used. The individual elements (8-mm in diameter) working at a central frequency of 1 MHz are driven by a multichannel transmit electronics. The phased array is spherically curved and is naturally focused at a focal depth of 140 mm. An ex vivo degassed human skull bone was placed in a water tank in front of the transducer. A needle hydrophone (PZT-Z44-0400 Onda Corp) was set at the focus of the array (see Fig. 1.a).

A short burst of 10µs was transmitted successively on each element and received on the hydrophone to determine the phase and amplitude aberrations. Then, the aberration correction technique was performed using the hydrophone: the appropriate combinations of signals were successively transmitted by the array and received by the hydrophone. The amplitudes of the received signals were determined, squared and used as the measurement of the acoustic intensity for the aberration process. After transmitting the 145x3 different emissions, the optimal phase was determined for each element of the array using the Eq (4). Fig. 1.b) shows an excellent agreement of the phase correction by this method and the real phase aberration measured by the hydrophone. A standard deviation of 0.28 radians was measured, which demonstrate the efficiency of the technique.

RADIATION FORCE BASED ABERRATION CORRECTION

In this part, it is shown that the acoustic radiation force can be used instead of the hydrophone to estimate the intensity of the beam for the aberration correction process. Because the electronics has only 64 channels working both in transmit and receive, only 64 elements of the phased array were used. A tissue mimicking phantom was placed at the focus of the array with a small stainless steel sphere (diameter 1.5 mm) embedded in the center of the phantom (Fig. 2). In this part, the skull bone was removed due to the high attenuation that prevents doing pulse echo imaging. However, it was simulated using a strong numerical aberrator set on each channel.

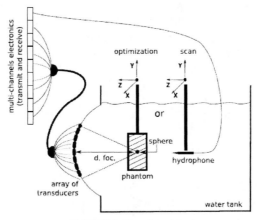

FIGURE 2. Experimental setup

The experiment consisted first in performing a pulse echo sequence in order to image the target position. Secondly, a burst of 400 µs of ultrasound at 1 MHz was transmitted using the appropriate combinations of signals computed from the Hadamard matrix. This burst generated enough radiation force to induce a small displacement of the sphere position (on the order of 10μm). Finally, following immediately the push a new pulse echo sequence was transmitted to image the new displacement of the target. A conventional speckle tracking technique was used on the consecutive echo signals to estimate the target displacement. The last step consisted in using these measurements in order to retrieve the phase aberrations form Eq.4. Figure 3.a shows the excellent agreement between the aberrator and the phase estimated by our technique. Fig.3.b displays a plot of the beam lateral profile, that shows that the focus is completely restored using our technique.

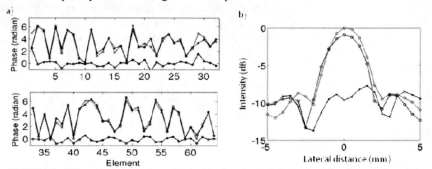

FIGURE 3. a) Numerical phase aberration (red line), estimated phase aberration (blue line), and the difference (black line). b) Lateral beam profile with no aberrations (red), with aberrations (black) and after correction (blue).

CONCLUSION

A new aberration correction technique was developed based on the estimation of the wave energy deposition at a target location. This method is very general and can be applied to many phase aberration problems in ultrasound, optics or other type of waves in medium where Green's functions are not accessible easily. In this paper, the problem of transcranial ultrasonic focusing was investigated. The feasibility of correcting the skull bone aberrations using acoustic radiation force was demonstrated. In practical situation, motion induced by the radiation force can be detected using motion sensitive MR sequences [4]. MR guided HIFU therapy of the brain should benefit greatly from this technique.

REFERENCES

1. FJ Fry and JE Barger Acoustical properties of the human skull *J. Acoust. Soc. Am.* **63** 1978 1576–90
2. M. Pernot, JF Aubry, M Tanter, JL Thomas and M Fink "High power transcranial beam steering for ultrasonic brain therapy." *Physics in medicine and biology*, 48 (3) 2003, pp. 2577-2589.
3. M. Urban, M. Bernal and JF. Greenleaf "Phase aberration correction using ultrasound radiation force and vibrometry optimization", *IEEE transactions Ultrasound ferroelec* freq, 54 (6) 2007
4. Sinkus R, Tanter M, Xydeas T, Catheline S, Bercoff J, Fink M. Viscoelastic shear properties of *in vivo* breast lesions measured by MR elastography. J. Magn. Reson. Imaging. 2005;23:159–65

Image-Based Refocusing of Dual-Mode Ultrasound Arrays (DMUAs) in the Presence of Strongly Scattering Objects

John R. Ballard, Andrew J. Casper, Yayun Wan and Emad S. Ebbini

Department of Electrical and Computer Engineering, University of Minnesota

Abstract. An advantage of imaging with DMUAs is the potential for identifying target and critical regions in the treatment field for avoidance. Refocusing of the therapeutic beam in the presence of strongly scattering objects, such as the ribs, while targeting liver tumors is of particular importance due to limited access and distortion of the HIFU beam. An image-based refocusing algorithm utilizing gray-scaled images obtained with single-transmit focus imaging allows for selection of control points to be taken from the visible target and ribs in the image. Using a two-step virtual array method to take advantage of the intercostal spacing of the ribs, the algorithm minimizes the power deposition over the critical regions while maintaining or improving the power deposition at the target location. The algorithm is verified experimentally with a 64-element 1MHz array, in an attenuating tissue mimicking phantom (.5 dB/cm/MHz) with Plexiglas ribs. Thermocouples are used to measure sub-therapeutic temperatures across the ribs and at the target location. An increase of temperature at the target location of 20% is measured, with a decrease of 30% across the ribs. In addition, the intensity of the gray-scaled images showed an improvement of 5 dB at the focus with a reduction of 2dB across the ribs. Image-based refocusing is shown to improve distortions of the HIFU beam experienced by strongly scattering objects that partially obstruct the target.

Keywords: DMUA, HIFU, Refocusing, Image-Guided Surgery
PACS: 85.70.yt

INTRODUCTION

Image based algorithms for refocusing phased arrays continues to attract attention as a means of monitoring and guidance for minimally-invasive HIFU therapy. Currently, MRI [1] and diagnostic ultrasound [2] are the most commonly used modalities for image guidance. Registration between the imaging and therapeutic coordinate system is often needed for many image-guided tasks including aberration correction and refocusing around obstacles. However, the recent advances in Piezocomposite technology have led to low cross coupling, high efficiency and larger bandwidth enabling therapeutic arrays to be used in pulse-echo mode [3, 4]. Images obtained with DMUAs have shown to provide suitable feeback for optimal refocusing of the HIFU beams while taking advantage of the inherent self registration of the imaging and therapeutic coordinate systems[5, 6]. These images will allow the attending physician to define critical and target point(s) to minimize and maximize power deposition respectively. In this paper, we outline a proposed constrained optimization methodology proceeded with a presentation of experimental results in a tissue mimicking phantom, including statistics to show the robustness and effectiveness of this approach.

CP1113, *8th International Symposium on Therapeutic Ultrasound*, edited by E. S. Ebbini
© 2009 American Institute of Physics 978-0-7354-0650-6/09/$25.00

MATERIALS AND METHODS

A DMUA system employing amplifier boards and matching circuitry for the DMUA prototype was built and is currently available in our laboratory. The array is a 64-element, 1-MHz, linear concave array on a spherical shell (100 mm radius) has been designed and fabricated using HI-1 Piezocomposite technology[3] for HIFU applications. A Spartan3 FPGA running at a system clock of 200 MHz is used to generate control signals and driving patterns for the DMUA prototype allowing for 100 different magnitude levels and 1.8 degrees of phase resolution for the driving signals. Array elements were connected to a transmitter and a receiver through a diplexer and a 4×64 matrix switch. A pulser/receiver was connected to the receive terminals on the matrix switch with the receiver connected to a 20 Msample/s 23-bit digitizer. Synthetic aperture imaging experiments were performed by connecting an arbitrary waveform generator and a power amplifier to the transmit terminal on the matrix switch.

Refocusing Algorithm design

The gray-scale image based feedback allows for determination of a target and critical points. The objective of refocusing is to maximize the array intensity gain at a target point(s), $\vec{r}_T$, while minimizing across a set of critical points, $\vec{r}_C(i)$, $i = 1, 2, ..., M_c$. This becomes an optimization problem which can be solved using Lagrange multipliers or a regularized minimum-norm least squares solution [7]. An excitation vector from an N-element array to the target location are defined by the array directivity vector at $\vec{h}_T$ as a row vector :

$$\mathbf{h}_t = [h_1(\vec{r}_T), h_2(\vec{r}_T), ..., h_N(\vec{r}_T)] \tag{1}$$

Excitation vectors from the array to each critical location, $\mathbf{h}_i$, are defined likewise. A matrix, $\mathbf{H}_C$ is the collection of the critical excitation vectors.

$$\mathbf{h}_i = [h_1(\vec{r}_C(i)), h_2(\vec{r}_C(i)), ..., h_N(\vec{r}_C(i))] \tag{2}$$

The weighting matrix $\mathbf{W}_C$ is formed with the matrix of critical excitation vectors and an appropriately chosen regularization parameter, γ as follows:

$$\mathbf{W}_C = [\mathbf{H}_C \mathbf{H}_C^{*t} + \gamma \mathbf{I}]^{-1} \tag{3}$$

The optimal complex array driver vecotr for the weighted minimum norm solution is:

$$\mathbf{u} = \mathbf{W}_c \mathbf{h}_T^{*t} (\mathbf{h}_T \mathbf{W}_C \mathbf{h}_T^{*t})^{-1} \tag{4}$$

The array is driven with unique magnitude and phases for each element as calculated from the driving vector solution to the optimization problem. The rationale to maintain driving the elements which were shadowed by the ribs was to take advantage of the coherence of the ultrasound emitted from each element which can be used for destructive or additive interference across the critical region and in intercostal spacing. The procedure for the image-based refocusing algorithm is as follows:

- Obtain B-mode STF and/or SA images to survey the target and critical regions in the therapeutic beam path.
- Determine the elements of $\mathbf{H}_C$ and $\vec{h}_T$ from the image(s) and evaluate for the optimal refocused vector.
- The optimal refocused vector is used to obtain a STF image for qualitative assessment of the refocusing result.
- Utilize the optimal refocused vector therapeutically and measure the direct effect of heating at the target and critical locations.

RESULTS

B-mode images are used for guidance of the therapeutic HIFU beam based on the aforementioned refocusing algorithm. The objective is to reduce the energy deposition across the critical locations (ribs) while maintaining (or improving) the energy deposition at the target region. Fig. 1 on the left shows the STF image of the phantom with geometric focusing while the right shows the STF image after the refocusing algorithm is completed. Once the location of the critical point(s) and the target region are determined from the

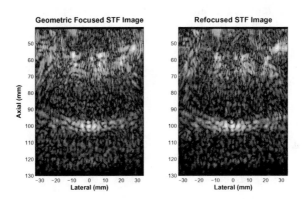

FIGURE 1. Comparison of STF images, 40 dB dynamic range

B-mode image the refocusing algorithm will determine the appropriate phase and magnitude to drive the array. By taking a STF image with the new magnitude and phase the performance of the algorithm can be seem qualitatively by noting the echogenicity across the critical structures and at the target region. The echogenicity of the gray-scale image across the ribs and at the focus are shown in Fig. 2.

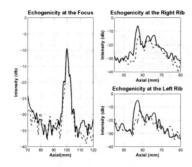

FIGURE 2. Comparison of Echogenicity of STF images: Geometric (solid line), Refocused (dotted line)

To demonstrate the feasibility of the constrained optimization method of maximizing the power at the target while minimizing the power deposition across critical objects, we designed a tissue mimicking phantom(0.45 dB/MHz/cm) with specular reflection modeling thoracic tissue and four embedded Plexiglas ribs (9.25mm in diameter) spaced 16mm apart to simulate the rib cage. A 1.5mm diameter needle thermocouple was used as a target at the geometric focus of the DMUA with an additional thermocouple placed on one of the middle ribs in the simulated rib cage to measure the effectiveness of the refocusing algorithm. The geometric and refocused array patterns were driven with normalized power to ensure that the same energy was being placed into the system. Furthermore, to show repeatability, each measurement was taken 5 times. In addition, robustness of the algorithm was considered by varying the critical point location in our algorithm by $\pm$ .5mm , and $\pm$ 1mm to account for human error in defining the critical structures.

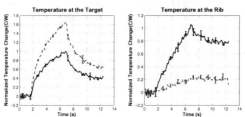

FIGURE 3. Normalized Temperature Measurements with Refocused (dotted line) and Geometric Case (solid line)

DISCUSSION AND CONCLUSION

The image quality currently available to DMUAs allows for recognizing large scattering obstacles, such as ribs, in the path of the therapeutic beam, which partially obstruct the target region thus distorting the HIFU beam. The experimental results shown in this

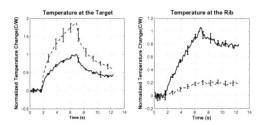

FIGURE 4. Normalized Temperature Measurments with Robustness shown over 5 different Refocused (dotted line) cases and Geometric (solid line) case

paper demonstrate the feasibility in using image based refocusing with DMUAs to avoid critical objects while maximizing power deposition at the target location. The refocusing optimization algorithm described assumes the knowledge of the array directivity at the target and critical location(s). However, these same assumptions are made in the image formation, thus the algorithm is quite robust against any distortions due to the inaccuracies in the speed of sound or other tissue properties. The only requirement is that the image used in the refocusing procedure provides a recognizable mapping of the treatment and critical region(s). The robustness of such an algorithm has been tested by varying the rib location slightly to account for human error when selecting the critical points. Comparison of the echogenicity of STF images and temperature before and after refocusing showed that the power deposition across critical locations decreased significantly while maintaining the power deposition at the target.

ACKNOWLEDGMENTS

The work presented here was funded by NIH Grant EB008191. The authors wish to acknowledge Dr. Yousry Botros , Dr. Hui Yao, Dr. Hanwoo Lee, Philip Van Barren , Dr. Claudio Simon, Dr. Jian Shen and Dalong Liu.

REFERENCES

1. C. M. Tempany, E. A. Stewart, N. McDannold, B. J. Quade, F. A. Jolesz, and K. Hynynen, *Radiology* **226**, 897 – 905 (2003).
2. N. T. Sanghvi, F. J. Fry, R. Bihrle, et al., *IEEE Trans. Ultrason., Ferroelect., Freq. Contr.* **43**, 1099–1110 (1996).
3. G. Fleury, R. Berriet, O. L. Baron, and B. Huguenin, "New piezocomposite transducers for therapeutic ultrasound," in *Proc. of the 2nd Int. Symp. on Therapeutic Ultrasound*, 2002, vol. 1, pp. 428 – 436.
4. E. S. Ebbini, H. Yao, and A. Shrestha, *Ultrasonic Imaging* **28**, 201–220 (2006).
5. H. Yao and E. S. Ebbini, "Dual-mode ultrasound phased arrays for imaging and therapy," in *IEEE Int. Symp. on Biomed. Imag.*, 2004, vol. 1, pp. 25–28.
6. H. Yao and E. S. Ebbini, "Refocusing dual-mode ultrasound arrays in the presence of strongly scattering obstacles," in *IEEE Ultrason. Symp.*, 2004, vol. 1, pp. 239–242.
7. Y. Botros, E. Ebbini, and J. Volakis, *IEEE Trans. Ultrason., Ferroelect., Freq. Contr.* **45**, 989 – 1000 (1998).

Cavitation bubble generation and control for HIFU transcranial adaptive focusing

J. Gâteau[a], L. Marsac[b], M. Pernot[a], J-F. Aubry[a], M. Tanter[a] and M. Fink[a]

[a]Laboratoire Ondes et Acoustique, ESPCI, Université Paris VII, INSERM, U.M.R. C.N.R.S. 7587, 10 rue Vauquelin, 75005 Paris, France
[b]SupersonicImagine ,510 rue René Descartes 13857 Aix en Provence, France

Abstract. Brain treatment with High Intensity Focused Ultrasound (HIFU) can be achieved by multichannel arrays through the skull using time-reversal focusing. Such a method requires a reference signal either sent by a real source embedded in brain tissues or computed from a virtual source, using the acoustic properties of the skull deduced from CT images. This non-invasive computational method allows precise focusing, but is time consuming and suffers from unavoidable modeling errors which reduce the accessible acoustic pressure at the focus in comparison with real experimental time-reversal using an implanted hydrophone. Ex vivo simulations with a half skull immersed in a water tank allow us to reach at low amplitude levels a pressure ratio of 83% of the reference pressure (real time reversal) at 1MHz. Using this method to transcranially focus a pulse signal in an agar gel (model for in vivo bubble formation), we induced a cavitation bubble that generated an ultrasonic wave received by the array. Selecting the 1MHz component, the signal was time reversed and re-emitted, allowing 97%±1.1% of pressure ratio to be restored. To target points in the vicinity of the geometrical focus, electronic steering from the reference signal has been achieved. Skull aberrations severely degrade the accessible pressure while moving away from the focus (~90% at 10mm in the focal plane). Nevertheless, inducing cavitation bubbles close to the limit of the primary accessible zone allowed us to acquire multiple references signal to increase the electronic steering area by 50%.

Keywords: ultrasonic adaptive focusing, non invasive method, cavitation bubble, transcranial brain therapy, ultrasonic array.
PACS: 43.20.-f, 43.30.Jx, 43.35.Wa, 43.60.Fg, 43.60.Mn, 43.60.Tj, 43.80.Sh

INTRODUCTION

The aberrations induced by the skull bone strongly degrade the focusing of an ultrasonic beam [1]. For transcranial brain HIFU therapy, an adaptive technique is then needed, and preferably a non-invasive one. Our team formerly proposed a time-reversal process based on a prior CT scan acquisition [2] to achieve these two goals. The technique is non-invasive due to a numerical simulation. This simulation, based on a 3D acoustic model of the skull (deduced from the CT images), computes the propagation through the skull of an acoustic pulse from a punctual virtual source to the

CP1113, 8th International Symposium on Therapeutic Ultrasound, edited by E. S. Ebbini
© 2009 American Institute of Physics 978-0-7354-0650-6/09/$25.00

ultrasound array using a finite-difference code. Thanks to the time-reversal technique, an aberration correction for the real experiment is then deduced. However, errors on modelling and repositioning lead to a suboptimal correction in comparison to what can be achieved using a hydrophone based time-reversal (invasive) technique [3]. To reach the optimum focusing non-invasively, an all-experimental time-reversal process has to be carried out. Such a process relies on the presence of a real acoustic source or a strong scatterer embedded in the brain case at the targeted location.

Pernot and al showed in [4] that intense ultrasound short pulses are able to create bubbles that immediately generate a characteristic signature. The signature was then successfully used for the time-reversal technique to correct strong aberrations. However, in their studies, two different arrays where involved, one to induce cavitation without any aberration in the beam path, and an other one to record the bubble signature, which had a strong aberrator glued on it. With only one ultrasonic array and through the skull, the use of such an acoustic source requires to concentrate enough energy in the brain case to induce cavitation, and also to control the location of the cavitation events. Conventional focusing (i.e. without any aberration correction) failed to provide such conditions. A non-invasive pre-focusing technique is then needed and is provided in this study by the CT images based time-reversal process.

OPTIMAL FOCUSING AT THE GEOMETIC FOCUS OF THE ARRAY

Using the experimental set-up presented on figure 1, we induced cavitation at the geometrical focus of the array and recorded a bubble signature. For this purpose, the aberration correction was computed from the CT images. The computed waveform were then emitted twice by the (real) ultrasound array, once at low power level (0.6 MPa peak pressure) and 10 second later, at high power level (3 MPa peak pressure). At low power level, the recorded pressure field consisted only of backscattered echoes from the gel itself, i.e speckle noise, while at high power level, a bubble appeared and generated a short pulse. Subtracting the two, the bubble signature was better selected.

With time reversal, the phase aberrations are corrected for every frequency of the recorded signal. For HIFU therapy, only a monochromatic component is back-propagated. The comparison of the focal spots obtained with the different emission laws is plotted on figure 2. The simulation-based emission law restores the focus location, but the focal spot is asymmetrical and the pressure at focus suboptimal. With the bubble-signature-based law, the symmetry of the focal spot is restored and the optimal pressure reached. The focus location with this law however depends on the cavitation event. By repeating 60 times the process to induce a bubble, and get the aberration correction from its signature, we found, as shown on Figure 3, that 82% of the cavitation events were actually distributed in the -1dB focal area.

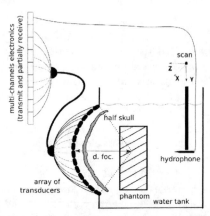

FIGURE 1. Experimental set-up. The array of transducers comprises 136 individual high-power transducers (1MHz central frequency, 20W.cm^{-2}), mounted on a spherical surface (aperture: 180 mm, focal distance: 140 mm) with a semi-random distribution. They are all driven by a fully programmable emission channel, and 54 of them also being able to receive. The phantom for *in vivo* bubble formation is a 1.75%w/v agar gel immersed in a 37°C water bath [6]. The half skull is a hydrated and degassed *ex vivo* human calvaria, mounted on a stereotactic positioning system. A needle hydrophone with a 3D positioning system is used to map the focal spots

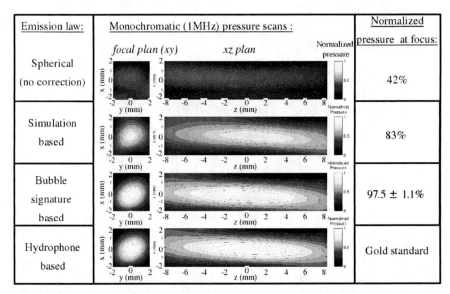

Emission law:	Monochromatic (1MHz) pressure scans :		Normalized pressure at focus:
Spherical (no correction)	focal plan (xy) ‖ xz plan		42%
Simulation based			83%
Bubble signature based			97.5 ± 1.1%
Hydrophone based			Gold standard

FIGURE 2. Monochromatic pressure fields measured in the geometrical focal zone of the array (the targeted position is the geometrical center, at (x,y,z)=(0,0,0) on the plots) for the spherical emission law, the simulation-based emission law, the bubble-signature-based and the hydrophone based time reversal. For each law, the pressure fields are shown along the focal plane of the array (xy), and the xz plane. The pressure values are normalized with respect to the maximum reached with the hydrophone based correction (gold standard). The peak pressure for each law is compared with the one obtained with the gold standard correction at the same exact position (right column).

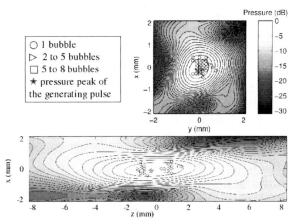

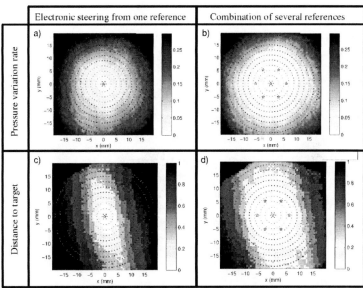

FIGURE 3. Estimated bubble locations within the initial impulse simulation-based focal spot, and their occurrence while the experiment is repeated 60 times on independent gel positions. The experiment consists in sending the impulse version of the simulation, recording a bubble signature, processing this signature, and back-propagating the extracted monochromatic aberration correction. The estimated locations are the locations of the pressure peak obtained in the final back-propagation. The projection of the positions on the focal plane (xy), and the xz plane are shown.

FIGURE 4. Error to the gold standard focusing, on positions surrounding the geometrical focus of the array in the focal plane, while targeting these positions using conventional electronic beam-steering from one optimally corrected location (a) & c)), and the combination of several references (b) & d)). For each position the peak pressure and peak position were measured. The error was then computed in term of variation rate of the peak pressure distribution with respect to the optimal distribution (a) & b)), and distance between the actual focal position and the targeted location (c) & d)). For b) and d) the minimum of the error at each location is shown here. The references, i.e. optimally corrected locations, are marked with stars.

EXTENDING THE ABBERATION CORRECTED ZONE

To treat a whole tumor, one could repeat the whole process of computing a pre-focusing emission law and correcting it optimally using an induced cavitation bubble, but the simulation part is time consuming. Conventional electronic steering can be used to extend the aberration corrected zone [5].

From one optimally corrected position, we extended the aberration correction in the immediate vicinity (figure 4 a) & c)). However, as the aberrations are not taken into account in conventional steering, the aberration correction and the accuracy of the targeting both degrade with the distance to the reference position. Nonetheless, conventional steering can also be used as a pre-focusing technique to induce cavitation bubbles and optimally correct new locations. Six new locations were corrected this way (marked with stars on Figure 4 b) & d)). Combining the conventional electronic steering capabilities in the immediate vicinity of each of these new locations plus the former one, both the area of low pressure variation rate with respect to the optimum (Figure 4 b)) and the area of zero positioning error (Figure 4 d)) were extended.

CONCLUSION

Cavitation bubbles, as punctual acoustic source for the time reversal technique, were efficiently induced non-invasively through the skull. The bubble's signature was successfully used to optimally correct the strong aberration induced by the bone, and to improve the correction provided by the CT images based simulation. Secondary bubbles were also generated away from the geometrical focus of the array to extend the electronic steering capabilities. This method should greatly benefit transcranical brain therapy.

REFERENCES

1. D.N. White, J.M. Clark, J.N. Chesebrough, M.N. White and J.K. Campbell, *J. Acoust. Soc. Am.* **44**, 1339-1345 (1968).
2. J.-F Aubry, M. Tanter, M. Pernot, J.-L Thomas, and M. Fink, *J. Acoust. Soc. Am.* **113** (1), 84-93 (2002).
3. J.L. Thomas and M. Fink, *IEEE Trans. On Ultrasonics, Ferroelectrics,* **43** (6), 1122-112 (1996)
4. Mathieu Pernot, Gabriel Montaldo, Mickael Tanter, and Mathias Fink, *Appl. Phys. Lett.* **88** (3), 034102 (2006).
5. M. Tanter, J.L. Thomas and M. Fink, *J. Acoust. Soc. Am.* **103** (5), 2403-2410 (1998).
6. S. Daniels, D. Blondel, L.A. Crum, G. Ter Haar and M. Dyson, *Ultrasound in Medicine and Biology* **13**, 527-539 (1987).

BIOLOGICAL EFFECTS

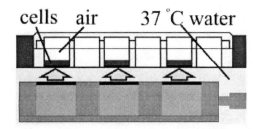

cells air   37 °C water

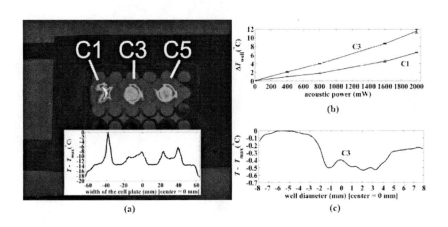

(a)

(b)

(c)

Bioeffective Ultrasound at Very Low Doses: Reversible Manipulation of Neuronal Cell Morphology and Function in Vitro

Robert Muratore, Ph.D.[a], Justine LaManna[b], Erin Szulman[b], Andrew Kalisz, M.S.[c], Michael Lamprecht[d], Melissa Simon, M.S.[d], Zhe Yu, M.S.[d], Nina Xu[e] and Barclay Morrison, Ph.D.[d]

[a]Ultrasonic Industry Association, 49 Cedar Dr, Huntington NY 11743-7101 USA
[b]Paul D. Schreiber High School, 101 Campus Dr, Port Washington NY 11050-3718 USA
[c]Frederic L. Lizzi Center for Biomedical Engineering, Riverside Research Institute,
156 William St Fl 9, New York NY 10038-5325 USA
[d]Department of Biomedical Engineering, Columbia University,
1210 Amsterdam Ave, New York NY 10027-7003 USA
[e]The Johns Hopkins University, 3400 N Charles St, Baltimore MD 21218-2608 USA

Abstract. Direct and safe manipulation of neurons by external means is an increasingly studied therapeutic modality with the potential to treat many neurological diseases. Anticipating such future applications, we investigated reversible bioeffects of very low dose focused ultrasound on neuronal cell morphology and function in vitro. To test morphological changes, undifferentiated PC12 cells were serum-cultured. The culture plates were placed on an inverted optical microscope. An f/1.1 ultrasound transducer with a water-filled coupling cone was focused on the culture and excited with 30-ms 4.67-MHz 100-kPa pulses. To test functional changes, rat hippocampal slices were cultured and individually transferred to the well of a 60-channel multi electrode array. An f/2.1 ultrasound transducer with a water-filled coupling cone was focused on a culture and excited with 100-µs 4.04-MHz 77-kPa pulses. The culture was stimulated before and after the ultrasonic stimulus with a 100-µs 100-µA biphasic electrical stimulus. Optical microscopy of PC12 cultures under insonification revealed that cells that were clustered near the ultrasound focal region elongated by approximately 2 µm during insonification and returned to approximately their original shapes following insonification. We conclude that the acoustic radiation force is capable of reversibly deforming cultured cells. In the rat hippocampal cultures, the ultrasonically and electrically evoked responses exhibited similar biphasic waveforms. In addition, robust electrically evoked responses following insonification indicated that the insonified cultures remained viable. We conclude that low-dose ultrasound can stimulate neurons; the mechanism is currently under investigation.

Keywords: ultrasonics, bioeffects, neuroscience, hippocampus, electrophysiology
PACS: 43.35.Wa, 43.80.Jz, 43.80.Sh, 87.50.yg, 87.50.yt

INTRODUCTION

Ultrasound attenuation imparts momentum to the attenuating medium [1]. The attenuating region of interest (e.g., bulk tissue, individual cells, or subcellular components) can exhibit three possible structural responses: translation, rotation, or deformation. Functionally, these responses can trigger surface and internal receptors (e.g., integrin-mediated and cytoskeletal responses) [2,3].

A considerable body of work exists on the use of acoustic tweezers for translation and rotation of cells [4-6]. Gavrilov and co-workers demonstrated a functional response in peripheral nerves from an acoustic radiation force stimulus [7-9]. Changes in electrically evoked neuronal responses in vitro and in vivo in response to ultrasonic stimuli have been studied also [10-12].

Sub-ablation therapeutic ultrasound has the potential to manipulate tissues remotely and safely. Possible neuroscience applications include non-invasive brain stimulus, plasticity studies [13], and the study of brain injury mechanisms [14]. In anticipation of such future applications, this study investigated reversible bioeffects of very low dose focused ultrasound on neuronal cell morphology and function in vitro.

METHODS

Structural Studies

Nondifferentiated PC12 cells [15] were serum-cultured in DMEM/F12 with 15% horse serum and 2.5% newborn calf serum on poly-L-lysine-coated polystyrene plates. The culture plates were placed on an inverted microscope (model IX71, Olympus America, Inc., Center Valley PA USA). An 80-mm diameter, 90-mm focal length f/1.1 PZT-4 spherical cap ultrasound transducer (model CST-100, Sonocare, Inc., Upper Saddle River NJ USA) [16] with a water-filled coupling cone, sealed at the distal end with a latex membrane, was focused on the culture plate at an approximately 45° angle-of-incidence, and excited with 30-ms 4.67-MHz pulses from a waveform generator (model 33250A, Agilent Technologies, Inc., Santa Clara CA USA) amplified by a radio-frequency amplifier (model 2100L, ENI, Rochester NY USA). Streaming was blocked by the latex membrane and by an intervening acetate sheet placed within 1 mm of the cell culture. The pressure within the focal region was estimated to be approximately 100 kPa, based on measurements with a needle hydrophone (model HNA-0400, Onda Corp., Sunnyvale CA USA). Brightfield digital images were recorded before, during, and after insonification with a 12-bit monochrome camera (model Photometrics CoolSNAP ES, Roper Industries, Inc., Sarasota FL USA) under the control of MetaMorph software (version 6.3r7, Molecular Devices, Downingtown PA USA).

Functional Studies

Hippocampal slices were prepared from 8-day-postnatal Sprague Dawley rats that had been sacrificed for other purposes under IACUC guidelines. The 400-μm thick slices were cultured for 6 days at 37°C on cellulose ester filter membranes (Millipore Corp., Billerica MA USA) in Neurobasal culture medium [17]. The mature slices were transferred to a glass-well 60-channel multi electrode array (Multi Channel Systems GmbH, Reutlingen Germany), secured by a stainless alloy ring with parallel wires spaced at 1-mm intervals, and irrigated with artificial cerebrospinal fluid saturated with a 0.95 O_2, 0.05 CO_2 gas mixture [18]. The location of the slice with respect to the electrodes was determined by optical microscopy. A custom-manufactured 42-mm diameter, 90-mm focal length f/2.1 PZT-4 spherical cap ultrasound transducer with a water-filled coupling cone, sealed at the distal end with a latex membrane, was focused on the culture plate at an approximately 45° angle-of-incidence (Figure 1), and excited with 100-μs 4.04-MHz pulses. The pressure within the focal region was estimated to be 77 kPa. Alternately, the slice culture was excited with a 100-μA 100-μs biphasic electrical stimulus applied across two adjacent electrodes. Waveforms from all electrodes were digitized at 20 kHz and recorded under the control of MC_Rack software (version 3.5.1.0, Multi Channel Systems); the recording period ranged from 100 ms pre-stimulus to 200 ms post-stimulus (excluding a 300-μs blanking period beginning with the stimulus onset).

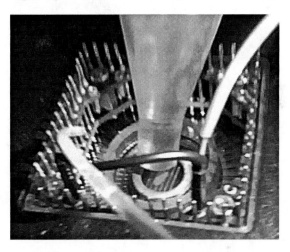

FIGURE 1. Apparatus for functional studies. The tip of the ultrasound coupling cone is immersed in a multi electrode array well. A rat hippocampal slice culture is just below the cone tip. The parallel wires securing the culture are spaced by 1 mm.

RESULTS

Optical microscopy of PC12 cultures under insonification revealed three cell populations: those which were stationary (apparently outside the effective force field region), those (seen in Figure 2) which elongated about 2 μm under radiation force and returned to approximately their original shapes when the force was removed (apparently adhered to the substrate), and those which moved about 50 μm with each pulse and did not return (apparently free-floating).

Multi electrode recordings of hippocampal cultures (Figure 3) demonstrated that ultrasonic stimuli elicited responses that were similar in their biphasic waveform to the electrically evoked responses. Typical amplitudes for electrically evoked responses before insonification were 500 μV; typical amplitudes for ultrasonically evoked responses were 100 µV. Post-insonification, electrically evoked responses exhibited waveforms similar to the ultrasonically evoked responses, with 1000-µV amplitudes.

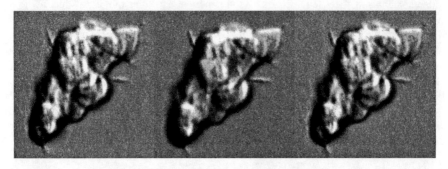

FIGURE 2. Optical microscopy image of a cluster of PC12 cells. The vertical field of view is 76 µm. (Left) Before insonification. (Center) During 30-ms insonification at 4.67 MHz, 100 kPa. The radiation force was applied diagonally from the upper right corner. (Right) After insonification. The cells reverted to their original positions.

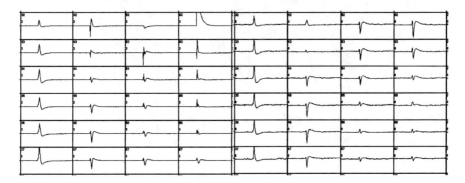

FIGURE 3. Multi electrode array recordings of evoked responses of rat hippocampal culture. Of the 60 channels recorded, the central 24 electrode recordings are presented here as average responses over multiple stimuli; the remaining channels exhibited similar behavior. The DG region (Dentate Gyrus, composed of granular cells) was located near the lower right electrodes, and the CA1 region (Cornu Ammonis, composed of pyramidal cells) was located near the central and upper left electrodes. (Left) Response to a 100-µA 100-µs biphasic electrical stimulus applied across the electrodes whose waveforms are represented by the two upper right plots. Individual waveform plots are 1 mV high and 300 ms wide. (Right) Response to a 100-µs 4.04-MHz 77-kPa ultrasonic stimulus, applied from the lower right. Individual waveform plots are 0.2 mV high and 300 ms wide.

DISCUSSION

The observed magnitude of motion of the cultured cells under insonification is consistent with earlier studies of bulk tissue motion under acoustic radiation force [19,20]. Stress-softening or -hardening of actin filaments [21], if present, did not mask the structural effects of the acoustic radiation force. The deformation of the cells and the minimization of streaming suggest that the acoustic radiation force is the mechanical cause of the observed structural changes. It is less clear that the acoustic radiation force is the mechanical cause of the observed functional effects. However, there is no evidence for competing mechanisms: stray electrical charge was not observed, and the heat deposited in the tissue by the 100-μs ultrasonic pulse is probably insignificant; further tests are planned.

CONCLUSIONS

The acoustic radiation force is capable of reversibly deforming cultured cells. Low-dose ultrasound can stimulate neurons in a rat hippocampal culture; the insonified cultures remain viable.

ACKNOWLEDGMENTS

This work was supported in part by the Riverside Research Institute Fund for Biomedical Engineering Research, and the Gatsby Initiatives in Brain Circuitry.

REFERENCES

1. H. Starritt, F. A. Duck et al., *Phys. Med. Biol.* **36**, 1465-1474 (1991).
2. F. G. Giancotti and E. Ruoslahti, *Science* **285**, 1028-1032 (1999).
3. D. E. Ingber, *J. Cell Sci.* **116**, 1397-1408 (2003).
4. J. R. Wu, *J. Acoust. Soc. Am.* **89**, 2140-2143 (1991).
5. A. Haake, A. Neild et al., *Ultrasound Med. Biol.* **31**, 857-864 (2005).
6. J. Lee and K. K. Shung, *Ultrasound Med. Biol.* **32**, 1575-1583 (2006).
7. L. R. Gavrilov, E. M. Tsirulnikov and I. A. Davies, *Ultrasound Med. Biol.* **22**, 179-192 (1996).
8. L. R. Gavrilov, J. W. Hand and E. M. Tsirulnikov, *J. Acoust. Soc. Am.* **123**, 3790-3791 (2008).
9. I. ab Ithel Davies, L. R. Gavrilov and E. M. Tsirulnikov, *Pain* **67**, 17-27 (1996).
10. P.C.. Rinaldi, J. P. Jones et al., *Brain Res.* **558**, 36-42 (1991).
11. M. R. Bachtold, P. C. Rinaldi et al., *Ultrasound Med. Biol.* **24**, 557-565 (1998).
12. N. I. Vykhodtseva and V. I. Koroleva, "Steady Potential Changes and Spreading Depression in Rat Brains Produced by Focused Ultrasound" in *Therapeutic Ultrasound: 5th International Symposium on Therapeutic Ultrasound*, edited by G. T. Clement et al., AIP Conference Proceedings 829, American Institute of Physics, Melville, NY, 2005; pp. 59-63.
13. M. O'Toole, P. Lamoureux and K. E. Miller, *Biophys. J.* **94**, 2610-2620 (2008).
14. B. Morrison III, H. L. Cater et al., *Stapp Car Crash J.* **47**, 93-105 (2003).
15. L. A. Greene and A. S. Tischler, *Proc. Natl. Acad. Sci. USA* **73**, 2424-2428 (1976).
16. R. Muratore, "A history of the Sonocare CST-100: The first FDA-approved HIFU device" in: *Therapeutic Ultrasound: 5th International Symposium on Therapeutic Ultrasound*, edited by G. T. Clement et al., AIP Conference Proceedings 829, American Institute of Physics, Melville, NY, 2005; pp. 508-512.
17. G. J. Brewer, J. R. Torricelli et al., *J. Neurosci. Res.* **35**, 567-576 (1993).
18. Z. Yu , T. E. McKnight et al., *Nano Lett.* **7**, 2188-2195 (2007).
19. F. L. Lizzi, R. Muratore et al., *Ultrasound Med. Biol.* **29**, 1593-1605 (2003).
20. K. Nightingale, R. Bentley and G. Trahey, Ultrasonic Imaging **24**, 129-138 (2002).
21. O. Chaudhuri, S. H. Parekh and D. A. Fletcher, *Nature* **445**, 295-298 (2007).

The Effect of High Intensity Focused Ultrasound Treatment on Metastases in a Murine Melanoma Model

Yifei Xing, Xiaochun Lu, Eric C. Pua, and Pei Zhong

Department of Mechanical Engineering and Materials Science
Duke University, Durham, NC 27708

Abstract. This study aims to assess the risk of high intensity focused ultrasound (HIFU) therapy on the incidence of metastases and to investigate the association of metastasis incidence with HIFU-elicited anti-tumor immunity using a melanoma model. Tumor-bearing legs were amputated immediately after or 2 days following HIFU treatment to influence the elicited anti-tumor immunity. Metastasis rates for groups undergoing amputation immediately after receiving mechanical or thermal HIFU and no treatment were comparable. However, with a 2-day delay in amputation, the corresponding metastasis rates were found to be 6.7% (1/15), 11.8% (2/17) and 40% (8/20), respectively. Animal survival rate was higher and CTL activity was enhanced in the HIFU treatment groups. Thus, HIFU treatment may elicit an anti-tumor immune response that has the potential to be harnessed to improve the overall effectiveness of cancer therapy.

Keywords: High intensity focused ultrasound; metastasis; anti-tumor immunity; bioluminescent imaging
PACS: 43.35.Wa, 87.50.ct

Introduction

Despite the advantages of high-intensity focused ultrasound, there has been a long-standing concern regarding whether HIFU-induced mechanical damage could lead to the dissemination of cancer cells into the blood circulation, and thus promote metastasis. Several groups have investigated the potential risk of metastasis induced by HIFU using animal models, but the results are contradictory [1, 2]. Because of the concern for mechanical damage outside the target region and the difficulty to control cavitation *in vivo,* traditionally, thermal coagulative necrosis has been the primary goal in HIFU therapy. However, using modern HIFU systems, cavitation is unavoidable in many therapeutic procedures, and in some instances, may even be beneficial. In fact, cavitation has been proposed and used to increase lesion size, thus reducing procedure time for HIFU ablations [3]. More importantly, our recent studies have demonstrated that HIFU-induced cavitation can cause lysis of tumor cells with concomitant release of a diverse array of endogenous danger signals, leading to a distinct host anti-tumor immune response [4]. These results suggest that HIFU-induced cavitation and associated mechanical damage may be harnessed to enhance the clinical outcomes of cancer therapy [4, 5]. Despite this potential benefit, the risk of mechanical HIFU on distant metastasis has yet to be investigated. Therefore, the goal of this study is to evaluate the potential metastasis risk induced by thermal and mechanical HIFU exposures and to monitor the time-course of metastasis development using a bioluminescent tumor model.

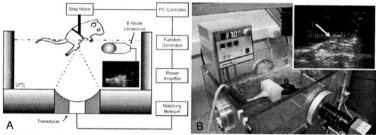

FIGURE 1. Experimental setup. (A) Schematic diagram, (B) photograph show a B-mode ultrasound image probe and two orthogonally placed CCD cameras. Alignment of the target tumor (arrow) was achieved under the guidance of B-mode ultrasound imaging (inset).

Materials and Methods

Tumor model. Murine melanoma cell line (B16-F10-Luc-G5) with stably transduced firefly luciferase gene was purchased from Xenogen Corporation (Alameda, CA). The tumor model was prepared by subcutaneous injection of 5×10^5 B16 tumor cells suspended in 50 µl of PBS into the right hind limbs of female C57BL/6 mice. Tumors were allowed to grow for 5-7 days to reach a maximum diameter of 4-6 mm before HIFU treatment. After HIFU treatment, tumor-bearing limbs were surgically amputated to ensure total eradication of the primary tumor. Amputation procedures were performed either immediately after or in 2 days following the HIFU treatment. Based on previous experience, the 2 day delay enables increased DC infiltration and maturation at the damaged tumor site, potentially leading to a boosted adaptive immune response. All animal studies were approved by the Duke University Institutional Animal Care & Use Committee.

HIFU Exposure System. The HIFU exposure system consists of a 3.3-MHz focused transducer (H-102, Sonic Concepts, Seattle, WA) as shown in Fig. 1A [4]. During the experiment, the anesthetized tumor-bearing mouse was fixed in a custom-designed animal holder, which was driven by a 3-D positioning system. To facilitate alignment of the tumor with the focus of the HIFU transducer, a portable ultrasound imaging system (Terason 2000, Terason, Inc., Burlington, MA) was employed in conjunction with two orthogonally positioned CCD cameras for visualization of the hind limb tumor (Fig. 1B). The pressure waveform and distribution in the focal plane of the HIFU transducer in water have been measured previously [6]. Progressive point-by-point scanning was employed for treatment of the tumor.

Metastasis Assessment. To assess the occurrence of metastasis, bioluminescent imaging (BLI) was performed weekly during a 4 week post-operative observation period. Animals were euthanized upon reaching either the observation endpoint at 4 weeks or humane endpoints. BLI was performed with a highly sensitive, cooled CCD camera mounted in a light-tight specimen box (IVIS, Xenogen, Alameda, CA), using protocols similar to those previously described [7]. Necropsies were performed at humane or observation endpoints. Heart, lungs, liver, spleen, kidneys, intestine, and lymph nodes were grossly examined, harvested, and examined for concordance with BLI results. Cytotoxic T-lymphocyte (CTL) assays were performed as previously described [8] as a means of analyzing immunological responses from HIFU.

Animal survival. Kaplan-Meyer analysis was performed to determine animal survival time on the basis that day 0 was set as the day of amputation and the endpoint was the day of euthanasia.

Statistical analysis. Statistical significance was evaluated with the Chi Square, Kaplan Meyer analysis and unpaired t-test, using p values of 0.05.

Results

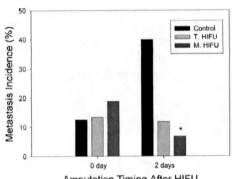

FIGURE 2. Endpoint data shows no significant different in metastasis incidence for 0 day amputation, but a significant reduction in metastasis for mice treated with mechanical HIFU 2 days before surgery.

When resection of the tumor-bearing leg was performed immediately following HIFU treatment, there was no statistically significant difference in metastasis rates among thermal HIFU, mechanical HIFU, and control groups (p>0.05) although the value for the mechanical HIFU group was slightly higher (Fig. 2). However, in mice whose tumors were removed 2 days after HIFU, providing the possibility for DC infiltration and maturation at the damaged tumor site [4], the metastasis incidence in mechanical HIFU-treated groups was 33% lower than in controls. In addition, metastasis incidence decreased when comparing mechanical HIFU treatment 2-days before and immediately before amputation, although the data is not statistically significant.

Examination of excised lungs and lymph nodes indicates a reduced severity of disease in HIFU-treated mice. The number of melanoma nodules and size of lymph nodes due to population of tumor cells was visibly lower in mechanical HIFU groups (Fig. 3A). Kaplan-Meyer analysis demonstrated that in mice treated with HIFU 2 days before amputation, animal survival time was significantly longer in both mechanical and thermal HIFU groups than in the control group ($p < 0.05$, Fig. 3B).

When amputation was performed 2 days after HIFU treatment, CTL activity was enhanced in the treatment group, particularly in the mechanical HIFU group when compared to the control group ($p < 0.05$, Fig. 4A). However, the difference in CTL activity between HIFU-treated and control groups was not statistically significant when amputation was performed immediately following HIFU (data not shown).

When amputation was performed 2 days following mechanical HIFU, the CTL activity was found to be notably higher than the corresponding data obtained immediately after HIFU treatment (Fig. 4B). EL4 cells were included as nonspecific target cells (10:1 and 5:1) for each cohort and cytotoxicity was < 5%.

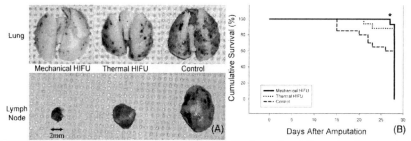

FIGURE 3. (A) Analysis of excised organs indicates reduced severity of disease in mice treated with HIFU 2 days before amputation. (B) Mechanical HIFU treatment 2 days before surgical resection prolonged survival time when compared with mice that did not receive HIFU.
($p < 0.05$, n=13-20 per group)

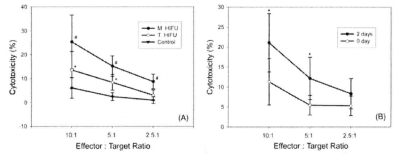

FIGURE 4. (A) CTL activity in treatment groups when amputation was performed 2 days after HIFU treatment. (B) Comparison of CTL activity in mice receiving amputation 0-days vs. 2 days after mechanical HIFU treatment. ($^{#}p < 0.0001$; $^{*}p < 0.05$)

Discussion

Recent studies have provided increasing evidence to suggest that HIFU can induce a systemic anti-tumor immune response [4, 5, 9, 10]. Our previous study demonstrated that HIFU-induced *in situ* tumor cell damage and associated release of endogeneous danger signals can lead to the activation of DC and a subsequently elicited anti-tumor immune response [4]. DC activation and migration is closely related to the HIFU-induced anti-tumor immunity, as DCs were observed to infiltrate into HIFU-treated tumors and migrate to the draining lymph node within 2 days after HIFU therapy [4]. Thus, in this study, it was observed that, when compared with control groups, metastasis incidence was lower with concomitantly prolonged survival time and elevated CTL activity in HIFU-treated mice with amputation performed 2 days after. This observation was more pronounced ($p < 0.05$) in mice treated with mechanical HIFU. However, when amputations were performed immediately following HIFU, no statistically significant difference in metastasis rates or CTL activity was observed compared to the control group.

The delayed time-point of amputation appeared to play a key role in eliciting an immune response in this study. Performing resection 2 days after HIFU resulted in improved resistance to the metastatic spread of melanoma, increased cytotoxic activity, and decreased severity of disease. However, the delayed time-point of surgery leads to a limitation in establishing an exact parallel control group. Specifically, tumor cell populations in control mice may be higher than in HIFU-treated mice, which may affect comparisons between the treatment groups. It is worth noting, though, that mice treated with mechanical HIFU two days before amputation exhibited a lower incidence of metastasis and higher cytotoxic activity than mice receiving HIFU treatment immediately before surgery, although the difference in metastasis rates is not of statistical significance. These results provide a strong indicator of an anti-tumor immunity induced by mechanical HIFU.

In summary, our results from the B16 melanoma model demonstrate that HIFU treatment itself will not increase the potential risk of metastasis. In contrast, HIFU may even elicit an anti-tumor immune response that can combat recurrence and metastasis. Furthermore, our findings suggest that new treatment strategies in HIFU should be explored to incorporate the immunotherapeutic effects of HIFU-produced mechanical damage. Such strategies to synergistically combine HIFU with immunotherapy may potentially improve the overall efficacy and quality of cancer therapy.

References

1. D. L. Miller and C. Dou, "The potential for enhancement of mouse melanoma metastasis by diagnostic and high-amplitude ultrasound," *Ultrasound in medicine & biology,* **32**, pp. 1097-101, Jul 2006.
2. G. O. Oosterhof, E. B. Cornel, G. A. Smits, F. M. Debruyne, and J. A. Schalken, "Influence of high-intensity focused ultrasound on the development of metastases," *European urology,* **32**, pp. 91-5, 1997.
3. P. M. Meaney, M. D. Cahill, and G. R. ter Haar, "The intensity dependence of lesion position shift during focused ultrasound surgery," *Ultrasound Med Biol,* **26**, pp. 441-50, Mar 2000.
4. Z. Hu, X. Y. Yang, Y. Liu, G. N. Sankin, E. C. Pua, M. A. Morse, H. K. Lyerly, T. M. Clay, and P. Zhong, "Investigation of HIFU-induced anti-tumor immunity in a murine tumor model," *J Transl Med,* **5**, p. 34, 2007.
5. Z. Hu, X. Y. Yang, Y. Liu, M. A. Morse, H. K. Lyerly, T. M. Clay, and P. Zhong, "Release of endogenous danger signals from HIFU-treated tumor cells and their stimulatory effects on APCs," *Biochem Biophys Res Commun,* **335**, pp. 124-31, Sep 16 2005.
6. Y. Zhou, L. Zhai, R. Simmons, and P. Zhong, "Measurement of high intensity focused ultrasound fields by a fiber optic probe hydrophone," *J Acoust Soc Am,* **120**, pp. 676-85, Aug 2006.
7. A. Rehemtulla, L. D. Stegman, S. J. Cardozo, S. Gupta, D. E. Hall, C. H. Contag, and B. D. Ross, "Rapid and quantitative assessment of cancer treatment response using in vivo bioluminescence imaging," *Neoplasia,* **2**, pp. 491-5, Nov-Dec 2000.
8. S. Radhakrishnan, L. T. Nguyen, B. Ciric, D. Flies, V. P. Van Keulen, K. Tamada, L. Chen, M. Rodriguez, and L. R. Pease, "Immunotherapeutic potential of B7-DC (PD-L2) cross-linking antibody in conferring antitumor immunity," *Cancer Res,* **64**, pp. 4965-72, Jul 15 2004.
9. F. Wu, Z. B. Wang, P. Lu, Z. L. Xu, W. Z. Chen, H. Zhu, and C. B. Jin, "Activated anti-tumor immunity in cancer patients after high intensity focused ultrasound ablation," *Ultrasound in medicine & biology,* **30**, pp. 1217-22, Sep 2004.
10. Q. Zhou, X. Q. Zhu, J. Zhang, Z. L. Xu, P. Lu, and F. Wu, "Changes in Circulating Immunosuppressive Cytokine Levels of Cancer Patients after High Intensity Focused Ultrasound Treatment," *Ultrasound in medicine & biology,* Sep 11 2007.

Ultrasound Induced Activation of Cell Signaling on Human MG-63 Osteoblastic Cells

Jarkko Leskinen[a], Anu Olkku[b], Mikko J. Lammi[c], Anitta Mahonen[b], Kullervo Hynynen[d]

[a]Department of Physics, University of Kuopio, Yliopistonranta 1F, 70210, Kuopio, Finland
[b]Institute of Biomedicine, Department of Medical Biochemistry, University of Kuopio, Yliopistonranta 1E, 70210, Kuopio, Finland
[c]Biocenter Kuopio and Department of Biosciences, Applied Biotechnology, University of Kuopio, Neulaniementie 2, 70210, Kuopio, Finland
[d]Department of Medical Biophysics, University of Toronto and Imaging Research, Sunnybrook Health Sciences Centre, 2075 Bayview Avenue, Toronto, ON, M4N 3M5, Canada

Abstract. Activity of Wnt/β-catenin signaling pathway associated to bone formation and maintenance was studied by exposing human MG-63 osteoblastic cells to ultrasound or heat.

The *in vitro* US system consisting of three planar PZT26 discs operating at frequency of 1.035 MHz was manufactured. The exposure type was very-near-field exposure with maximal standing wave effect. The culture medium volume and exposure distance were accurately controlled, and the temperature elevations and distributions were measured using fine wire thermocouples and IR-camera. The acoustic power (TA) varied between 0.2 to 2 W (dc = 0.2 and PRF = 1 kHz).

Using this set-up, MG-63 osteoblastic cells were exposed to US with varying acoustic powers. Based on the temperature measurements the cells were also exposed to bare heat using heat exposures. With both methods the treatment was 10 minutes long single exposure.

Clear temperature variance between exposed wells was detected implicating that the set-up type used in this experiment is vulnerable to uneven exposure unless this variation is taken into account.

Wnt-specific TOPflash reporter was found to be activated after US exposure, and the best activation was reached with acoustic power of 2 W. Similar behavior was seen with heat treatment. The effects with heat and US stimulation were convergent suggesting that the US-induced temperature rise is one of the cell stimulating factors in our study. To our knowledge, this is the first time Wnt signaling is shown to be activated using US stimulation.

Keywords: ultrasound, heat, bone, MG-63 osteoblasts, Wnt.
PACS: 43.80.Jz, 87.50.Y-, 87.50.yg

INTRODUCTION

Ultrasound (US) as a one form of mechanical energy has been found to promote bone regeneration [1]. The stimulation factor of US on bone has been detected with various US parameters and intensity levels, many of them capable to also produce substantial heat rises [1-2]. However, in many US bone studies both *in vitro* and *in vivo* the temperature rise in US stimulations has been simply ignored or estimated based on studies using nearly similar set-up or US parameters. Respectively, also temperature elevation alone has been found to be favorable to fracture healing [3-4].

CP1113, *8th International Symposium on Therapeutic Ultrasound*, edited by E. S. Ebbini
© 2009 American Institute of Physics 978-0-7354-0650-6/09/$25.00

The beneficial effects of US on bone repair are apparent, however, the precise mechanism or mechanisms by which US interacts with cells inducing these biological responses, are still not fully understood.

Many signaling cascades that originate from the cell membrane have been reported to impact bone formation. Recently, the Wnt/β-catenin signaling pathway has been identified as one of these central pathways regulating e.g. bone accrual and maintenance [5], bone mass [6] and osteoblastogenesis [7]. Wnt is also linked to apoptotic behaviour on e.g bone cells [8] implying its pleiotropic nature of function.

In this study, an *in vitro* US set-up type, which is widely used on bone studies was manufactured and systems temperature rise uniformity was verified. Since the importance of Wnt signaling pathway for bone health is inevitable and, according to our knowledge, there are no previous studies on the effects of therapeutic US on Wnt signaling, the effects of US on the activity of Wnt signaling in human osteoblast-like cells was tested using this US set-up.

MATERIAL AND METHODS

Ultrasound Set-Up, Heat Set-Up and Parameters

US device consist of six PZT26 elements (Ø25 mm, Ferroperm Piezoceramics A/S, Denmark), of which three operates at frequency of 1.035 MHz (Fig.1). The device is modification of our previously used exposure system [9]. Independent driving signals to transducer were generated using three function generators (Agilent 33120A, Agilent Technologies Inc., USA) and amplified with three RF amplifiers (ENI 240L 50dB RF Electronic Navigation Industries, USA). Transducers and 50 Ω driving electronics were matched using LC circuits. The US device was connected to 3D linear slides (Unislide®, Time and Precision Ltd., UK). The culture well (24-well plate, Greiner Bio-One International, Austria) was positioned on top of the transducer using a special stand. With linear slides the transducer can be operated accurately under specific culture plate wells. The distance to the cells was 7.7 mm. The transducer and the plate stand are positioned inside acrylic water tank, and tank is filled with deionized and degassed water. The temperature of the water is regulated using immersion thermostat (Grant GP200, Grant Instruments Ltd., UK), which also circulates the water inside the tank. The accuracy of the bath was better than 0.1°C.

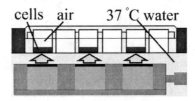

FIGURE 1. Operation principle of the US system. Strong standing wave is formed between the transducers and culture-medium-air interface. Cells are in monolayer inside the wells.

The heat exposure system consist of stainless steel water bath (Memmert WB22, Memmert GmbH + Co.KG, Germany) equipped with immersion pump to mix the water. The system has a similar plate stand as US system allowing direct contact of the 24-well plate with bath water. The accuracy of the bath was better than 0.1°C. Temperature values between 37°C to 50°C were tested.

Acoustic powers used in this study were 200, 400, 800, 1600, and 2000 mW (Temporal-Average). The temporal parameters for the US were $f = 1.035$ MHz, PRF = 1 kHz, and duty cycle = 0.2. The acoustic power values were measured using radiation force balance with absorbing target in free-field set-up. These values do not directly tell the actual power values during the sonications due to non-free-field behavior of actual exposure system, but can be used as repeatable values to estimate the circumstances during exposures. The electro-acoustic efficiencies for the transducer elements were found to be 74%, 78%, and 81%, and this variation was compensated in exposures. Forwarded and reflected electric power was measured during cell exposures so that the value for net electric power fed to the transducer using set-up was also quantified. When the electric power values between radiation force measurements (free-field) and exposure conditions was compared the net forwarded power was as an average 8% higher in radiation force measurements with free-field circumstances. When the bath US set-up was heated from 25°C to 37°C, the net electric power declined less than 5% as an average with the powers we used.

The temperature rise and distribution inside the wells was measured using digital multimeter (Keithley 2000 and TCSCAN 2001, Keithley Instruments Inc., USA) with fine wire thermocouples (75 μm, Omega Engineering Inc., UK) and infrared camera (IRTIS-200, Irtis Ltd., Russia).

Cells and Protocol

Human MG-63 osteoblast-like cell line was obtained from the American Type Culture Collection. The cells were maintained in DMEM (Gibco, Invitrogen Co., USA) supplemented with 7% fetal bovine serum (HyClone, Thermo Fischer Scientific Inc., USA), 2 mM L-glutamine, 100 U/ml penicillin, and 0.1 mg/ml streptomycin at 37°C in a humidified atmosphere of 5% CO_2 in air. For the experiments, MG-63 cells were seeded into 24-well plates (monolayer of 35000 cells/well) in medium containing 7% FBS. After overnight incubation, the medium was changed to one containing 2% charcoal-treated FBS and 2 mM L-glutamine. The cells were transiently transfected four hours later (1 μg of plasmid DNA per 24-well, FuGENE HD transfection reagent, Roche Ltd., Switzerland), and exposed the next day. TCF-binding site reporter plasmid TOPflash, was purchased from Upstate Biotechnology Inc., USA.

The medium was changed after overnight incubation, and an exact amount of medium was added to each well so that volume was exactly 510 μl/well. The cells were then exposed to single treatment of US or heat for 10 min, and then moved inside the incubator to wait for further analysis. Firefly luciferase activities were measured 24 h after treatments with Luciferase Assay System (Promega Co., USA).

37

RESULTS

Temperature Rise in Set-Up is Substantial and Non-Uniform

The system was first imaged using infrared camera to see whether the heating in all wells was identical and uniform. As Fig. 2a shows, large variation between the wells and also inside the certain well (C1) was obvious. The polystyrene border of well was found to heat up the most. At the center of the well, there was significant difference in temperature rises with varying acoustic powers between C1 and C3 (Fig. 2b). When the temperature distribution at the bottom of the well C3 was measured using thermocouple (Fig. 2c) it was observed that the center of the well is the coolest place on well bottom. However, the variation inside the well was approximately only 0.5°C.

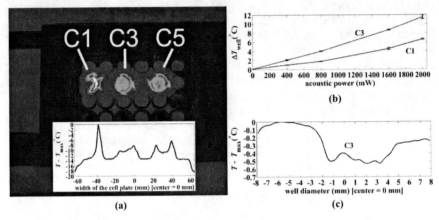

FIGURE 2. (a) IR-image and its lateral profile visualizing the heating of the three wells on a 24-well plate. The polystyrene border of the wells is heated most due the absorption of US and lack of cooling effect of the water bath. (b) The difference in maximum temperature elevations ΔT in wells C1 and C3 as a function of acoustic power measured at the center of the well. (c) Thermocouple measurement in contact of the well C3 bottom ($\varnothing_{well}$ = 15.8 mm). The bath water's cooling effect smoothes the temperature distribution at the position where the cells are located.

Wnt Activation using US or Heat – Preliminary Results

After system characterizations, only the wells in which the temperature distribution was found to be uniform were chosen for Wnt activation tests. US was found to activate Wnt signaling with acoustic powers of 400 and 800 mW, but the best activation was reached when the power was the highest which we used, i.e., 2000 mW (Fig. 3a).

The similar activation was also seen with heat exposure, peaking at 48°C and declining at higher temperatures (Fig. 3b). Despite the relatively high temperature rise, no immediate cell death and significant detachment from the well bottom could be observed at the used US exposures or heat treatments to comparable temperatures.

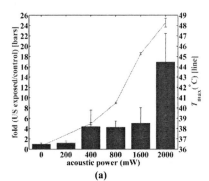 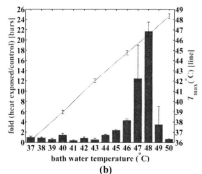

(a)   (b)

FIGURE 3. (a) TOPflash activation after single US stimulation with varying US powers. T_{max} is the maximum temperature rise inside the well (bottom contact) at the end of the 10 minutes long exposure. (b) TOPflash activation using single heat exposure. Clear systematic difference between T_{max} and bath water temperature is evident. Error bars = ± SD.

DISCUSSION

It was observed that in our transducer cell-plate combination the US induced temperature rise and distribution was substantial and uneven. Thereby, at least *in vitro* set-ups like this should be carefully characterized/heat controlled and the use of set-up should be standardized to avoid possible misinterpretations of biological results.

Our preliminary results indicate that Wnt signaling can be activated using US stimulation. To our knowledge, this is the first time US stimulation has been found to activate Wnt signaling. Our results also indicate that the stimulating factor of US is elevated temperature, since the same activation was present in heat-exposed cells. Other reporters, such as HSP70 and osteocalcin, were also activated (data not shown). This study gives new information of cellular level effect on bone cells after US stimulation with varying intensity levels. Further studies are required to get information, e.g., about cell viability and possible other interaction mechanisms.

ACKNOWLEDGEMENTS

Academy of Finland (#206113). Ms. Eija Korhonen for her technical assistance.

REFERENCES

1. L. Claes and B. Willie, *Prog Biophys Mol Biol* **93**, 384-398 (2007).
2. W.H. Chang, J. Sun et.al., *Bioelectromagnetics* **23**, 256-263 (2002).
3. S.A. Leon, S.O. Asbell et.al., *Int J Hyperthermia* **9**, 77-87 (1993).
4. C. Shui and A. Scutt, *J Bone Miner Res* **16**, 731-741 (2001).
5. J.J. Westendorf, R.A. Kahler et.al., *Gene* **341**, 19-39 (2004).
6. V. Krishnan, H.U. Bryant et.al., *J Clin Invest* **116**, 1202-1209 (2006).
7. P.V.N. Bodine and B.S. Komm, *Rev Endocr Metab Disord* **7**, 33-39 (2006).
8. P.V.N. Bodine, *Cell Res* **18**, 248-53 (2008).
9. J.J. Leskinen et.al., *Biorheology*, **45**, 345-354 (2008).

CAVITATION AND BUBBLES

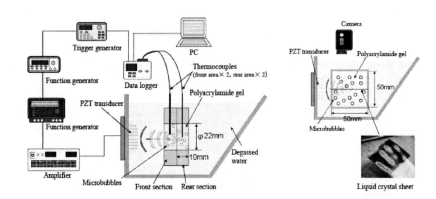

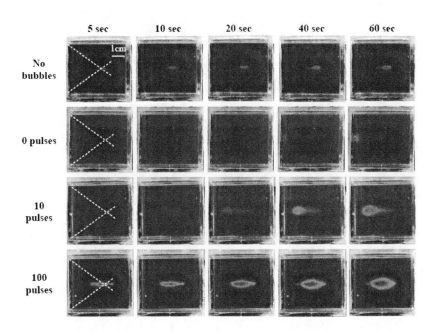

Role of Cavitation in Bulk Ultrasound Ablation: A Histologic Study

Chandra Priya Karunakaran, Mark T. Burgess, Christy K. Holland, and T. Douglas Mast

Department of Biomedical Engineering, University of Cincinnati, Cincinnati, Ohio

Abstract. The role of cavitation in bulk ultrasound ablation has been evaluated in a series of *in vitro* experiments. Fresh bovine liver tissue was ablated with a 3.1 MHz ultrasound image-ablate probe at 31 W/cm^2 for 20 minutes under normal and elevated ambient pressures. A 1 MHz passive cavitation detector recorded acoustic emission signals which were quantified by computation of average subharmonic, broadband, and low-frequency emission levels. After ablation, tissue was sliced and stained with 2% TTC to evaluate thermal damage. Emission levels were quantified and correlated with tissue ablation histology. The results indicate that bubble activity significantly affects heat deposition in ultrasound bulk ablation, in a manner different from high-intensity focused ultrasound (HIFU) ablation.

Keywords: Bulk ultrasound ablation, passive cavitation detection, TTC staining.
PACS: 43.80.Sh, 43.35.Ei, 43.80.Gx

INTRODUCTION

Liver and intrahepatic bile duct cancer is a major public health problem, with 21,370 new cases and 18,410 deaths estimated to occur during 2008 (National Cancer Institute, 2008). Ultrasound ablation techniques have potential advantages for liver cancer treatment compared to radiofrequency and microwave ablation, including reduced invasiveness and greater treatment selectivity (Fry 1993). The therapy modality considered here is bulk ultrasound ablation, in which tissue is exposed to unfocused or weakly-focused ultrasound at acoustic intensities lower than HIFU (<100 W/cm^2), resulting in thermal ablation at volumetric rates of ~1 ml/min or higher (Mast 2005, 2008).

Therapeutic ultrasound is known to produce acoustic cavitation, defined as the formation and destruction of microbubbles due to alternating compressional and rarefactional pulses of ultrasound (ter Haar 1981, Rabkin 2001). Effects of cavitation in therapeutic ultrasound include tissue fragmentation (Xu 2005), enhancement of thermal lesion depth (Melodelima 2003), and alteration of thermal lesion geometry (Fry 1993, Watkin 1996, Bailey 2001, Reed 2003). Suppression of cavitation during HIFU ablation, achieved by use of overpressure, has been shown to reduce "tadpole" shaped distortions of thermal lesions (Bailey 2001) and to increase HIFU lesion size (Reed 2003).

Here, the role of cavitation in ultrasound bulk ablation was studied in a series of *in vitro* ablation experiments, performed at elevated pressure to suppress bubble activity and at normal pressure. Similar to a previous study (Mast 2008), passive cavitation

CP1113, *8th International Symposium on Therapeutic Ultrasound*, edited by E. S. Ebbini
© 2009 American Institute of Physics 978-0-7354-0650-6/09/$25.00

detection was performed throughout ablation exposures to quantify subharmonic, broadband, and low-frequency emissions caused by acoustic cavitation and vaporization. Tissue damage was quantified by TTC vital staining and then correlated with measured acoustic emission levels. The results indicate significant differences in acoustic emission and ablation results between the two pressure levels.

MATERIALS AND METHODS

The constructed pressure chamber and experimental setup is shown in Figure 1. A pressure chamber was constructed using a polyethylene terepthalate (PET) bottle (9.3 length, 3.3 cm diameter, 0.8 mm wall thickness) which was threaded onto a galvanized iron pipe reducer, and in turn connected to a hydraulic hand pump (Ralston Instruments). Bovine liver tissue was obtained from a local slaughterhouse, immediately placed in 0°C phosphate buffered saline (PBS), and used within 12 hours *post mortem*. Immediately before each exposure, tissue blocks were cut to 8.5×3.5×3 cm^3 and placed in the pressure chamber, which was then filled with degassed PBS. The pressure chamber was placed in a glass tank filled with degassed, deionized water and its surface was cleaned with a soft brush to remove any adhering bubbles.

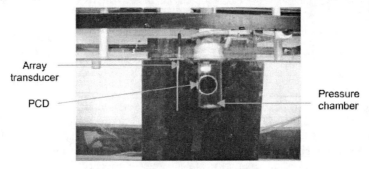

FIGURE 1. Photograph of experimental setup showing the transparent pressure chamber, 3.1 MHz image-ablate ultrasound array, and 1 MHz PCD.

The setup for ablation experiments, similar to a previous study (Mast 2008) except for the pressure chamber, employed sonication by a 3 mm diameter, 32 element, 3.1 MHz image-ablate ultrasound array (Makin 2005; THX 3N, Guided Therapy Systems). Passive cavitation detection (PCD) was performed by a 1 MHz, 25 mm circular unfocused receiver (C302, Panametrics). The image-ablate array was placed at a distance of 8 mm from the bottle surface (13-15 mm from tissue surface) with the active surface facing the liver capsule. The PCD was placed perpendicular to the direction of sound propagation, 10-15 mm from the bottle surface. The chamber was then pressurized to 175 psi (1.1 MPa) through the PBS-filled hand pump for 11 overpressure experiments, and was not pressurized for 11 control experiments.

Ultrasound exposures were programmed and controlled using the Iris imaging and ablation system (Makin 2005; Guided Therapy Systems). For all exposures, the 16 center array elements, comprising an unfocused 2.3×24.5 mm^2 active aperture, were

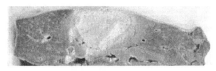
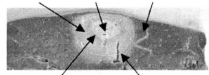

Partial TTC uptake   No TTC uptake   Complete TTC
(Partially viable)   (nonviable)   uptake (viable)

Ablation boundary   Treatment boundary

FIGURE 2. Representative TTC-stained cross sections of bovine liver tissue after ultrasound bulk ablation. Left: control (normal pressure) conditions. Right: overpressure conditions, with annotations showing segmentation of ablated and treated regions based on TTC uptake.

fired at 3.1 MHz to produce a beam of 30 W/cm^2 estimated *in situ* intensity (1.0 MPa pressure amplitude) for 20 minutes. PCD signals of length 1 s were amplified by a low-noise preamplifier (SR 560, Stanford Research Systems) with an amplitude gain of 200, and recorded by a digital oscilloscope (Lecroy Waverunner 6050A) with a sampling rate of 1 MHz at 2.6 s intervals. Power spectra for each PCD signal were estimated by the periodogram method using 1000-point FFTs with rectangular windowing and 1000 averages over the 1 s signal duration.

For each treatment, acoustic emission levels were quantified as the total spectral energy within three distinct frequency bands: subharmonic (1.55 MHz), broadband (0.3-0.75 MHz), and low-frequency (10-30 kHz). Average emission levels were determined by computing the average dB-scaled power spectrum level, relative to the measured frequency-dependent noise floor, for each 20 minute exposure.

After each treatment, treated tissue was cut at the center of the image/treatment plane. Ablation histology was evaluated by triphenyl tetrazolium chloride (TTC) vital staining (2% TTC, 45 min). Stained sections were scanned at 1500 dpi using a flatbed scanner (Canonscan 8800F). The scanned images were segmented using ImageJ (National Institutes of Health) as illustrated in Figure 2. The segmented images show three distinct regions based on level of TTC uptake. An inner bleached region shows no TTC uptake due to cessation of enzymatic activity and is considered nonviable or ablated. Surrounding the ablated area is a region staining pink due to reduced metaboltic activity resulting in partial TTC uptake. Normal untreated liver takes up TTC completely, causing a dark red appearance, and is considered viable. Areas of tissue ablation (no TTC uptake) and tissue treatment (no or partial TTC uptake) were quantified using ImageJ for the 11 control and 11 overpressure runs.

RESULTS

TTC-stained tissue cross sections for control and overpressure experiments (runs 1 and 2) are shown in Figure 2. Consistent with the overall results given below, the inner ablated area is smaller under overpressure conditions, while the area of partial TTC uptake is larger. The total treated area is comparable.

Time-dependent, dB-scaled power spectra of acoustic emissions for representative control and overpressure experiments (runs 1 and 2) are shown in Figure 3. Consistent with the overall results, these time-frequency surface plots show that the 1.55 MHz subharmonic component decreased in the presence of overpressure. Also consistent

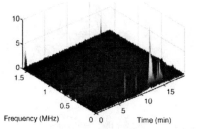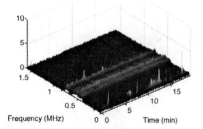

FIGURE 3. Time-dependent power spectra for representative control (left) and overpressure (right) ablation experiments. Each surface plot shows the power spectrum level in dB as a function of time throughout each 20 minute ablation exposure.

with overall results, low-level broadband emissions increased in the presence of overpressure.

Figure 4 summarizes statistics for treatment areas and emission levels for the 11 control and 11 overpressure experiments. Comparison of ablated and treated areas indicates that overpressure reduced the area of ablation in a statistically significant manner (Student t test, $t = -3.03$, $p = 6.65 \cdot 10^{-3}$). Though the overall treated area was slightly smaller under overpressure conditions, this difference was not statistically significant ($t = 1.39$, $p = 0.18$). Overpressure significantly decreased time-average subharmonic emission levels ($t = -2.45$, $p = 2.32 \cdot 10^{-3}$), but significantly increased broadband emission levels ($t = 4.12$, $p = 5.31 \cdot 10^{-4}$), while low-frequency emissions were not significantly altered.

Ablation areas and acoustic emission levels were correlated using regression analysis for each of the control and overpressure experiments. For the control (normal pressure) experiments, the total treated area correlated significantly ($p < 0.05$) with all three defined acoustic emission levels, including subharmonic ($r = 0.630$, $p = 0.0378$), broadband ($r = 0.632$, $p = 0.0369$), and low-frequency emissions ($r = 0.693$, $p = 0.0181$). For the overpressure experiments, the overall treated area was anticorrelated with the time-averaged broadband emission level ($r = -0.608$, $p = 0.0471$). Other correlations between treatment areas and mean acoustic emission levels were not statistically significant ($p > 0.05$).

DISCUSSION

The results reported here suggest that bubble activity significantly influences ultrasound bulk ablation. Application of overpressure suppressed subharmonic emissions associated with stable cavitation, but caused an increase in low-level broadband emissions. This increase in low-level broadband activity is not completely understood, but may be associated with an overpressure-induced change in the size distribution of cavitation nuclei.

Notably, overpressure significantly decreased the area of tissue ablation in these experiments, suggesting that suppression of microbubble activity may decrease heat deposition by bulk ultrasound ablation in liver tissue. This trend is opposite to trends previously observed for HIFU ablation, in which overpressure caused an increase in

46

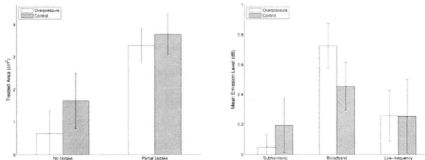

FIGURE 4. Comparison of acoustic emission and ablation results for control and overpressure experiments. Left: comparison of ablated and treated areas. Right: comparison of time-averaged subharmonic, broadband and low frequency emission levels.

thermal lesion size, possibly due to suppression of cavitation-induced focus aberration (Reed 2003). The present study suggests that cavitation plays a different role in bulk ultrasound ablation. For the lower ultrasound intensities employed in ultrasound bulk ablation, the primary effect of cavitation may be an effective increase in tissue absorption due to scattering and microbubble oscillations.

Acknowledgments: This research was supported by a University of Cincinnati Summer Graduate Student Research Fellowship and by NIH grants R43-CA124283 and R01-NS047603. The authors thank Ronald Burrage (Measurement Technologies Inc.) for his help in hand pump construction.

REFERENCES

Bailey MR, Couret LN, Sapozhnikov OA, Khokhlova VA, ter Haar G, Vaezy S, Shi X, Martin R, Crum LA. Use of overpressure to assess the role of bubbles in focused ultrasound lesion shape *in vitro*. Ultras Med Biol 2001; 27:695-708.

Fry FJ. Intense focused ultrasound in medicine. Eur Urol 1993; 23:2-7.

Makin IRS, Mast TD, Makin IRS, Faidi W, Runk MM, Barthe PG, Slayton MH. Miniaturized ultrasound arrays for interstitial ablation and imaging. Ultras Med Biol 2005; 31:1539-1550.

Mast TD, Makin IRS, Faidi W, Runk MM, Barthe PG, Slayton MH. Bulk ablation of soft tissue with intense ultrasound: modeling and experiments. J Acoust Soc Am 2005; 118:2715-2724.

Mast TD, Salgaonkar VA, Karunakaran CP, Besse JA, Datta S, Holland CK. Acoustic emissions during 3.1 MHz ultrasound bulk ablation *in vitro*. Ultras Med Biol 2008; 34:1434-1448.

Melodelima D, Chapelon JY, Theillère Y, Cathignol D. Combination of thermal and cavitation effects to generate deep lesions with an endocavitary applicator using a plane transducer: *ex vivo* studies. Ultras Med Biol 2004; 30, No.1: 103-111.

National Cancer Institute, http://www.cancer.gov/cancertopics/types/liver/, accessed September 2008.

Rabkin BA, Zderic V, Vaezy S. Hyperecho in ultrasound images of HIFU therapy: involvement of cavitation. Ultras Med Biol 2001; 27: 1399-1412.

Reed JA, Bailey MR, Nakazawa M, Crum LA, Khokhlova LA. Separating nonlinear propagation and cavitation effects in HIFU. IEEE Ultrasonics Symposium 2003; 728-731.

ter Haar GR, Daniels S. Evidence for ultrasonically induced cavitation in vivo. Phys Med Biol 1981; 26: 1145-1149.

Watkin NA, ter Haar GR, Rivens I. The intensity dependence of the site of maximal energy deposition in focused ultrasound surgery. Ultras Med Biol 1996; 22:483-491.

Xu Z, Fowlkes JB, Ludomirsky A, Cain AC. Investigation of intensity thresholds for ultrasound tissue erosion. Ultras Med Biol 2005; 31: 1673-1682.

Development of HIFU treatment in which the heating location is controlled using microbubbles

Kenichi Kajiyama[1], Naoyuki Iida[1], Keisuke Hasegawa[1], Shin Yoshizawa[3], Kiyoshi Yoshinaka[2], Shu Takagi[1], and Yoichiro Matsumoto[1]

[1] *Department of Mechanical Engineering, The University of Tokyo*
7-3-1 Hongo, Bunkyo-ku, Tokyo 113-8656, JAPAN
[2] *Department of Bio Engineering, The University of Tokyo,*
7-3-1 Hongo, Bunkyo-ku, Tokyo 113-0033, JAPAN
[3] *Department of Electrical and Communication Engineering, Tohoku University*

Abstract:

High-intensity focused ultrasound (HIFU) treatment that employs microbubbles to provide enhanced heating has been investigated in order to develop a less invasive and more rapid tumor therapy. Previous studies by us have demonstrated that ultrasound propagation is disturbed when there are microbubbles in front of the focus. In this study, we develop a method for obtaining enhanced heating by using microbubbles just at the focus, thus avoiding heating on the transducer side. In this method, microbubbles are destroyed in front of the HIFU focus (on the transducer side) by irradiating a very short burst wave of microsecond order, before irradiating the ultrasound waves for heating the focus. The experiment is conducted in a medium of a gel containing microbubbles, and a temperature-sensing liquid crystal sheet is set in the focus to observe the temperature distribution. The ultrasound frequency was 2.2 MHz and the intensity was 5000 W/cm^2, and 20 burst wave waves were irradiated at pulse repetition frequency of 1 kHz. The number of wave pulses was varied. The continuous-wave frequency, intensity and irradiation time are 2.2 MHz, 1000 W/cm^2 and 60 sec, respectively. As the number of pulses increased, the heating region moves from the transducer side to the focus. This is because microbubbles in front of the focus are destroyed and the ultrasound propagates around the target position effectively. These results suggest that the microbubble distribution and the heating position in the developed HIFU system can be controlled.

Keywords: HIFU, microbubble, gel, temperature rise

INTRODUCTION

High-intensity focused ultrasound (HIFU) therapy is receiving considerable attention since it is an attractive and non-invasive means of providing thermal therapy. HIFU treatment has been applied to tumors such as prostate and breast tumors. However, targets that are behind bone (e.g., brain tumors) or that lie deep inside the body (e.g., liver tumors) are difficult to treat since the ultrasound beam is reflected, refracted, and attenuated by the intervening tissue and/or bone. In order to resolve this problem, microbubble-enhanced HIFU has been investigated [1]. In this method, microbubbles in the HIFU field oscillate greatly and generate heat. However, previous studies by our group have revealed that ultrasound propagation is disturbed when there are microbubbles in front of the focus [2-3]. In addition, the destruction of

CP1113, *8th International Symposium on Therapeutic Ultrasound*, edited by E. S. Ebbini
© 2009 American Institute of Physics 978-0-7354-0650-6/09/$25.00

encapsulated microbubbles has been reported [4]. So, we developed a method for destroying microbubbles on the transducer side by irradiating burst waves having durations of the order of microseconds with the goal of achieving accurate position control of heating in microbubble-enhanced HIFU. The objective of this study is to analyze the relationship between the microbubble distribution in a gel and the heating profile by varying the number of burst waves.

EXPERIMENTAL SETUP

Figure 1 shows the experimental setup. Figure 1(a) shows the setup for the temperature rise experiment. The piezoelectric transducer is 40 mm in diameter and its focal length is 40 mm. A container consisting of two sections separated by a PET film is filled with a polyacrylamide gel that contains microbubbles. The case is positioned such that its rear section lies in the HIFU focus. Two thermocouples are used to measure the temperatures in front of the focus (i.e., the transducer side of the focus) and two are used to measure the temperature at the focus. Figure 1(b) shows the setup for the temperature distribution experiment. The devices used to generate the ultrasound waves (i.e., the function generator, amplifier, etc.) are the same as those depicted in Fig. 1(a). The container (50 mm × 50 mm × 50 mm) is filled with a polyacrylamide gel containing microbubbles. A thermal liquid-crystal sheet, which changes color for temperatures in the range 50 to 60°C, is positioned in the plane containing the ultrasound beam axis. A camera is used to record the color changes of this sheet.

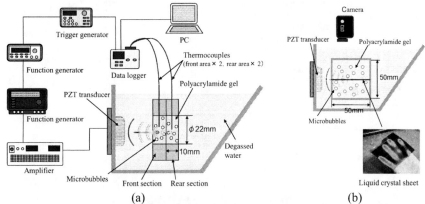

FIGURE 1. Experimental setups (a) Temperature-rise setup
(b) Temperature-distribution setup

EXPERIMENTAL CONDITIONS

Table 1 shows the ultrasound parameters for destroying microbubbles, and Table 2 shows the ultrasound parameters for heating. Figure 2 depicts the burst wave used to destroy microbubbles on the transducer side. In this experiment, we observe how the heating location shifts on varying the number of burst waves; the other burst wave parameters are kept constant. The microbubbles occupied a constant void fraction (10^{-5}). Levovist® microbubbles were used in this study.

TABLE 1. Ultrasound parameters for microbubble destruction

Frequency	2.2 [MHz]
Intensity	5000 [W/cm²]
Peak-to-peak pressure	29.7 [MPa]
No. of cycles	20
Pulse repetition freq. (PRF)	1 [kHz]
No. of pulses	0 - 10000

TABLE 2. Ultrasound parameters for heating

	Temperature rise	Temperature distribution
Frequency	2.2 [MHz]	
Intensity	1000	300 [W/cm²]
Peak-to-peak pressure	11.8	6.3 [MPa]
Exposure time	60 [s]	

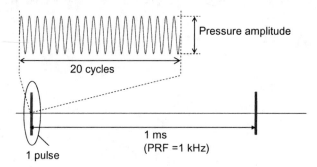

FIGURE 2. Burst wave used to destroy microbubbles on the transducer side

RESULTS AND DISCUSSION

First, the temperature rise as a function of time was measured three times by thermocouples for each number of pulses. Figure 3 shows the average temperature rise as a function of time at the focus for each number of pulses. The temperature rise increases as the number of pulses increases, except for 10000 pulses, which give only a slight temperature rise relative to the case of 0 pulses. The temperature rise is greatest when 100 pulses are used. This is because 100 pulses destroy most of the microbubbles in front of the focus enabling ultrasonic energy for heating to reach the focus. Next, Fig. 4 shows snapshots of the temperature distribution when each pulse is irradiated. In the case of no pulses, the microbubbles in front of the focus absorb ultrasonic energy resulting in heating in front of the focus, which is undesirable. As the number of pulses increases, the heating region moves towards the focus and increases in size. Compared to when there are no pulses, 100 pulses result in very good heating at the focus. This shows that applying 100 pulses does not produce undesirable heating but does enable enhanced heating due to microbubbles.

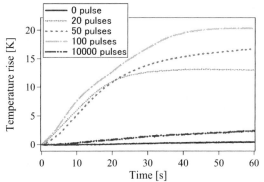

FIGURE 3. Average temperature rise for different pulse numbers

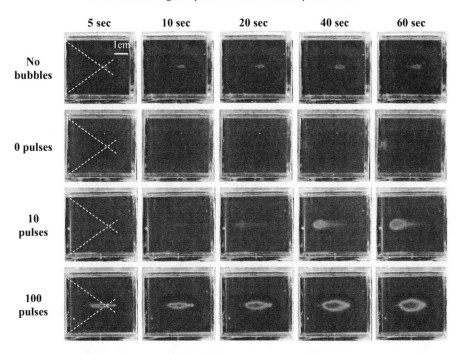

FIGURE 4. Snapshots of temperature distribution profile for different pulse numbers

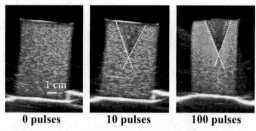

| 0 pulses | 10 pulses | 100 pulses |

FIGURE 5. Ultrasound images of the gels after ultrasound irradiation showing the degree of bubble destruction for different pulse numbers.

Finally, we used a medical ultrasound scanner to examine the gels after ultrasound irradiation for microbubble destruction. Figure 5 shows ultrasound images for each burst pulse number. These results reveal that as the number of pulses increases more microbubbles are destroyed on the transducer side. Particularly in the case of 10 pulses, the heating region appears in front of the focus (Fig. 4). The reason for this may be that the microbubbles are not completely eliminated, and the remaining microbubbles cause heat generation. These results indicate that the degree of microbubble destruction depends on the number of pulses of very short, high-intensity ultrasound. When a sufficient number of ultrasound pulses are applied to a gel containing microbubbles, most of the microbubbles in front of the focus can be destroyed, thus altering the distribution of microbubbles in the gel, and allowing effective heating at the focus to be achieved.

CONCLUSION

In this study, in order to suppress heating on the transducer side, burst waves for destroying microbubbles are irradiated into a gel containing microbubbles and the temperature rise and the temperature distribution are investigated by varying the number of pulses. The heating location depends on the number of pulses. This suggests by irradiating a sufficient number of burst waves and controlling the microbubble distribution in a gel the microbubbles can be used to achieve heating at the focus. In the future, in order to realize microbubble-enhanced HIFU treatment, it is important to investigate the effectiveness of this method for different microbubbles such as Sonazoid® and biomedical tissue.

REFERENCES

1. Razansky D., Einziger P. D., et al., Enhanced heat deposition using ultrasound contrast agent-modeling and experimental observations, 2006, IEEE Trans. UFFC, vol. 53, pp. 137-147.
2. Kaneko Y., Ph. D. thesis, The University of Tokyo, 2007.
3. Kaneko Y., Iida N., et al., Effective heat therapy controllling heat deposition of microbubbles in the ultrasound field, 2006, Proc. 6th ISTU, pp. 157-163.
4. Poster T.M., Smith D.A.B., et al., Acoustic techniques for assessing the Optison destruction threshold, 2006, Journal of Ultrasound in Medicine,vol.25, pp. 1519-1529

Lowering Cavitation Threshold Using Bifrequency Excitation: Nonlinear Aspect And Influence Of The Difference Frequency

Izella Saletes[a,b], Bruno Gilles[a,b] and Jean-Christophe Béra[a,b]

[a]*Inserm Unité 556, 151 cours Albert Thomas, 69424 Lyon Cedex 03, France.*
[b]*Université Lyon 1, Lyon, F-69003, France ; Université de Lyon, Lyon, F-69003, France.*

Abstract. The control of cavitation phenomena is a challenge in ultrasound therapy. Within the scope of investigating the influence of the excitation waveform on the cavitation activity, we have shown that using a signal combining two neighbouring frequencies (f_1 and f_2) instead of a pure sine wave excitation (f_0), a reduction of more than 40% of the power needed to initiate inertial cavitation can be obtained. The present work focused on the influence of such parameters as dissolved gas concentration and the difference frequency $\Delta f = f_2 - f_1$, on cavitation thresholds and cavitation activity. Experiments were carried out in a water tank, using a piezoelectric transducer focused on targets of controlled roughness. The acoustic signal diffused, either by the target or by the cavitation bubbles, was filtered using a spectral and cepstral-like method enabling the extraction of a broadband criterion for inertial cavitation. The pulsed excitations (center frequency f_0=550 kHz) were 1.8 ms long. For experimental conditions where low intensities were needed to trigger cavitation (high dissolved gas concentration), cavitation thresholds measured using bi-frequency excitation were higher than when using mono-frequency excitation. This result indicates that the mechanism responsible for the effect should be the nonlinear combination of two neighbouring frequency components f_1 and f_2. Concerning the influence of the difference between frequency components for bifrequency excitations, cavitation activity just beyond the threshold was much higher when using bi-frequency signals and was increased when $\Delta f = f_2 - f_1$ was increased.

Keywords: cavitation threshold, multifrequency excitation, nonlinearity.
PACS: 43.35.Ei, 87.50.Y-

INTRODUCTION

A better control of the cavitation phenomenon in tissues is a key requirement for the improvement of the existing ultrasonic therapies and the emergence of new therapeutic applications [1]. The challenge is to take advantage of the phenomenon to enhance the therapeutic efficiency of ultrasound while limiting the damage that could be done to the surrounding tissues.

In a previous paper [2], we showed that the inertial cavitation threshold could be significantly lowered using a bifrequency excitation composed of two similar frequencies. This could be very useful to limit heating in applications where strong mechanical effects of cavitation bubbles are required, like in the field of transcutaneous ultrasonic thrombolysis in the absence of pharmacological thrombolytic agent [3].

CP1113, *8th International Symposium on Therapeutic Ultrasound,* edited by E. S. Ebbini
© 2009 American Institute of Physics 978-0-7354-0650-6/09/$25.00

In this study, the nonlinear origin of the effect is discussed and the evolution of the cavitation activity beyond the threshold, as well as the influence of the difference frequency, is studied.

EXPERIMENTAL SETUP AND PROCEDURE

The experimental setup is sketched on **FIGURE 1(a)**. A more detailed description can be found in [4]. Experiments were carried out in a 60-liter tank full of degassed filtered water. A cavitation target is placed at the focus of a piezoelectric spherical broadband transducer (focal length: 10 cm; aperture diameter: 10 cm). The resonant frequency of the device is 550 kHz, and at this frequency, the −3dB focal volume is 20 mm long and 3 mm wide. Its transfer function is plotted on **FIGURE 1(b)**. The cavitation target is made of fine-grain sandpaper whose mean grain size is 46 μm unless otherwise specified [5].

The acoustic signal scattered by bubbles is measured using a low-frequency hydrophone (Reson TC4034, bandwidth: [1 ; 500 kHz]) set outside the direct field of the focused transducer.

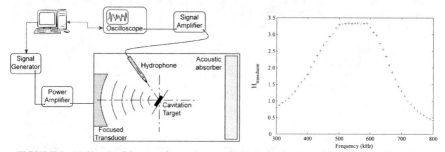

FIGURE 1. (a) Sketch of the experimental setup. (b) Transfer function of the broadband transducer.

Two types of signal were used, in order to compare their respective effects in terms of cavitation generation:

- The first one consists of a 1.8 ms long wave train composed of a pure sine wave at frequency f_0=550 kHz, and will be called the *monochromatic excitation*.
- The second one is a 1.8 ms long wave train consisting of the sum of 2 sine waves of respective frequencies $f_1 = f_0 - \Delta f /2$ and $f_2 = f_0 + \Delta f /2$ with the same pressure amplitude. It will be called the *dichromatic excitation*. Unless otherwise specified, the difference frequency Δf is equal to 30 kHz. Other Δf values between 5 kHz and 90 kHz are also studied in order to investigate the influence of this parameter on the cavitation threshold and activity.

The acoustic signal scattered by bubbles on the target is recorded and filtered using a cepstral-like method that enables to extract the broadband noise component, characteristic of the presence of inertial cavitation activity. This broadband noise is integrated in the [1-500 kHz] frequency domain, to obtain an inertial cavitation activity measurement. Plotting this cavitation activity as a function of the intensity at the focal point enables us to obtain the inertial cavitation threshold intensity $I_{T\,mono}$ (*resp.* $I_{T\,di}$) for a monochromatic (*resp.* a dichromatic) excitation, and for any set of experimental conditions [2].

The ratio between mono- and di-chromatic thresholds, as well as the cavitation activity slightly beyond the threshold, can thus be obtained for different dissolved gas concentration, different difference frequencies Δf, and different target rugosities.

RESULTS

Nonlinear Aspect of the Threshold Reduction

The ratio of the threshold intensities $R_{mono/di} = \dfrac{I_{T\,mono}}{I_{T\,di}}$ is plotted on **FIGURE 2(a)** for different dissolved gas concentrations. When oxygen concentration increases, both threshold intensities are reduced, but not in the same way for mono- and di-chromatic excitations: despite a clear tendency for the ratio $R_{mono/di}$ to decrease when the oxygen concentration increases, there is a strong dispersion on the data. This dispersion is mainly due to the one that can be observed on monochromatic threshold intensities $I_{T\,mono}$ for a given oxygen concentration. This suggests that $I_{T\,mono}$ could be better suited than the oxygen concentration to describe $R_{mono/di}$ variations. $R_{mono/di}$ is thus plotted as a function of the *reference* intensity $I_{T\,mono}$ on **FIGURE 2(b)**. The correlation between both parameters is much better, and $R_{mono/di}$ is an increasing function of $I_{T\,mono}$. This means that the reduction of the threshold when a dichromatic excitation is used becomes even more pronounced as the threshold intensity increases, which shows the nonlinear origin of the phenomenon.

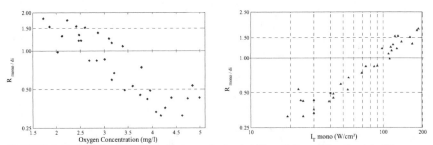

FIGURE 2. Ratio of the mono- over di-chromatic threshold intensities as a function (a) of the oxygen concentration; (b) of the threshold intensity measured for the monochromatic excitation ($I_{T\,mono}$).

Influence of the Difference Frequency

Different values of Δf have been used between 5 kHz and 90 kHz in order to investigate the influence of the difference frequency on the threshold reduction. All the experiments are realized in the same conditions of temperature and dissolved gas concentration. It has been checked that the monochromatic threshold intensity is equal to 170 W/cm^2 throughout this set of dichromatic experiments. **FIGURE 3(a)** shows the ratio of the threshold intensities $R_{mono/di}$ as a function of Δf. The ratio R_{5000} of the mono- over di-chromatic intensities needed to reach a given strong cavitation activity (a value of 5000 a.u. for the inertial cavitation activity measurement described above is chosen) is also plotted. No significant evolution of $R_{mono/di}$ can be observed, but this is not the case for R_{5000}, which becomes significantly higher than $R_{mono/di}$ for lowest and highest values of Δf. This means that those experiments show an influence of Δf only beyond the threshold. This influence can be seen more clearly on **FIGURE 3(b)** where the slope of the cavitation activity as a function of the acoustic intensity just beyond the threshold has been plotted for different values of Δf. If the evolution of the cavitation activity beyond the threshold is the same for mono- and di-chromatic excitation at 40 kHz, the increasing rate is 3 times higher with dichromatic excitation at 5 kHz, and 5 times higher at 90 kHz. The evolution of the cavitation activity beyond the threshold is linked to bubbles dynamics and resonance effects of the low frequency component Δf with some characteristic length in the target could be partly responsible for these observations. In order to check this point, several targets have been used.

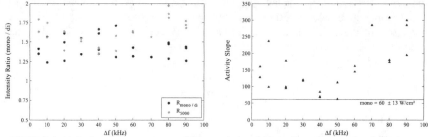

FIGURE 3. (a) Ratios of the mono- over di-chromatic intensities at the cavitation threshold, $R_{mono/di}$, (red circles) and of the mono- over di-chromatic intensities needed to achieve a cavitation activity of 5000 a.u., R_{5000}, (green diamonds) as a function of Δf.
(b) Activity slope beyond threshold as a function of Δf for dichromatic (red triangles) excitation; the corresponding activity slope for monochromatic excitation in the same conditions of temperature and dissolved gas concentration is equal to 60 ± 13 W/cm^2 (black line).

Influence of Target Sandpaper Grain Size

TABLE 1. Different types of target sandpaper.

Paper Type	P80	P180	P320	P600	P1200
Grain Size (µm)	201	82	46.2	25.8	15.3

Typical grain sizes range from 15.3 µm for P1200 paper type to 201 µm for P80 paper type, as shown on **TABLE 1**. The ratios $R_{mono/di}$ and R_{5000} are plotted on **FIGURE 4** for all the types of paper used. There are strong variations of the measurement dispersion, depending of the type of sandpaper used, but no significant evolution of $R_{mono/di}$ and R_{5000} can be observed while typical grain size has been changed by a factor 13. This suggests that the effect of changing Δf is not to be linked to any characteristic length of the target.

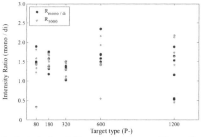

FIGURE 4. $R_{mono/di}$ (red circles) and R_{5000} (green diamonds) as a function of the target type.

CONCLUSION

Enhancing cavitation activity with lower intensities could be interesting in a variety of therapeutic applications where mechanical effects of cavitation are needed with minimal heating of tissues. For that purpose, a dichromatic excitation made of two similar frequency components is used to trigger inertial cavitation on a fine grain sandpaper target. The cavitation threshold is reduced only for sufficiently high threshold intensities, which shows that the effect results from the nonlinear combination of the components of the dichromatic signal. The value of the difference frequency Δf affects the cavitation activity beyond the threshold, and the use of well-chosen bifrequency excitation can also reduce the additional intensity beyond threshold needed to achieve a strong cavitation activity. No link between this Δf dependence and the typical target grain size could be observed. This suggests that the effect observed is not specific to the target used, but can be applied in a very wide range of applications.

REFERENCES

1. C . E. Brennen, "Cavitation in biological and bioengineering contexts" in *Proceedings of the Fifth International Symposium on Cavitation (CAV2003)*, Osaka (2003).
2. B. Gilles, J. C. Béra, J. L. Mestas, D. Cathignol, *Appl. Phys. Lett* **89(9)**, 094106 (2006).
3. U. Rosenschein, V. Furman, E. Kerner, I. Fabian, J. Bernheim and Y. Eshel, *Circulation* **102(2)**, 238-245 (2000).
4. B. Gilles, I. Saletes and J. C. Béra, "Influence of a bifrequency excitation on the ultrasonic cavitation threshold" in *Acoustics for the 21st Century*, edited by A. Calvo-Manzano, A. Perez-Lopez, J.S. Santiago, Proceedings of the 19th International Congress on Acoustics, ISBN: 84-87985-12-2, CD-Rom paper NLA-03-001-IP (2007).
5. J. L. Mestas, P. Lenz and D. Cathignol, *J. Acoust. Soc. Am.* **113(3)**, 1426-1430 (2003).

The Dependence of the Ultrasound-Induced Blood-Brain Barrier Opening Characteristics on Microbubble Size *In Vivo*

James J. Choi[a], Jameel A. Feshitan[b], Shougang Wang[a], Yao-Sheng Tung[a], Babak Baseri[a], Mark A. Borden[b], Elisa E. Konofagou[a,c]

[a]*Department of Biomedical Engineering, Columbia University, New York, NY 10027 USA*
[b]*Department of Chemical Engineering, Columbia University, New York, NY 10027 USA*
[c]*Department of Radiology, Columbia University, New York, NY 10032 USA*

Abstract. Recent neuropharmaceutical developments have led to potent disease-modifying drugs. In spite of these advancements, most agents cannot traverse the blood-brain barrier (BBB) and deposit in the brain. Focused ultrasound (FUS) with microbubbles has been shown to induce noninvasive, localized, and transient BBB opening. Although promising, safety and efficacy concerns still remain. Previously reported experiments used conventional imaging contrast agents that have a wide size distribution. In this study, we hypothesize that BBB opening characteristics are dependent on bubble diameter. A 25 µl bolus of in-house manufactured, lipid-shelled bubbles with either 1-2 or 4-5 µm diameter ranges was injected intravenously. Pulsed FUS (frequency: 1.5 MHz, peak-negative pressure: 146-607 kPa, duty cycle: 20%, duration: 1-min) was then applied to the left hippocampus of mice ($n=16$) *in vivo* through the intact skin and skull. MRI or fluorescence microscopy was used to determine BBB opening. Contrast-enhanced (Omniscan™; 0.75 mL; molecular weight: 574 Da) MRI (9.4-T) was acquired on multiple days after sonication to determine BBB opening and closing. Fluorescence microscopy was also used to determine the feasibility of delivering large, 3 kDa dextran compounds through the BBB. The BBB opening acoustic pressure threshold for the 4-5µm bubbles was in the 146-304 kPa range while the threshold for the 1-2µm bubbles was higher. In conclusion, FUS-induced BBB opening and closing was shown to be dependent on the bubble diameter indicating the possibility of specifically designing bubbles to enhance this therapeutic application.

Keywords: Blood-brain barrier; Ultrasound; FUS; Brain drug delivery; MRI; dextran
PACS: 87.50.Yt

INTRODUCTION

One of the major impediments to treatment of central nervous system diseases is the inability to deliver large, pharmacologically relevant sized compounds to the brain. This is mainly due to the low permeability of the brain's specialized microvasculature known as the blood-brain barrier (BBB). The intact BBB excludes compounds greater than 400 Da, and, as a result, neuropharmaceuticals, including inhibitors (~1 kDa) and antibody fragments (~30 to 300 kDa), cannot reach their desired target.

Focused ultrasound (FUS) has been shown to deliver large pharmacologically relevant sized compounds noninvasively, locally, and transiently to the BBB[1-3]. However, efficacy and safety concerns remain. Our previous work indicated that FUS-

CP1113, *8th International Symposium on Therapeutic Ultrasound*, edited by E. S. Ebbini
© 2009 American Institute of Physics 978-0-7354-0650-6/09/$25.00

induced BBB opening induced a variety of effects. Systemic injection of dextrans depicted regions with both homogenous and inhomogenous distributions of compounds[2]. Concentration differences varied not only spatially, but also with the administered compound's molecular weight. They accumulated near large vessel branches (e.g., transverse hippocampal arteries and veins), indicating a possible dependency of BBB opening on the vascular geometry[2]. Several studies have tested for safety and have observed petechial red blood cell extravasations within the sonicated region. However, certain regions depicted opening without extravasations. These studies have used polydispersed bubbles, which have a wide size distribution ranging from nanometers to up to 10 μm in diameter. They circulated microvessels that ranged between 4 and 8 μm and arterioles and venules that ranged between 10 and 60 μm diameter[4]. Since the safety and efficacy of BBB opening varied spatially, there may be a correlation between bubble size and the different BBB opening behaviors.

The purpose of this paper is to determine the BBB opening dependence on microbubble size. Feshitan et al. (2008) developed a technique that could generate monodispersed microbubbles, which are bubbles size-fractionated to a narrow range of diameters. BBB opening pressure threshold differences between 1-2 and 4-5 μm in diameter bubbles will be determined. Thus, we will be able to determine the bubbles responsible for BBB opening at acoustic pressures close to the threshold of opening.

MATERIALS AND METHODS

A FUS transducer (frequency: 1.5 MHz) was confocally aligned with a pulse-echo diagnostic transducer (frequency: 7.5 MHz) (Fig. 1A). A water-filled cone was mounted onto the transducer and attached to a positioning system (Velmex Inc., Lachine, QC, CAN). The FUS transducer was connected to a matching circuit and driven by a function generator (Agilent, Palo Alto, CA) and a 50-dB power amplifier (ENI Inc., Rochester, NY). The diagnostic transducer was driven by a pulser-receiver system (Panametrics, Waltham, MA) connected to a digitizer (Gage Applied Technologies, Inc., Lachine, QC, CAN). Pressure measurements of the FUS transducer were made with a needle hydrophone in a water tank as previously described[3,5]. The full-width-at-half-maximum intensities of the lateral diameter and axial length of the beam were calculated to be 1.32 and 13.0 mm, respectively.

All animal procedures were approved by the Columbia University Institutional Animal Care and Use Committee. Each mouse (n=16, strain: C57BL/6, sex: male) was anesthetized with isoflurane, placed prone, and immobilized by a stereotaxic apparatus (Fig. 1A). The hair was removed, ultrasound coupling gel was applied on the skin, and a water-filled container sealed at the bottom was placed on the head (Fig. 1A). The transducers were submerged in the water and their foci were positioned to overlap with the left hippocampus of the brain using a previously described targeting method that utilized the diagnostic transducer[3]. The right hippocampus was not targeted and acted as the control.

Prior to each sonication, monodispersed bubbles were manufactured in-house at either a 1-2 or 4-5 μm diameter range (Fig. 1BC)[6]. A 25 μl bolus of bubbles was intravenously injected 1 min prior to sonication. Pulsed FUS (pulse rate: 10 Hz, pulse duration: 20 ms, duty cycle: 20%) was then applied at select acoustic pressure between the range of 146 and 607 kPa peak-rarefactional in two 30 s sonication intervals at the left hippocampus[3,5]. Between each interval, a 30-s window allowed for residual heat to dissipate and microbubbles to reperfuse the vasculature undisturbed[5].

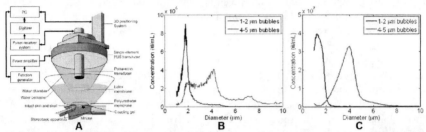

FIGURE 1. (A) Experimental setup. (BC) Size distribution of bubbles intravenously injected prior to sonication. Different bubbles were used in the (A) MRI and (B) fluorescence microscopy experiments.

A 9.4-Tesla MRI system (Bruker Medical, Boston, MA) acquired T_1-weighted horizontal slices (TR/TE: 246.1 ms / 10 ms, bandwidth: 50,505.1 Hz, matrix size: 256×256, field of view: 1.8×1.8 cm, slice thickness: 0.6 mm, number of averages: 5) of the brain in two sessions: day 1 (3-hrs post-sonication) to depict BBB opening and day 2 (24-hrs post-sonication) to depict closure. In each session, MR images were acquired before (m=3) and after (n=21, duration: 90 min) BBB-impermeable, MRI contrast agent (Omniscan™, Amersham Health, AS Oslo, NOR, amount: 0.75 ml, molecular weight: 574 Da) was administered intraperitoneally.

The delivery of pharmacologically-relevant sized compounds was evaluated using fluorescence microscopy. Following sonication, 3 kDa dextran tagged with Texas Red®, or tetramethylrhodamine, was intravenously injected and allowed to circulate for 20 min. The mice were transcardially perfused with 30 ml of PBS and 60 ml of 4% paraformaldehyde. The brain was then post-fixed in 4% paraformaldehyde, soaked in 30% sucrose overnight, embedded in optimum cutting temperature compound (Sakura Tissue-Tek O.C.T. Compound; Torrance, CA), frozen, and sectioned into horizontal 200-μm thick slices using a cryostat. Images were acquired using an inverted light and fluorescence microscope (IX-81; Olympus, Melville, NY). The sections were excited at 568±24 nm while emissions were filtered for 610±40 nm.

RESULTS

The MRI study used monodispersed bubbles as depicted in Fig. 1B. Omniscan™ was injected intraperitoneally to determine BBB opening. With 1-2 μm bubbles, no opening was observed at 146 or 304 kPa while opening was observed at 456 kPa (Table 1; Fig. 2AC). With 4-5 μm bubbles, no opening was observed at 146 kPa while opening was observed at 304 and 456 kPa (Table 1; Fig. 2DF). BBB closure was observed for both bubbles at pressures close to their respective thresholds (Fig. 2BG).

The fluorescence microscopy study used monodispersed bubbles as depicted in Fig. 1C. Dextran was injected intravenously to determine BBB opening. With 1-2 μm bubbles, no opening was observed at either 456 or 607 kPa (Table 1; Fig 3A-D). No higher acoustic pressures were tested. With 4-5 µm bubbles, no opening was observed at 146 kPa, while opening was observed at 304 and 607 kPa (Table 1; Fig 3E-H).

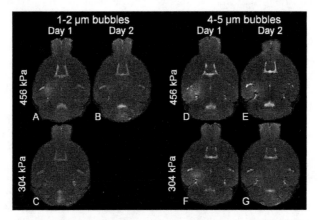

FIGURE 2. MRI determined BBB opening in four mice by injecting Omniscan™. The left hippocampus was sonicated and the right acted as a control. MRI was obtained 3-hrs (day 1; ACDF) or 24-hrs (day 2; BEG) post-sonication. At 456 kPa, Omniscan™ was trans-BBB delivered with both 1-2 (A) and 4-5 (D) µm bubbles. At 304 kPa, BBB opening was only observed with 4-5 (F) µm bubbles.

TABLE 1. Determination of BBB opening experimental results with different monodispersed bubbles.

	1-2 µm bubbles				4-5 µm bubbles			
	MRI		Dextran		MRI		Dextran	
Pressure (kPa)	Open	Not Open	Open	Not Open	Open	Not Open	Open	Not Open
607	--	--	--	1	--	--	1	--
456	1	1	--	1	1	--	--	--
304	--	2	--	--	2	1	2	1
146	--	1	--	--	--	1	--	1

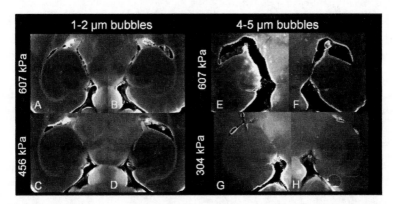

FIGURE 3. Fluorescence images of the left (sonicated; ACEG) and right (control; BDFH) hippocampi. Fluorescence in the sonicated hippocampus was not observed at 456 or 607 kPa for 1-2 µm bubbles (AC), but was observed at 304 and 607 kPa for 4-5 µm bubbles (EG).

DISCUSSION AND CONCLUSIONS

Focused ultrasound with monodispersed microbubbles noninvasively and locally opened the BBB in the left hippocampus of the mouse brains. The right hippocampus was not sonicated and acted as the control. Two methods were used to determine trans-BBB delivery or large compounds: MRI and fluorescence microscopy.

Both MRI and fluorescence microscopy determined that BBB opening is dependent on the bubble size (Table 1). In particular, 4-5 µm bubbles have a lower pressure threshold for BBB opening than 1-2 µm bubbles (Fig. 2, 3). Assuming no significant interactions between the 1-2 and 4-5 µm bubbles, these results imply that, at acoustic pressures close to the threshold of BBB opening, 1-2 µm bubbles may not induce opening. However, it remains to be shown that lower pressures are more desirable since BBB closing was observed for both bubble sizes studied (Fig. 2ABFG). Ongoing studies will determine the dependence of safety on these two bubble sizes.

The BBB opening acoustic pressure threshold for 1-2 µm bubbles differed in the two imaging studies (Table 1). In fact, no opening was observed in the fluorescence microscopy study at the acoustic pressures tested. This may be due to several reasons. First, differences between the bubble size distributions of the two studies existed (Fig. 1BC). Bubbles labeled as 1-2 µm in the MRI study included bubbles larger than that range while the 4-5 µm had an overall wider range. The size distribution and stability of bubbles were better in the fluorescence microscopy study, but clear differences between the 1-2 and 4-5 µm bubbles existed in the MRI study. Second, the compounds administered had different chemical compositions and injection routes. A 574 Da contrast agent was injected intraperitoneally in the MRI study while a 3 kDa compound, with a 2.33 ± 0.38 nm diameter, was injected intravenously in the fluorescence microscopy study.

In conclusion, BBB opening was determined to be dependent on microbubble size. The pressure threshold for opening was lower for 4-5 µm than for 1-2 µm bubbles. As a result, when using polydispersed bubbles and acoustic pressures near the threshold of BBB opening, smaller bubbles may not play as significant a role in opening as larger bubbles. Underlying reasons for these findings are part of an ongoing study.

ACKNOWLEDGMENTS

NSF CAREER 0644713, NIH R21 EY018505, and Kinetics Foundation supported this study. We thank Riverside Research Institute (New York, NY) for the transducers, Jennifer Hui for bubble characterization and Eugenia Kwon for *in vivo* experiments.

REFERENCES

1. K. Hynynen, N. McDannold, N. Vykhodtseva and F. A. Jolesz, Radiology **220** (3), 640-646 (2001).
2. J. J. Choi, S. Wang, Y.-S. Tung, B. Morrison III and E. E. Konofagou, Acoustics 2008 (Paris, France).
3. J. J. Choi, M. Pernot, S. A. Small and E. E. Konofagou, Ultrasound Med Biol **33** (1), 95-104 (2007).
4. B. V. Zlokovic, Neuron **57** (2), 178-201 (2008).
5. J. J. Choi, M. Pernot, T. R. Brown, S. A. Small and E. E. Konofagou, Phys Med Biol **52** (18), 5509-5530 (2007).
6. J. A. Feshitan, C. C. Chen, J. J. Kwan and M. A. Borden, Journal of Colloid and Interf Sci (2008).

Dependence of Cavitation Bubble Size on Pressure Amplitude at Therapeutic Levels

Kelsey J. Carvell and Timothy A. Bigelow

Department of Electrical and Computer Engineering, Iowa State University, Ames, IA, USA

Abstract High-intensity, focused ultrasound therapy is a minimally invasive therapy technique that is effective and relatively safe. It can be used in areas including histotripsy, thermal ablation, and administering medication. Inertial cavitation is used to improve these therapy methods. The purpose of this study was to determine the effect of pressure amplitude on cavitation resonance frequency/bubble size at therapeutic field levels. Earlier work has indicated that the resonance size depends on pressure amplitude; however, the investigation only considered pressure amplitudes up to 1 MPa [1]. Our study was conducted by simulating the response of bubbles to linearly propagating sine waves using the Gilmore-Akulichev formulation to solve for the bubble response. The frequency of the sine wave varied from 1 to 5 MHz while the amplitude of the sine wave varied from 0.0001 to 9 MPa. The resonance size for a particular frequency of excitation and amplitude was determined by finding the initial bubble size that resulted in the maximum bubble expansion for an air bubble in water. The simulations demonstrated a downshift in resonance size with increasing pressure amplitude. Therefore, smaller bubbles will have a more dramatic response to ultrasound at therapeutic levels..

Keywords: Cavitation, Bubble Resonance Size, Amplitude Dependence
PACS: 43.35.Ei, 43.80.Sh

INTRODUCTION

For years ultrasound has shown remarkable potential as a tool for minimally invasive therapy. Recently, ultrasound thermal ablation of tissue has successfully treated some cancers and uterine fibroids. Ultrasound thermal ablation uses the energy in the ultrasound waves to heat and kill targeted tissue and has been extensively studied [2-14]. In addition to killing tissue, ultrasound therapies are being successfully developed to enhance thrombolysis [15,16], improve drug and gene delivery [17-22], control bleeding and hemorrhaging from severe trauma [13,24], and erode or liquefy tissue by controlled technique [7,25-30]. Many of these developing therapies have been found to depend upon or be significantly enhanced by the cavitation of microbubbles. Therefore, it is critical to understand the interaction of microbubbles with high intensity sound waves. Fully understanding the interaction will better ensure effective ultrasound therapy.

In this paper, the response of a spherically symmetric air bubble in an unbounded water media to ultrasound waves was simulated. The goal was to determine how the bubble responded to pressure amplitudes at therapeutic levels. The hypothesis was that as the pressure amplitude increased the resonant bubble size would decrease where resonance size was defined as the initial bubble size that results in the greatest bubble expansion relative to the initial size. Earlier work has indicated that the resonance size depends on pressure amplitude; however, the investigation only considered pressure amplitudes up to 1 MPa [1].

CP1113, *8th International Symposium on Therapeutic Ultrasound*, edited by E. S. Ebbini
© 2009 American Institute of Physics 978-0-7354-0650-6/09/$25.00

SIMULATION PARAMETERS

The response of the bubbles to the acoustic wave was simulated by solving the Gilmore-Akulichev (eq1) formulation for bubble dynamics [30-34]. The calculations assumed that the ultrasound waves were not corrupted by nonlinear propagation distortion and that the bubble remained spherical throughout the simulation.

$$R\left(1 - \frac{U}{c}\right)\frac{dU}{dt} + \frac{3}{2}\left(1 - \frac{U}{3c}\right)U^2 = \left(1 - \frac{U}{c}\right)H + \frac{U}{c}\left(1 - \frac{U}{c}\right)R\frac{dH}{dR} \quad (1)$$

Equation 1 represents the response of a single bubble with respect to time. The R corresponds to the initial radius, U is the first derivative with respect to time, C is the speed of sound of the liquid that the bubble is in, and H is the enthalpy of that liquid. Equation 1 is dependent on four basic equations (2-5).

$$P = (C_0^2\rho/P_0m)(\rho/\rho_0)^m - \left(\frac{C_0^2\rho}{P_0m} - 1\right) \quad (2)$$

$$H = \int_{P_\infty}^{P(R)} \frac{dP}{\rho} \quad (3)$$

$$P(R) = P_g - 2\sigma/R - (4\mu/R)U \quad (4)$$

$$C = [C_0^2 + (m - 1)H]^{1/2} \quad (5)$$

Equations 2-5 define parameters accounted for while simulating a bubble using the Gilmore-Akulichev formulations. P is the pressure of the fluid around the bubble, the equilibrium liquid density is ρ_0, and the time varying density of the fluid is ρ. C_0 is the infinitesimal speed of sound in the liquid, and P_0 is the ambient pressure of the liquid surrounding the bubble and the variable m is seven [34]. The enthalpy of the liquid (H) is described by equation 3, where P_∞ is the pressure of the sound wave and P(R) is the pressure at the bubble wall. P(R) in equation 4, depends on P_g, the pressure of the gas inside the bubble, the surface tension σ, and the coefficient of shear viscosity, μ. C in equation 5 is the speed of sound at the bubble wall.

The frequency for each set of simulations was chosen as well as a set of pressure amplitudes. The amplitudes ranged 100 Pascals up to 9 MPa in varying step size depending on areas of interest, and three frequencies were selected; 1, 3, and 5 MHz because of their relevance to therapeutics. The function in MATLAB scanned initial bubble sizes searching for the maximum expansion relative to initial size, prior to inertial collapse. An inertial collapse was defined as when the bubble radius dropped below 1/10th of its initial radius. The simulation ran for a maximum of fifty cycles in the absence of an inertial collapse to insure that any transients present in the stable cavitation cases would not impact the results. After the resonance size was found, it was used to find the maximum expansion of the bubble relative to the initial size.

RESULTS

The results for the simulation are shown below. For the 3 and 5 MHz cases, there is a consistent decrease in resonance size with increasing pressure amplitude. There is also a corresponding increase in maximum expansion relative to initial size. For the 1 MHz case, there is also a decrease in resonance size with increasing pressure amplitude, but there is a discontinuity at 0.49-0.50 MPa which needs to be investigated further.

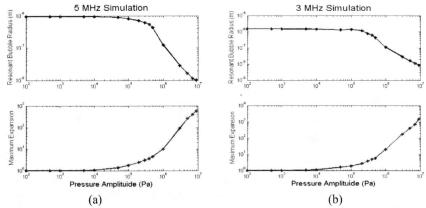

(a)   (b)

FIGURE 1: The simulation results for 5 MHz 1(a) and 3MHz 1(b) illustrate the dramatic decrease in resonance size with increasing pressure. The top graph represents a decrease in bubble size as the pressure increases and the bottom graph corresponds to the maximum expansion relative to initial size.

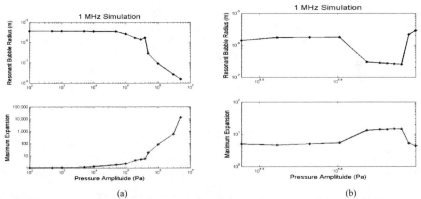

(a)   (b)

FIGURE 2: The simulations driven at 1MHz generally displayed a linear downshift except in the region of the discontinuity. Graph 2(b) magnifies the discontinuity. The top graphs represent a decrease in bubble size as the pressure increases and the bottom graphs correspond to the maximum expansion relative to initial size.

65

CONCLUSIONS

Simulation results show pressure amplitudes of 1MPa through 9MPa correspond to a drastic downshift in resonance size. The discontinuity shown in Fig. 2(b) is probably an artifact of the minimization routine used in the simulated search for the resonance bubble size perhaps resulting from a transition from stable to inertial cavitation. Fig. 3(a) shows the oscillation of a bubble during stable cavitation driven at low pressure amplitudes. During higher amplitude excitation, as seen in Fig. 3(b), the bubble is undergoing inertial cavitation. This hypothesis needs to be further explored in the future. In all cases, the growth of bubble expansion normalized to initial size is dramatic and may mean an increase the effectiveness or efficiency of cavitation at therapeutic treatment levels.

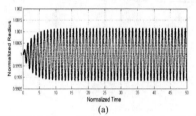 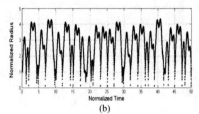

(a)   (b)

FIGURE 3: Figure 3(a) demonstrates a bubble oscillating at low pressure levels (10KPa) displaying stable cavitation and a bubble oscillating at high pressure levels (1MPa) displaying inertial cavitation is shown in 3(b).

ACKNOWLEDGMENTS

Special thanks to Charles Church (Associate Research Professor, University of Mississippi, Oxford, MS) for providing code that could be modified to calculate the bubble response. This work is supported by NSF grant Award ECCS-0643860 "CAREER: Ultrasound Histotripsy System Development to Improve Cancer Treatment" and overseen by Dr. Timothy Bigelow (Assistant Professor, Iowa State University, Ames, IA.)

REFERENCES

1. MacDonald, C.A., Sboros, V., Gomatam, J. et al., *Ultrasonics* **43**, 113-122 (2004).
2. Wu, F., Wang, Z.-B., Chen, W.-Z. et al., *Ultrasound in Medicine & Biology* **30**, 245-260 (2004).
3. Damianou, C., Pavlou, M., Velev, O. et al., *Ultrasound in Medicine & Biology* 30, 397-404 (2004).
4. Lizzi, F.L., Driller, J., Lunzer, B. et al., *Ultrasound in Medicine & Biology* 18, 59-73 (1992).
5. Mast, T.D., Makin, I.R.S., Faidi, W. et al., *The Journal of the Acoustical Society of America* **118**, 2715-2724 (2005).
6. Otsuka, R., Fujikura, K., Hirata, K. et al., *Ultrasound in Medicine & Biology* **31**, 109-114 (2005).

7. Roberts, W.W., *Urologic Oncology: Seminars and Original Investigations* **23**, 367-371 (2005).
8. Wang, Z., Bai, J., Li, F. et al., *Ultrasound in Medicine & Biology* **29**, 749-754 (2003).
9. Wu, F., Wang, Z.-B., Lu, P. et al., *Ultrasound in Medicine & Biology* **30**, 1217-1222 (2004).
10. Foley, J.L., Little, J.W., Starr III, F.L. et al., *Ultrasound in Medicine & Biology* **30**, 1199-1207 (2004).
11. Held, R.T., Zderic, V., Thuc Nghi, N. et al., *Ultrasonics, Ferroelectrics and Frequency Control, IEEE Transactions on* **53**, 335-348 (2006).
12. Christopher, T., *Ultrasonics, Ferroelectrics and Frequency Control, IEEE Transactions on* **52**, 1523-1533 (2005).
13. Fry, F.J. and Eggleton, R.C., *Technical Communication* 33-37 (1972).
14. Goss, S.A. and Fry, F.J., *IEEE Transactions on Sonics and Ultrasonics* **SU-31**, 491-496 (1984).
15. Everbach, E.C. and Francis, C.W., *Ultrasound in Medicine & Biology* **26**, 1153-1160 (2000).
16. Xie, H., Kim, K., Aglyamov, S.R. et al., *Ultrasound in Medicine & Biology* **31**, 1351-1359 (2005).
17. Kamaev, P.P., Hutcheson, J.D., Wilson, M.L. et al., *The Journal of the Acoustical Society of America* **115**, 1818-1825 (2004).
18. Van Wamel, A., Bouakaz, A., Bernard, B. et al., *Ultrasonics* **42**, 903-906 (2004).
19. Guzman, H.R., McNamara, A.J., Nguyen, D.X. et al., *Ultrasound in Medicine & Biology* **29**, 1211-1222 (2003).
20. Christiansen, J.P., French, B.A., Klibanov, A.L. et al., *Ultrasound in Medicine & Biology* **29**, 1759-1767 (2003).
21. Zarnitsyn, V.G. and Prausnitz, M.R., *Ultrasound in Medicine & Biology* **30**, 527-538 (2004).
22. Carmen, J.C., Roeder, B.L., Nelson, J.L. et al., *American Journal of Infection Control* **33**, 78-82 (2005).
23. Zderic, V., Keshavarzi, A., Noble, M.L. et al., *Ultrasonics* **44**, 46-53 (2006).
24. Martin, R.W., Vaezy, S., Kaczkowski, P. et al., *Ultrasound in Medicine & Biology* **25**, 985-990 (1999).
25. Xu, Z., Fowlkes, J.B., Ludomirsky, A. et al., *Ultrasound in Medicine & Biology* **31**, 1673-1682 (2005).
26. Xu, Z., Fowlkes, J.B., Rothman, E.D. et al., *The Journal of the Acoustical Society of America* **117**, 424-435 (2005).
27. Xu, Z., Ludomirsky, A., Eun, L.Y. et al., *Ultrasonics, Ferroelectrics and Frequency Control, IEEE Transactions on* **51**, 726-736 (2004).
28. Xu, Z., Fowlkes, J.B., and Cain, C.A., *Ultrasonics, Ferroelectrics and Frequency Control, IEEE Transactions on* **53**, 1412-1424 (2006).
29. Parsons, J.E., Cain, C.A., Abrams, G.D. et al., *Ultrasound in Medicine & Biology* **32**, 115-129 (2006).
30. Flynn, H.G. and Church, C.C., *The Journal of the Acoustical Society of America* **84**, 985-998 (1988).
31. Church, C.C., *The Journal of the Acoustical Society of America* **83**, 2210-2217 (1988).
32. Chavrier, F., Chapelon, J.Y., Gelet, A. et al., *The Journal of the Acoustical Society of America* **108**, 432-440 (2000).
33. Yang, X. and Church, C.C., *The Journal of the Acoustical Society of America* **118**, 3595-3606 (2005).
34. Church, C.C., *The Journal of the Acoustical Society of America* **86**, 215-227 (1989).

Localization and Interpretation of Bubble Activity during HIFU Exposure

Peter Kennedy[a], Manish Arora[a] and Constantin-C. Coussios[a]

[a]Biomedical Ultrasonics & Biotherapy Laboratory (BUBL), Institute of Biomedical Engineering, Department of Engineering Science, University of Oxford, Headington, Oxford OX3 7DQ, U.K.

Abstract. Bubble activity has been found to play a key role in many HIFU applications, ranging from thermal ablation to histotripsy. A combined active-passive cavitation detection system is presented, which enables localization of bubble activity with respect to the HIFU focus during HIFU exposure. The system consists of a high-frequency detector positioned coaxially with the therapy transducer, either driven in pulse-echo mode or used passively. Spectral analysis of the received signal makes it possible to distinguish between inertial cavitation and thermally induced bubble activity, and to track the evolution of either bubble population during HIFU exposure. Inertial cavitation is found to play a key role in the early stages of HIFU exposure, beyond which it gradually shuts down under the effect of heating. Thermal bubbles appear in the later stages of HIFU exposure, are most readily tracked by the active detection scheme, and gradually migrate towards the pre-focal region. This dual active-passive cavitation system could provide an invaluable tool for ensuring both treatment safety and efficacy during clinical HIFU application.

Keywords: HIFU, inertial and stable cavitation, active and passive detection, broadband noise, harmonics.
PACS: 43.35.Wa, 47.55.dp, 64.70.fh.

INTRODUCTION

Bubble activity has been previously shown to play a key role in a broad range of therapeutic ultrasound applications [1]. In the context of non-invasive cancer therapy by HIFU, the occurrence of inertial cavitation can potentially be highly beneficial under moderate HIFU exposure conditions, since it can result in greatly enhanced rates of heat deposition [2]. By contrast, the occurrence of stable cavitation, and in particular of larger, thermally induced bubbles, can be detrimental as it may result in asymmetric (or 'tadpole-shaped') lesion formation, overtreatment and undesirable prefocal damage [3, 4]. Exploitation of the potential benefits of cavitation-enhanced HIFU therapy is presently hindered by difficulties in detecting, localizing and characterizing bubble activity during HIFU exposure.

All types of bubble activity re-radiate part of the incident HIFU field at frequencies far removed from the main HIFU excitation frequency, making it possible to detect and qualify cavitation via spectral analysis of the noise emissions acquired passively during HIFU exposure. In particular, the onset of inertial cavitation is associated with a sudden increase in broadband noise, whilst larger cavities oscillating stably will result in increased emissions at harmonics, subharmonics and superharmonics of the main HIFU excitation frequency (collectively qualified as 'harmonics' hereafter).

CP1113, *8th International Symposium on Therapeutic Ultrasound*, edited by E. S. Ebbini
© 2009 American Institute of Physics 978-0-7354-0650-6/09/$25.00

Furthermore, certain types of bubble activity induce a change in the local characteristic impedance of the target medium, resulting in a well-documented increase in the scattering and reflection of an actively generated incident diagnostic pulse that has become known as 'hyperecho' in B-mode images [5].

The objective of the present work is to introduce a system that combines passive and active cavitation detection schemes to provide real-time detection, classification, and localization of cavitation activity. The ability of active and passive schemes to identify particular types of cavitation activity is also explored.

EXPERIMENTAL METHODS

The experimental apparatus used in the present work is shown in Fig. 1. A 1.1 MHz HIFU transducer with central opening (Sonic Concepts H102) is driven at a 95% duty cycle using a function generator (Agilent 33220A) and a 55dB fixed gain power amplifier (Electronics and Innovation A300). A previously described polyacrylamide-based tissue-mimicking material containing dissolved bovine serum albumin was used as the target [6]. In order to enable co-axial cavitation detection during HIFU exposure, a high-frequency, single-element diagnostic transducer (Panametrics V319) is placed inside the central opening of the HIFU transducer and positioned so that its focus overlaps with that of the therapy transducer. The diagnostic transducer is driven in pulse-echo mode using a pulser-receiver (JSR Ultrasonics DPR300) ensuring that the transmitted pulse is incident upon the HIFU focal region during the 5% off-time of the HIFU excitation. A second cavitation detection transducer was positioned transversely to the HIFU focus to enable independent validation of the observations yielded by the axial detector.

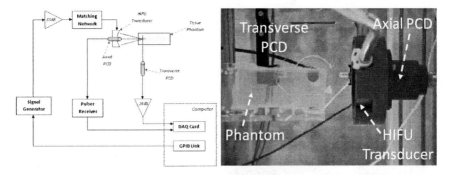

FIGURE 1. Diagrammatic representation (left) and photograph (right) of the experimental apparatus used for combined active and passive cavitation detection along the HIFU axis during 1.1 MHz exposure of tissue and tissue-mimicking materials.

A 400-microsecond time trace of the signal received by the axial cavitation detector was recorded every 50 ms throughout the HIFU exposure, the first 200 microseconds coinciding with the HIFU off-time, and the last 200 microseconds with the HIFU on-time. This makes it possible to utilize a single trace to reap the benefits of both an active and a passive detection scheme. The active scheme enables localization of bubble clouds by tracking the position of large reflections of the transmitted pulse. The passive scheme also provides information as to the position of the bubble cloud front nearest to the HIFU transducer, which can be identified by tracking the time-of-flight of the leading edge of the passively received signal. More importantly, however, the passive scheme also enables classification of the type of cavitation activity being detected by using the spectral analysis technique described hereafter.

In order to distinguish between the presence of inertial and stable cavitation, a Fast Fourier Transform (FFT) is applied to each passively received signal, which enables separation of its harmonic and broadband noise components by digital filtering. This is achieved by applying bandpass filters of bandwidth 0.18 MHz around all multiples and sub-multiples of the HIFU excitation frequency: taking an inverse FFT of this signal provides the 'harmonic' time trace that only captures activity due to stable cavitation and, to a lesser extent, non-linear propagation through the phantom (the latter was not found to be significant in the tissue-mimicking material in the absence of bubbles). The signal remaining after applying 0.18 MHz notch filters to the original signal is purely representative of broadband noise. Similarly, its inverse FFT therefore provides a 'broadband' time trace that solely captures inertial cavitation activity.

Prior to experimentation, the inertial cavitation threshold in the tissue phantom was determined and found to be in the region of 1.5 MPa peak negative focal pressure. All pressures used in subsequent exposures were chosen to be well above this value.

RESULTS

Passive Localization Scheme

The principle of localization of inertial cavitation activity using a passive detection scheme is illustrated in Fig. 2, which shows the time traces corresponding to the broadband component of the passively received signal during 1.1 MHz HIFU exposure of a tissue phantom at two different peak negative pressure amplitudes, chosen to be greater than the cavitation threshold.

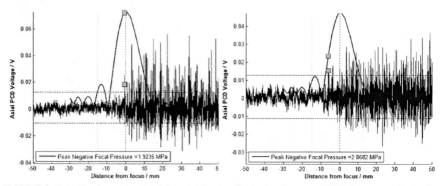

FIGURE 2. Broadband component of the axial Passive Cavitation Detector (PCD) time traces obtained during HIFU exposure of a tissue-mimicking material at two different peak negative focal pressures.

The overlaid continuous line represents the axial pressure profile of the HIFU transducer measured using a hydrophone in water, whilst the leftmost dotted vertical line indicates the position of the phantom edge nearest to the HIFU transducer. The x-axis is converted into relative axial distance by using the speed of sound through the phantom and the square markers indicate the earliest occurrence of inertial cavitation activity. At the lower peak negative focal pressure amplitude (1.92 MPa), which is close the cavitation threshold, inertial cavitation activity is seen to onset at the position of maximum HIFU pressure. However, at the higher pressure amplitude (2.86 MPa), inertial cavitation is seen to onset some 10mm ahead of the HIFU focus.

Passive Detection - Based Classification of Cavitation Activity

Continuous monitoring of the variance of passively received noise emissions during HIFU exposure has been previously shown to provide a good indication of the evolution of bubble activity. Application of the digital filtering techniques described in the experimental methods prior to computing this variance makes it possible to qualify the different types of cavitation activity during HIFU exposure. This is illustrated in Fig. 3, which shows the broadband and harmonic components of the original, unfiltered passively received signal. At this high peak negative pressure amplitude (8.3 MPa), the broadband noise emissions associated with inertial cavitation activity occur immediately, but decay rapidly. This is most probably due to heat deposition in the phantom resulting in an increase in vapour pressure that inhibits bubble collapse, as described previously [2]. By contrast, stable cavitation activity is present throughout the exposure but increases dramatically beyond 4 seconds. This is likely due to the formation of boiling bubbles due to excessive heating of the phantom, which result in a sharp increase in the harmonic component of the passively received signal.

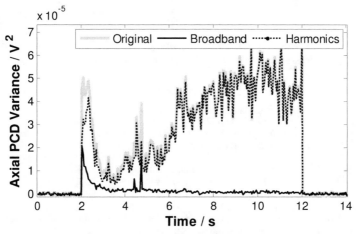

FIGURE 3. Unfiltered ('Original'), broadband and harmonic components of the variance of the signal detected by the axial Passive Cavitation Detector (PCD) during a 10 second HIFU exposure of a polyarcylamide tissue-mimicking material at a peak negative focal pressure amplitude of 8.3 MPa.

Combined Passive-Active Cavitation Detection

Lastly, the benefits of combining active and passive localization techniques are illustrated in Fig. 4, which shows the variance of the passively received signal during a 30 second HIFU exposure (starting at t = 2s) at 3.5 MPa peak negative focal pressure (top), and the corresponding active trace at two different time instants over the course of the HIFU exposure (bottom), indicated by arrows on the passive trace. At t = 2.80 s, passively detectable emissions are clearly present, but there is no signal detectable on the active trace. At t = 5.05 s, the passively detectable emissions are considerably higher than at t = 2.80 s, but there is now a large reflection visible on the active trace from the region coincident with the HIFU focus. The active scheme therefore seems more apt at detecting and localizing stable cavitation activity that tends to occur in the latter stages of HIFU exposure, whilst the passive scheme provides a more reliable indicator of inertial cavitation activity.

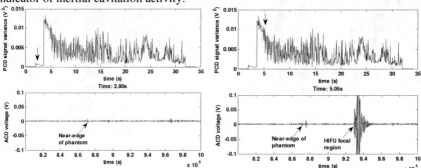

FIGURE 4. Combined passive (top) and active cavitation detection at two different time instants (t = 2.8 s & t = 5.05 s) during a 30 s, 1.65 MHz HIFU exposure at 3.5 MPa peak rarefaction pressure.

ACKNOWLEDGMENTS

The authors gratefully acknowledge support from the UK's Engineering and Physical Sciences Research Council under grant EP/D06127X/1.

REFERENCES

1. Coussios, C.C. and R.A. Roy, *Applications of acoustics and cavitation to non-invasive therapy and drug delivery.* Annual Review of Fluid Mechanics, 2008. **40**: p. 395–420.
2. Coussios, C.C., et al., *Role of acoustic cavitation in the delivery and monitoring of cancer treatment by HIFU.* International Journal of Hyperthermia, 2007. **23**(2): p. 105 - 120.
3. Bailey, M.R., et al., *Use of overpressure to assess the role of bubbles in focused ultrasound lesion shape in vitro.* Ultrasound in Medicine and Biology, 2001. **27**(5): p. 695-708.
4. Khokhlova, V.A., et al., *Effects of nonlinear propagation, cavitation, and boiling in lesion formation by high intensity focused ultrasound in a gel phantom.* Journal of the Acoustical Society of America, 2006. **119**(3): p. 1834-1848.
5. Rabkin, B.A., et al., *Biological and physical mechanisms of HIFU-induced hyperecho in ultrasound images.* Ultrasound in Medicine & Biology, 2006. **32**(11): p. 1721-1729.
6. Lafon, C., et al., *Gel phantom for use in high-intensity focused ultrasound dosimetry.* Ultrasound in Medicine and Biology, 2005. **31**(10): p. 1383-1389.

Passive imaging of cavitational acoustic emissions with ultrasound arrays

Vasant A. Salgaonkar,[a] Saurabh Datta,[b] Christy K. Holland,[a] and T. Douglas Mast[a]

[a]*Department of Biomedical Engineering, University of Cincinnati, Cincinnati, OH*
[b]*Siemens Medical Solutions USA Inc., Mountain View, CA*

Abstract. A method is presented for imaging emissions from active microbubbles using an ultrasound array. Since bubble activity plays a role in ultrasound ablation, monitoring cavitation may assist in therapy guidance. This is often achieved by listening passively for bubble emissions with a single-element transducer. Such schemes do not capture the variation in cavitation in form of a two dimensional (2D) map or image. The technique presented here obtains spatial information by creating images solely from the beamformed cavitational-emission energy received by an array, dynamically focused at multiple depths. An analytic expression was derived for these passive images by numerically solving the Rayleigh-Sommerfield integral under the Fresnel approximation. To test accuracy in mapping of localized emissions, a 192-element array was employed to passively image scattering of 520-kHz ultrasound by a 1-mm steel wire. The wire position was estimated from the passive images with rms error 0.9 mm in azimuth and 17.2 mm in range. Bubbles created in air-saturated saline sonicated at 520-kHz were imaged passively from both ultraharmonic and broadband emissions. Good agreement was found between azimuthal brightness distributions of the passive images and B-scan images of the bubble cloud. Broadband emission images from *ex vivo* bovine liver sonicated with 2.2-MHz focused ultrasound were also recorded. The image brightness along the array azimuth was consistent with the source beam profile. This indicates the possibility of mapping therapeutic ultrasound beams *in situ*.

Keywords: acoustic cavitation, array beamforming, acoustical medical instrumentation
PACS: 43.35.Ei, 43.60.Fg, 43.80.Vi

INTRODUCTION

A method to spatially resolve acoustic emissions from active bubbles using ultrasound arrays is presented. Acoustic cavitation is known to play an important role in ultrasound-based therapies including shock-wave lithotripsy [1], thrombolysis [2], targeted drug delivery [3], and thermal ablation [4]. During ultrasound ablation, cavitation results in enhanced tissue heating [5], but also complicates energy deposition and distorts ablative lesion shapes [6]. Monitoring of ablation by measuring bubble activity, typically with single-element transducers [7], could be improved if spatial variation in cavitation was captured. Ultrasound arrays have been employed with some success in imaging bubbles during high-intensity focused ultrasound (HIFU) exposures in B-mode imaging [8] and as passive cavitation detectors [9]. In this paper, a method for passive cavitation imaging using ultrasound arrays is introduced, analyzed, and illustrated by example simulations and experiments.

CP1113, *8th International Symposium on Therapeutic Ultrasound*, edited by E. S. Ebbini
© 2009 American Institute of Physics 978-0-7354-0650-6/09/$25.00

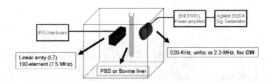

FIGURE 1. Experimental setup: CW ultrasound sources sonicate a 1 mm steel wire, PBS solution, and bovine liver, while a 192-element linear array captures passive images.

THEORY

In the passive cavitation imaging method presented here, acoustic emissions from cavitating bubbles are detected by a linear ultrasound array. These passively received signals are then beamformed in real time by delay-and-sum methods common to clinical B-scan imaging systems. To model this imaging method, a bubble is represented as a point source at position $\mathbf{r_s}$. The frequency-domain signal received by an array subaperture is modeled as an integral of the point-source field over the receiver surface S_0,

$$S(\omega) = \oint \frac{e^{ik|\mathbf{r_0}-\mathbf{r_s}|}}{|\mathbf{r_0} - \mathbf{r_s}|} dS_0. \tag{1}$$

The brightness of a passive cavitation image at the coordinate (Y,Z) is then given by the beamformed acoustic emission energy received by a subaperture focused at that point. For an array subaperture modeled as a continuous receiver with a fixed focus in the elevation (x) direction and a width $2b$ in the array (y) direction, the beamformed emission for a single source is given under the Fresnel approximation [10] as

$$S(\omega,Y,Z) = \frac{f(x_s,z_s)}{\sqrt{1-\frac{z_s}{Z}}} \left(\mathbf{F}\left[\frac{k[(y_s-Y)-(\frac{z_s}{Z}-1)b]}{\sqrt{\pi k(\frac{z_s}{Z}-1)z_s}} \right] - \mathbf{F}\left[\frac{k[(y_s-Y)+(\frac{z_s}{Z}-1)b]}{\sqrt{\pi k(\frac{z_s}{Z}-1)z_s}} \right] \right), \tag{2}$$

where (x_s,y_s,z_s) is the bubble position, k is the wavenumber ω/c, $\mathbf{F}$ is the complex Fresnel integral, and terms not dependent on the image coordinate (Y,Z) have been incorporated into the function $f(x_s,z_s)$. The final point-spread function (passive cavitation image for a single point source) is then given by the total beamformed emission energy for all frequencies of interest,

$$I(Y,Z) = \sum_i |q(\omega_i) S(\omega_i,Y,Z)|^2, \tag{3}$$

where $q(\omega_i)$ is the source strength at each frequency ω_i. Alternatively, passive cavitation images can be simulated by computing the emission signal received by each element using the Fresnel approximation, and synthetically focusing the received signals by standard delay and sum methods.

EXPERIMENTS

Passive cavitation imaging was tested here in a series of *in vitro* experiments. A glass tank was filled with deionized, degassed ($\%O_2 < 35$), filtered (particle size $< 0.2 \ \mu$m) water. Passive images were obtained using a 192-element linear array with a 7.5 MHz center frequency and a total aperture size of 42×7 mm^2 (L7 array and Iris imaging system, Guided Therapy Systems). For an image frame, 192 beamformed RF emission signals, each obtained by real-time focusing at 16 equally-spaced depths, were sampled at 33.3 MHz by a 14-bit, PC-based A/D card (Compuscope CS 14200, Gage Applied). For each exposure, 38 sequential frames were acquired at 28 fps and stored. To form passive cavitation images, power spectra were computed for each receive focal zone and filtered to create separate images for distinct frequency bands, including ultraharmonic emissions due to stable cavitation and broadband emissions due to inertial cavitation [11]. The filtered energy was summed in each focal zone over all 38 frames to obtain a single passive image with 192×16 points.

Passive imaging performance was first evaluated using ultrasound scattered from a 1 mm steel wire. Continuous-wave sonication was performed by a 520 kHz, 1" diameter source (Panametrics C302) with peak-negative pressure amplitude 0.123 MPa (0.241 MPa peak-to-peak). The wire was placed orthogonal to the image plane to approximate a point source. Scattering of the source (520 kHz) harmonics between 5.2–9.36 MHz (covering the bandwidth of the L7 array) was passively imaged using subapertures designed to maintain a constant f-number (subaperture width divided by focal depth) of 7.1. The passive image is consistent with the corresponding simulated image of a point source, for both the "idealized" subaperture and time-delay focusing formulations (Figure 2). To assess spatial resolution of the passive images, the wire was moved to 21 distinct positions distributed throughout the image plane. To estimate the target position, energy of each beamformed signal was integrated over all depths, and the target azimuth was estimated as the position of peak integrated energy (rms error 0.9 mm). The target range was estimated as the position of peak signal amplitude at this azimuth (rms error 17.2 mm).

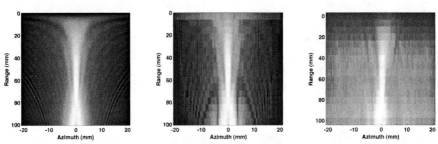

FIGURE 2. Simulated and experimental passive images of a point source at position (0 mm, 55 mm), obtained using a constant f-number and shown with 40 dB dynamic range. Left: simulated image for idealized aperture. Center: simulated image for linear array with time-delay focusing. Right: measured image of scattering from 1-mm wire.

In order to test the spatial correlation of passive cavitation images with confirmed bubble activity, cavitation was created by sonicating phosphate-buffered saline (PBS) solution in a 30-mm latex condom with 520-kHz, CW ultrasound (Panametrics C302). No bubbles were evident by B-scan imaging until the peak-negative sonication pressure exceeded 0.125 MPa (0.245 MPa peak-to-peak pressure), after which echogenic bubbles would accumulate on the distal wall of the condom. Passive images were formed, using a constant 64-element subaperture size, from ultraharmonic and broadband frequency components (Figure 3). The azimuthal position of the bubble cluster is seen to correspond with the region of greatest bubble activity. For quantitative comparisons, a region of interest (ROI) containing the bubble cluster on the B-scan was selected, spanning 15 mm in depth and the entire image in the array direction. The depth-integrated signal energy within this ROI was computed for both the B-scan and broadband-emission images. The spatial correlation between these two 192-point energy distributions was > 0.85 for each of 10 trials. It should be noted that the B-scan did not show a visible change in the size and position of the bubble cloud during the image acquisition.

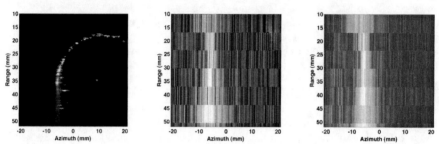

FIGURE 3. Passive cavitation imaging in saline solution for sonication at 520-kHz with 0.137 MPa peak negative pressure (0.31 MPa peak-to-peak). Left: B-scan showing a cavitating bubble cloud. Center: co-registered passive cavitation image formed from ultraharmonic emissions (6.5 MHz, or 12.5 times the fundamental frequency). Right: co-registered passive cavitation image formed from broadband emissions (6.3-6.7 MHz).

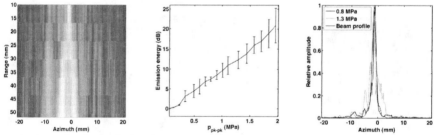

FIGURE 4. Passive cavitation imaging using broadband emissions from bovine liver tissue sonicated at 2.2 MHz. Left: passive image at 0.8 MPa peak-to-peak pressure (0.38 MPa peak negative pressure). Center: spatially-integrated emission energy as a function of sonication amplitude (mean ± standard deviation, $N = 4$). Right: representative comparison of emission amplitude at 20 mm depth with measured beam profile.

Finally, *ex vivo* bovine liver was exposed to a 2.2-MHz, 4×15 mm^2 focused source (UTX IX327), aligned with the propagation direction orthogonal to the image plane. The source focus was aligned to the image plane on the array axis at a depth of 20 mm using a pulse-echo technique. The sonication amplitude was increased from 0–1.96 MPa peak-to-peak pressure, corresponding to 0–0.58 MPa peak-negative pressure, and passive images were captured with a constant 64-element subaperture for 4 tissue samples of size $7 \times 3 \times 3$ cm^3 (FIgure 4). While emissions detected by the linear array did not show a significant signal at ultraharmonics of the source frequency, the broadband energy (8–10 MHz) increased monotonically with the sonication amplitude. The azimuthal position of the source focus could be visually identified from the broadband emission images. The passive image brightness pattern at the source focus depth was consistent with the beam profile along the array azimuth, as measured by a scanning hydrophone system. The passive image brightness pattern is seen to broaden with sonication amplitude, possibly because of cavitation activity within sidelobes in the transducer beam pattern.

CONCLUSIONS

A method for passive cavitation imaging using linear ultrasound arrays has been introduced and its analytic point-spread-function has been derived. Experiments substantiate that passively detected acoustic emissions can be spatially resolved into separate images for different frequency ranges. Acoustic emission sources can be localized more accurately in the array direction than in the range direction. In experiments with tissue, the broadband energy distribution along the azimuth corresponded with the beam shape of the focused source. Passive cavitation imaging could potentially enable direct visualization of therapeutic ultrasound beams *in situ*.

Acknowledgments: This research was supported by a University of Cincinnati College of Medicine Dean's Bridge Funding Program Award and NIH grant R01-NS047603. Jonathan Kopecheck, Mark Burgess, and Eileen Slavin are thanked for help during the experiments.

REFERENCES

1. Cleveland RO. Acoustics of shock wave lithotripsy. Renal Stone Disease, 1st Annual International Urology Research Symposium 2007; 311–316.
2. Datta S, Coussios CC, McAdory LE, Tan J, Porter T, De Courten-Myers G, Holland CK. Correlation of cavitation with ultrasound enhancement of thrombolysis. Ultras Med Biol 2006; 32:1257–1267.
3. Hynynen K. Ultrasound for drug and gene delivery to the brain. Adv Drug Del Rev 2008; 60:1209–1217.
4. ter Haar GR, Daniels S. Evidence for ultrasonically induced cavitation *in vivo*. Phys Med Biol 1981; 26:1145–1149.
5. Coussios CC, Farny CH, ter Haar GR, Roy RA. Role of acoustic cavitation in the delivery and monitoring of cancer treatment by high-intensity focused ultrasound (HIFU), Int J Hyperthermia 2007; 23:105–120.
6. Watkin NA, ter Haar GR, Rivens I. The intensity dependence of the site of maximal energy deposition in focused ultrasound surgery. Ultras Med Biol 1996; 22:1690–1698.
7. Mast TD, Salgaonkar VA, Karunakaran C, Besse JA, Datta S, Holland CK. Acoustic emissions during 3.1 MHz ultrasound bulk ablation *in vitro*. Ultras Med Biol 2008; 34:1434–1448.
8. Rabkin BA, Zedric V, Vaezy S. Hyperecho in ultrasound images of HIFU therapy: Involvement of cavitation. Ultras Med Biol 2005; 31:947–956.
9. Farny CH. *Identifying and monitoring the roles of cavitation in heating from high-intensity focused ultrasound* (PhD dissertation, Boston University, 2007).
10. Mast TD. Fresnel approximations for ultrasonic fields of rectangularly symmetric sources. J Acoust Soc Am 2007; 121:311–3322.
11. T. G. Leighton, *The Acoustic Bubble* (Academic Press, 1994), ch. 4.

CLINICAL AND PRE-CLINICAL STUDIES

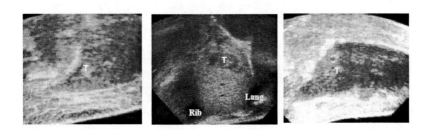

type of tumor	no of patients	tumor contour	patient posture		shading by rib and lung	duration of sonication from first to final shot
A	3	clear	prone		0 %	80 - 160 min.
B	4	clear	right lateral		35, 50, 60, 60	160 - 240
C	5	obscure	prone	3	0, 50, 50	240 -
			right lateral	2	40, 70	

Usefulness of contrast-enhanced ultrasonography in assessing therapeutic response in hepatocellular carcinoma treated with HIFU

Hiroyuki Fukuda, Masao Ohto , Ryu Ito, Yasushi Shinohara, Akio Sakamoto*, Eii Karasawa[†], Hui Zhu[‡] and Zhi-Biao Wang[¶]

* *International HIFU center, Naruto General Hospital, Naruto167,Sanbu-shi, Chiba 289-1326, Japan*
[†] *IUHW Atami Hospital, Higashikaigan 13-1, Atami-shi, Shizuoka 413-0012, Japan*
[‡] *Clinical Center of Tumor Therapy of 2nd Affiliated Hospital, Chongqing University of Medical Sciences, Chongqing, China*
[¶]*Institute of Ultrasonic Engineering in Medicine, Chongqing University of Medical Sciences, Chongqing, China*

Abstract.
PURPOSE: We evaluated the efficacy and change of contrast-enhanced ultrasonography after HIFU, and decided on the best timing for contrast-enhanced ultrasonography to evaluate the response of hepatocellular carcinoma with HIFU.
MATERIALS AND METHODS: HIFU ablation was carried out without rib resection and the aid of transcatheter arterial chemoembolization (TACE) or percutaneous ethanol injection (PEI) in 11 patients with small hepatocellular carcinoma ($\leq$ 3 lesions, $\leq$ 3 cm in diameter). The HIFU system (Chongqing Haifu Tech) was used under ultrasound guidance. Assessment of contrast-enhanced (Sonazoid, CHA mode, MI 0.8) ultrasonography (Logic7, GE) was performed.
RESULTS: HIFU treatments were successfully performed in all patients. After HIFU, treated lesions showed decreased vascular area with peripheral rim enhancement in the border of the ablated area at 30 seconds after the injection of Sonazoid in all cases. 7 days after the treatment, peripheral rim enhancement persisted in 6 of 11 lesions. The rim enhancement was completely resolved in all lesions after 3 months. During 6 months follow-up, the ablated lesions showed a gradual decrease in diameter.
CONCLUSDION: The 7 days after HIFU is most appropriate and practical for the performance of contrast-enhanced ultrasonography to evaluate the therapeutic response.

Key words: liver carcinoma, HIFU

PACS: 87.50.yt

INTRODUCTION

Hepatocellular carcinoma (HCC) is one of the most common malignancies in the world. High-intensity focused ultrasound (HIFU) is a conformal extracorporeal treatment method that can noninvasively cause complete coagulation necrosis without surgical exposure or insertion of instruments. The purpose of this study is to evaluate the efficacy and change of contrast-enhanced ultrasonography after HIFU, and decided on the best timing for contrast-enhanced ultrasonography to evaluate the response of hepatocellular carcinoma with HIFU.

MATERIALS AND METHODS

The Tumor Therapy System (Chongqing Haifu Tech Co., Ltd, Chongqing, China) used in this study is guided by means of real-time ultrasonographic imaging. The Diagnostic Ultrasound Imaging System was Logic7 (GE). Ultrasound contrast agent was Sonazoid. The maximum diameters of treated lesions were measured at each follow-up study.

Between July 2007 and August 2008, 11 patients with HCC were enrolled for this clinical study. 10 of all HCC patients were HCV-Ab positive. The patients consisted of 6 men and 5 women, with a mean age of 74.2 ± 5.6 (mean $\pm$ SD) years. The average tumor diameter was 16.4 ± 3.0 mm (mean $\pm$ SD). Epidural anesthesia was used. No TAE or PEI was performed before HIFU. No costectomy was performed before HIFU treatment.

RESULTS

Figure1 shows the results of contrast enhanced US Imaging. Before HIFU treatment, tumor stain clearly detected. 1 day after HIFU, treated lesions showed decreased vascular area with peripheral rim enhancement in the border of the ablated area at 30 seconds after the injection of Sonazoid. This rim enhancement disappeared 1 month after HIFU. The size of the treated area after HIFU decreased in diameter.

Figure2 shows the results of contrast enhanced MPR 3D-US Imaging. It was difficult to evaluate the efficacy of the HIFU treatment only by using the two dimensional enhanced ultrasonography because of the presence of the peripheral rim enhancement. So the ablated zones were evaluated on the three different planes depicted on sagital, axial and coronal sections according to the relationship between the location of the original tumor and surrounding parameters, such as portal veins and arteries.

Figure3 shows the contrast enhanced pair imaging. Left side is the monitor mode, which can detect the tumor contour clearly. On the other hand, right side is the CHA mode, which can detect the ablated area clearly. The combination of the both mode is useful to evaluate the efficacy of the HIFU treatment.

Figure4 shows the frequency of peripheral rim enhancement. 7days after HIFU, a peripheral rim enhancement persists 6 of 11 (54.5%). This persists 1 of 11 (9%) lesions 1 month after HIFU. Rim enhancement disappeared in all lesions 3 months after HIFU.

Figure5 reports the change in size of ablated lesion. During 6 months follow-up, the ablated lesions showed a gradual decrease in diameter. The mean percentage of size change was 51%±5.

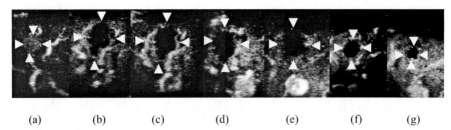

(a)　　　　(b)　　　　(c)　　　　(d)　　　　(e)　　　　(f)　　　　(g)

FIGURE 1. The results of contrast enhanced US Imaging. (a) Before, (b) 1 day after HIFU, (c) 3 days after HIFU, (d) 7 days after HIFU, (e)1 months after HIFU, (f) 3 months after HIFU, (g) 6 months after HIFU

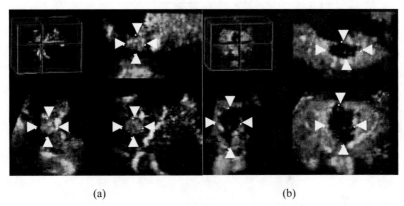

(a)　　　　　　　　　　　　(b)

FIGURE 2. The results of contrast enhanced MPR 3D-US Imaging. (a) Before, (b) 7 days after HIFU

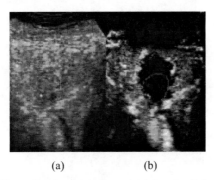

(a)　　　　　　(b)

FIGURE 3. The results of contrast enhanced pair imaging. 7 days after HIFU.
(a) Monitor mode, (b) CHA mode

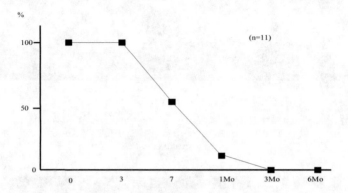

FIGURE 4. Frequency of peripheral rim enhancement after HIFU

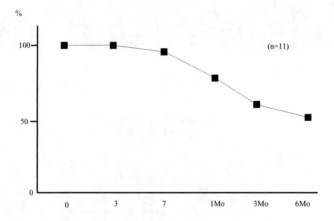

FIGURE 5. The change in size of ablated lesion

DISCUSSION

It is reported that rim enhancement surrounding the ablated lesion in patients who underwent RFA, PEI and microwave coagulation therapy, representing inflammatory reaction to the thermal injury, frequently occurred at short-term follow-up CT performed 1 month after treatment (1-3). Sometimes it is very difficult to differentiate rim enhancement from residual tumor. Peripheral rim enhancement that results from reactive hyperemia is uniform in thickness and envelopes the ablated lesion, whereas residual tumor shows focal and irregular peripheral enhancement. And it is reported that the nontumorous enhancing lesions produced by reactive hyperemia and arteriovenous shunt have usually resolved within 1-3 months (4). In this study, rim enhancement disappeared 3 months after the treatment. On the other hand, the ablated lesions showed a gradual decrease in diameter. Considering the presence of the rim enhancement and the change in size of the ablated lesion, the best timing to evaluate the efficacy of HIFU is thought to be 7 days after treatment by using the MPR 3D-US and contrast-enhanced pair imaging.

CONCLUSION

The best timing for contrast-enhanced ultrasonography to evaluate the response of hepatocellular carcinoma with HIFU is 7 days after the treatment. It is recommended to use the 3D contrast-enhanced ultrasonography.

Footnote

Address correspondence to: Dr. Hiroyuki Fukuda, International HIFU center, Naruto General Hospital, Naruto167,Sanbu-shi, Chiba 289-1326, Japan, Japan. Phone: +81-475-82-2521, Fax: +81-475-82-3354 E-mail: fukuhiro1962@hotmail.com

REFERENCES

1. Lim HK, Choi D, Lee WJ, et al. Hepatocellular carcinoma traeted with percutaneous radio-frequency ablation: evaluation with follow-up multiphase helical CT. Radiology 2001;221:447-454.
2. Ebara M, Kita K, Sugiura N, et al. Therapeutic effect of percutaneous ethanol injection on small hepatocellular carcinoma: evaluation with CT. Radiology 1995;195:371-377.
3. Mitsuzaki K, Yamashita Y, Nishiharu T, et al. CT appearance of hepatic tumors after microwave coagulation therapy. AJR 1998;171:1397-1403.
4. Filippone A, Iezzi R, Di Fabio F, et al. Multidetecter-row computed tomography of focal liver lesions treated by radiofrequency ablation: spectrum of findings at long-term follow-up. J Comput Assist Tomogr 2007;31:42-52

Contrast-Enhanced Three Dimensional Ultrasonography supporting HIFU treatment of Small Liver Cancer

Masao Ohto[a], Hiroyuki Fukuda[a], Ryu Ito[a], Yasushi Shinohara[a], Akio Sakamoto[a] and Eii Karasawa[b]

[a]Internationl HIFU Therapy Center, Naruto General Hospital, 167 Naruto, Sammu-shi, Chiba 289-1326, Japan
[b]IUHW Atami Hospital, 13-1 Higashimati, Atami-shi, Shizuoka 413-0012, Japan

Abstract. HIFU was carried out in the 12 patients with small hepatocellular carcinoma (small HCC) as a extracorporeal ablation therapy, and clinical availability was studied from the results. In carrying out the HIFU therapy, contrast enhanced (CE) three dimensional (3D) ultrasound imaging played an important role to clarify the tumor nature , to monitor the sonication procedure and to assess the tumor ablation and was almost indispensable for the treatment. All the patient had no serious side effects and they are all alive with no local tumor progression for 3 to 14 months after the treatment. Ultrasound supporting HIFU therapy could be usefully available for the treatment of small HCC.

Keywords: three dimensional ultrasound imaging, ultrasound supporting HIFU therapy, small hepatoma
PACS: 87.50.yt, 87.57.-s

INTRODUCTION

With the advance of modern imaging modalities, the number of patients with small HCC less than 3 cm in size is greatly increased in Japan, and now occupies almost one of the fourth in the number. A safer and more reliable extracorporeal ablation therapy is still requested in clinical practice.

So, we have started to carry out ultrasound supporting HIFU therapy as a hopeful clinical treatment modality of small HCC, and are intending to clarify clinical utility of the HIFU therapy. Up to now, the 12 patients with small HCC have received the HIFU therapy.

3D ultrasound imaging with and without contrast enhancement was applied in planning the HIFU therapy, in monitoring the sonication procedure, and in assessing the ablation zone.

From the results, utility of 3D ultrasound imaging was evaluated, and at the same time, clinical availability of the HIFU therapy was studied based on the safety and the therapeutic effects.

CP1113, 8th International Symposium on Therapeutic Ultrasound, edited by E. S. Ebbini
© 2009 American Institute of Physics 978-0-7354-0650-6/09/$25.00

METHODS

The HIFU therapy system (new model, HAIFU, Chongqing, China) was used in this study. Ultrasound imaging apparatus was Logiq 7 (GE-Yokogawa, Tokyo, Japan). Ultrasound contrast agent was Sonazoid (Daiichi-Sankyo, Tokyo, Japan).

The 12 patients with small HCC were treated without rib resection and without adjuvant therapy.

Informed consent from all the patients at the time of enrollment and approval of Ethical Committee of Naruto General Hospital, Japan were essential.

RESULTS

In planning the treatment, the tumor location, the tumor contour, the blood vessels around the tumor, the image shading by rib and lung were minutely studied with relation to the patient posture in the treatment.

Images in monitoring the sonication (FIGURE 1.)

When the tumor had the sonication, two characteristic echo signs such as hyperechoic shot spot and hyperechoic dot-thread one, appeared instantly at the sonication zone. The shot spot sign was accompanied by acoustic back shadowing and soon disappeared in several minutes. The dot-thread sign was seen along the blood vessels around the tumor and continued to retain for a longer period. When the both signs covered the whole tumor including the peritumor zone, the sonication procedure was regarded to finish.

Images in assessing the ablation zone (FIGURE 2.)

Following the sonication procedure, non contrast 3D ultrasound imaging was carried out to confirm the ablation zone including the whole tumor. When a group of hyperechoic dot-thread signs covered the ablation zone in total, the tumor ablation was thought to be in success. Then, CE 3D ultrasound imaging was carried out to confirm ablation zone from the perfusion defect in the contrast dynamics.

When the sonicated tumor was located inside the perfusion defect and further distinctly separated from the perfusion rim on the pair images of ultrasound B mode and contrast mode, the sonication procedure could be finished at all.

Type of tumor on simulation image (FIGURE 3.)

At the beginning, the tumor was classified into three types A, B, and C according to the tumor contour, the patient posture and the grade of image shading by rib and lung on the images in the simulation. Type A had the clear tumor contour, the prone patient posture, and 0 % of the image shading. Type B did the clear tumor contour, the right lateral patient posture, and various % of the image shading. Type C did the obscure tumor contour, the prone or right lateral patient posture, and various % of the image shading by rib and lung.

Relation between tumor type and duration of sonication from first to final shot (FIGURE 4.)

Duration of the sonication was dependent on the tumor type. Type A had a short duration, Type B a intermediate duration, and Type C a long duration. So, difficulty in the sonication procedure was varied dependent on the tumor type in the simulation.

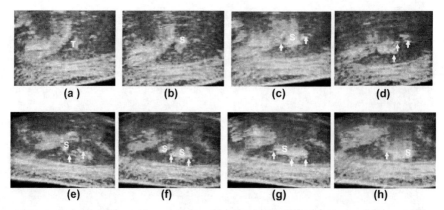

FIGURE 1. Images in monitoring the sonication procedure showing hyperechoic shot spot sign and hyperechoic dot-thread sign. (a)pre shot (b)3rd shot (c)9th shot (d)32nd shot (e)122nd shot (f)135th shot (g)138th shot (h) 146th shot (final shot)
T: tumor S: hyperechoic shot spot sign ▲: hyperechoic dot-thread sign

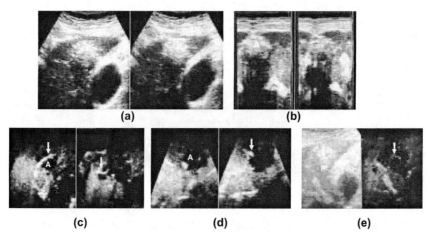

FIGURE 2. Images in assessing the ablation zone. The upper images with non CE 3D ultrasound imaging show a collection of hyperechoic dots, covering the whole tumor and the peritumor zone. (a) A plane-3D images (b) B plane-3D images The bottom images with CE 3D ultrasound imaging delineate the perfusion defect zone due to the ablation. (c) A plane-3D images in arterial dynamic phase (d) B plane -3D images in the same phase (e) pair image of B mode and contrast mode showing the position of treated tumor   A: ablation zone ▲ retained artery P: position of ablated tumor

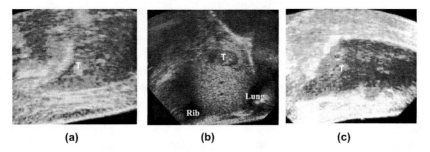

(a)   (b)   (c)

FIGURE 3.. Tumor type on images in ultrasound monitoring. (a)tumor type A: clear tumor contour, prone patient position and 0 % of image shading by rib and lung (b)Tumor type B: clear tumor contour, right lateral patient position and various % of image shading by rib and lung (c)Tumor type C: obscure tumor contour, prone or right lateral patient position, and various % of image shading by rib and lung

type of tumor	no of patients	tumor contour	patient posture	shading by rib and lung	duration of sonication from first to final shot
A	3	clear	prone	% 0	→ 80 - 160 min.
B	4	clear	right lateral	35, 50, 60, 60	→ 160 - 240
C	5	obscure	prone 3	0, 50, 50	→ 240 -
			right lateral 2	40, 70	

FIGURE 4. Relation between tumor type and duration of sonication from first to final shot in the 12 patients with HIFU therapy

DISCUSSION

HIFU therapy has been applied mainly in advanced hepatoma as a palliative method in combination with trasncatheter arterial embolization. In this study, HIFU therapy was performed as a radical cure method in the 12 patients with small HCC who had no previous rib resection and no combination therapy.

From the results, the application of 3D ultrasound imaging was essential for carrying out successfully the HIFU therapy. Each of tumor types on the simulation image was closely related with duration of the sonication procedure. It was understood that the HIFU therapy was deeply affected from the tumor type and the feasibility could be predicted from the tumor image beforehand obtained in the simulation.

During the sonication procedure, two hyperechoic signs such as hyperechoic shot spot sign and hyperechoic dot-thread one were observed. The former sign appeared promptly corresponding to the sonication accompanying by acoustic back shadowing, then disappeared soon within several minutes.

The later sign occurred at the same time in combination with the former sign and the distribution was more widely along the blood vessels around the shot spot.

The dot corresponded with the cross section of the vessel and the thread did with the vertical section of the vessel on the images. The dot-thread sign lasted for a while after the shot spot sign disappeared.

According to the figure, the distribution and the lasting time, the both signs were thought to possess a different origin. The shot spot sign seemed to be due to the cavitation, while the dot-thread sign did to be due to the thermal.

Assessment of the ablation zone also needed the help of 3D ultrasound imaging to delineate exactly the ablation zone. The position of the ablated tumor was clearly demonstrated relating with the periablation zone on the pair images of B mode and contrast mode by CE 3D imaging.

As a whole, 3D ultrasound imaging was essential for carrying out the HIFU therapy.

CONCLUSION

1. Three dimensional ultrasound imaging is essential for carrying out ultrasound supporting HIFU therapy.

2. Ultrasound supporting HIFU therapy could be available clinically as a radical cure method of small hepatoma.

REFERENCES

1. Wu F, Wang ZB, .Chen WZ, et al. Advanced hepatocellular carcinoma: treatment with high-intensity focused ultrasound ablation combined with transcatheter arterial embolization. Radiology 2005; 235: 659-667
2. Fukuda H, Yamaguchi T, Yukisawa S, etal. Animal and clinical studies for the treatment of liver carcinoma with high-intensity focused ultrasound (HIFU). 6th International Symposium on Therapeutic Ultrasound edited by C.-C. Coussios and G. ter Haar. American Institute of Physics. 2007, 375-381.

Producing Uniform Lesion Pattern in HIFU Ablation

Yufeng Zhou[a], Steven G. Kargl[b], and Joo Ha Hwang[a,b]

[a]Division of Gastroenterology, School of Medicine, University of Washington, 1959 NE Pacific Street, Seattle, WA, 98195
[b]Center for Industrial and Medical Ultrasound, Applied Physics Laboratory, University of Washington, 1013 NE 40th Street, Seattle, WA, 98105

Abstract. High intensity focused ultrasound (HIFU) is emerging as a modality for treatment of solid tumors. The temperature at the focus can reach over 65°C denaturing cellular proteins resulting in coagulative necrosis. Typically, HIFU parameters are the same for each treated spot in most HIFU control systems. Because of thermal diffusion from nearby spots, the size of lesions will gradually become larger as the HIFU therapy progresses, which may cause insufficient treatment of initial spots, and over-treatment of later ones. It is found that the produced lesion pattern also depends on the scanning pathway. From the viewpoint of the physician creating uniform lesions and minimizing energy exposure are preferred in tumor ablation. An algorithm has been developed to adaptively determine the treatment parameters for every spot in a theoretical model in order to maintain similar lesion size throughout the HIFU therapy. In addition, the exposure energy needed using the traditional raster scanning is compared with those of two other scanning pathways, spiral scanning from the center to the outside and from the outside to the center. The theoretical prediction and proposed algorithm were further evaluated using transparent gel phantoms as a target. Digital images of the lesions were obtained, quantified, and then compared with each other. Altogether, dynamically changing treatment parameters can improve the efficacy and safety of HIFU ablation.

Keywords: HIFU ablation, uniform lesion generation, parameters, scanning pathway, energy exposure

PACS: 43.80.Sh

1. Introduction

   High intensity focused ultrasound (HIFU) is emerging as a new modality for ablating solid tumors, such as uterine fibroids and cancers of the prostate, kidney, liver, breast, and pancreas [1-4]. In China and Europe more than 100,000 cases have already been carried out in clinics. Despite its uniqueness and encouraging preliminary clinical results, HIFU is still a developing technology yet to be accepted as a therapeutic modality by both patients and physicians. Since tumors are typically several centimeters in diameter, much larger than the focal zone of a HIFU transducer (which is on the order of millimeters in diameter and approximately 1 cm in length), treatment of the entire volume of tumor requires multiple treatment spots. Individual treatment spots are administered in a raster pattern in a treatment layer. Subsequent layers are treated moving proximal to the HIFU source. Because of thermal diffusion from nearby treatment spots, the lesion size of individual treatment spots will gradually become larger as the HIFU therapy progresses, which may cause insufficient treatment of the initial spots and over-treatment of later ones. In this study, two new scanning pathways are proposed and compared with the conventional raster scanning method with the same HIFU parameters (acoustic power and exposure duration). It is found that the scanning pathway affects the lesion production with the new pathways producing more uniform lesions.

   From the viewpoint of the physician, there are 3 basic requirements for the HIFU ablation: 1) ability to generate a predictable lesion for every treatment spot; 2) all generated lesions need to be uniform; 3) complete coverage of the entire treated volume. In order to achieve these goals, an algorithm was developed to generate uniform lesions using different scanning pathways. The uniform lesion production was confirmed in both the gel phantom and *ex vivo* experiments. Furthermore, the number of pulses delivered for each spot and the total number of pulses applied using these scanning pathways are compared. Altogether, it is suggested that the HIFU energy needs to be adjusted dynamically in order to achieve uniform lesions and to guarantee the subsequent therapeutic effect.

CP1113, *8th International Symposium on Therapeutic Ultrasound*, edited by E. S. Ebbini
© 2009 American Institute of Physics 978-0-7354-0650-6/09/$25.00

2. Methods

A conventional scanning approach used in clinical HIFU therapy is raster scanning (Fig. 1a). Here, only one treatment layer is considered for simplicity. Besides the raster scan, two new scanning pathways, spiral scanning from the center of the treatment area to the outside (Fig. 1b) and spiral scanning from the outside to the center (Fig. 1c) are evaluated. In this study, there are total 25 treatment spots arranged in the shape of a diamond with a grid size of 4 mm. The treatment parameters are the same for each spot: the HIFU on time is 150 ms, the HIFU off time is 150 ms, there are 60 pulses per spot with an interval time between treatment spots of 6 s.

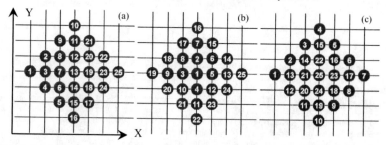

FIGURE 1. Schematic illustration of different high-intensity focused ultrasound scanning pathways, (a) raster scanning, (b) spiral scanning from the center to the outside, and (c) spiral scanning from the outside to the center.

The mathematical model for temperature elevation in the tissue is based on the BioHeat transfer equation (BHTE) [5],

$$\frac{\partial T}{\partial t} = k\Delta T - \frac{T - T_0}{t_p} + \frac{Q}{c_v}, \qquad (1)$$

where t is the time, t_p is the perfusion time, $T(r, t)$ is the tissue temperature, T_0 is the equilibrium temperature, $k = K/c_v$ is the local tissue temperature conductivity, K is the heat conductivity, C_v is the heat capacity of a unit volume, and Δ is the Laplacian operator. The pressure waveform through sample was measured using a fiber optic probe hydrophone (FOPH) [6], and the absorbed ultrasound energy, Q, was calculated as

$$Q = 4\sum_{n=0}^{\infty} \alpha_n |C_n|^2 / c_0 \rho_0, \qquad (2)$$

where C_n is the amplitude of the nth harmonic in the measured pressure waveform, $\alpha_n = (n\omega_0)^2 b / 2c_0^3 \rho_0$ is the attenuation coefficient, which exhibits quadratic frequency dependence.

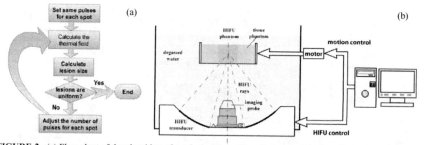

FIGURE 2. (a) Flow chart of the algorithm of producing the uniform lesions and (b) the schematic diagram of the experimental setup for generating multiple lesions in the gel phantom using a HIFU system.

The HIFU system used in this study (FEP-BY02, Yuande Bio-Engineering, Ltd., Beijing, China) consists of 251 individual PZT elements, driven all in phase and arranged in a concave spherical holder. The HIFU transducer has a center frequency of ~1 MHz, an outer diameter of 33.5 cm and an inner diameter of 12 cm with integrated ultrasound imaging probe (S3, Logiq 5, GE, Seongnam, Korea) mounted in the central hole co-axial to the HIFU beam. An optically transparent gel phantom (L×W×H=5.5 cm×5.5 cm×5 cm), composed of polyarylamide hydrogel and bovine serum albumin (BSA) that becomes optically opaque when denatured by heat [7], was surrounded by a tissue phantom that contains 6.5% Alginate (Jeltrate, Dentsply International, York, PA). The center of the transparent gel phantom was aligned with the HIFU focus under the guidance of B-mode ultrasound imaging. A LabVIEW (National Instruments, Austin, TX) program was written and run on a PC to control the motion of the treatment table and delivery of HIFU pulses. After the treatment, the HIFU phantom was taken out and the lesions were recorded photographically for comparison. Furthermore, the projected lesion areas and maximum lesion lengths were calculated by processing the images in Photoshop (Adobe Systems Inc., San Jose, CA).

An algorithm was developed to generate uniform lesions according to the different scanning pathways (Fig. 2a). First, the same number of pulses was used to calculate the thermal field and the subsequent lesion sizes. Then the number of pulses for each spot was adjusted in order to obtain 4 mm diameter lesions using a linear extrapolation model. Such an iteration was repeated, usually 5~10 times, until uniform lesions were obtained in the simulation.

3. Results

The lesions generated in the gel phantom were found to have similar pattern and characteristics as predicted by the theoretical simulations (data not shown). By using the raster scanning method, the lesion can only be visualized beginning with the 3rd treatment spot (Fig. 3a). In addition, two other spots on the boundary of the treatment area, 5th and 10th treatment spots, were not visible. With the progress of the HIFU treatment the lesion size became larger because of the thermal diffusion from nearby spots. Merging of lesions occurred toward the end of the treatment. However, the change of lesion size was not monotonic in nature. For example, the largest spot was not the last treatment spot, rather it is the 3rd to last spot. When using the spiral scanning pathway from the center to the outside, only the first lesion was not visible (Fig. 3b). However, the other lesions were smaller in comparison to those generated in raster scanning pathway, and no merging of lesions was observed. The lesion pattern using the spiral scanning, from the outside to the center, had different characteristics (Fig. 3c) with all treatment spots along the outside boundary (first 12 spots) not being visible. Since thermal energy is concentrated toward the center of the treatment area, the last few lesions merged to form a large lesion. The lesion areas are calculated to be 96.8 mm^2, 26.1 mm^2, and 67.1 mm^2, respectively, using these scanning pathways. The patterns of lesion production and their characteristics can also be assessed by observing the lesions from the lateral direction. The maximum lesion lengths using these scanning pathways were 10.1 mm, 6.9 mm, and 12.2 mm, respectively.

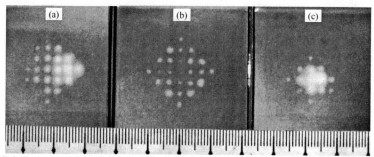

FIGURE 3. Comparison of the generated lesions in the phantom from the top view by using different scanning pathways, (a) raster scan, (b) spiral scanning from the center to the outside, and (c) spiral scanning from the outside to the center.

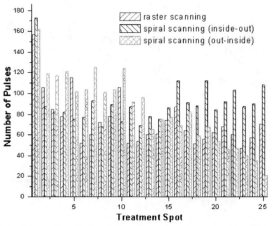

FIGURE 4. Comparison of the number of pulses delivered to each treatment spot using different scanning pathway.

In order to generate uniform lesions the number of pulses delivered to each treatment spot should be adjusted using our proposed algorithm. It is found that at the first spot the maximum energy (largest number of pulses) should be used, ~ 160 (Fig. 4) in comparison to 60 in Fig. 3. The trend of adjusting the energy exposure is complicated and also dependent on the specific scanning pathway. The generated lesions are shown in Fig. 5. The total numbers of pulses delivered using the 3 scanning pathways are: 1832, 2261, and 2105, respectively. In addition, uniform lesions can also be generated in the bovine liver to validate the application of our algorithm in tissue (data not shown).

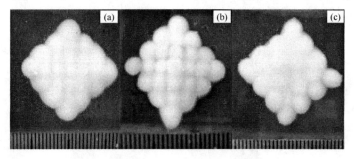

FIGURE 3. Comparison of the generated lesions in the phantom by using the dynamically adjusted energies and different scanning pathways, (a) raster scanning, (b) spiral from the center to the outside, and (c) spiral from the outside to the center.

4. Discussion

HIFU has been used in the clinical setting in China and Europe with promising results. However, it remains a developing technology. Currently, the HIFU focus is scanned throughout the tumor in either discrete points/spots as with the FEP-BY02 system or pre-determined scanning trajectories as with the model JC system (Chongqing

Haifu Technology Co., Ltd., Chongqing, China) [1]. Treatment parameters are typically not adjusted during the treatment unless adjustment is necessary for patient tolerance. Because of the thermal accumulation and diffusion effects, the lesion size will increase as the HIFU therapy progresses. Therefore, the lesions produced at the beginning of the HIFU therapy may be insufficient to cause tissue necrosis while those areas treated toward the end of the therapy may be overexposed, increasing the potential of unintended collateral thermal injury. This asymmetric lesion production pattern has been observed in our *ex vivo* studies (data not shown). Although no *in vivo* study has been performed to confirm this phenomenon, it is reasonable to extrapolate this lesion production pattern to the clinical environment. From the viewpoint of the physician, predictable uniform lesion formation is desired. In this study, two new pathways, spiral scanning from the center to the outside and from the outside to the center, are evaluated and compared with the conventional raster scanning. It is found that more uniform lesions are produced by using these new spiral pathways, although resulting in different lesion patterns and requiring more energy to achieve uniform lesions. Therefore, the scanning pathway has a great impact on the lesion production. However, the consequences on HIFU therapy outcomes require further investigation.

A considerable body of research has been undertaken to understand the mechanisms of HIFU lesion production [9-12]. In these experiments, usually a single lesion was studied. However, clinically, HIFU treatment of tumors requires multiple lesions for effective ablation. Multi-lesion production is more complex than simply summing multiple single lesions. Tissue at the focal region of the HIFU transducer absorbs the acoustic energy and then converts it into thermal energy. Owing to the thermal diffusion phenomenon the thermal energy at the focal region will spread towards the surrounding space and the ambient temperature will be raised. It has already been shown that larger lesions are formed with the same delivered energy at a higher background temperature. Therefore, the lesion size will gradually increase as the HIFU therapy progresses. If the lesion size is larger than the interval distance between spots, lesions may coalesce. All together, it is illustrated that thermal accumulation and diffusion effects are critical in multi-lesion treatments. Accounting for thermal accumulation and diffusion effects is of importance in HIFU planning in order to produce uniform lesions and minimize the total acoustic energy used during the treatments. In addition, lesion formation by HIFU in tissue depends on the physical properties of the tissue, such as perfusion time and heat capacity. A hyper-vascular tumor, such as hepatocellular carcinoma, has a short perfusion time. Its thermal accumulation and diffusion effects may not be as significant as in hypo-vascular tissues, such as pancreatic cancer. Thus tissue type also needs to be considered in HIFU therapy planning.

In order to generate uniform lesions, delivered acoustic energies should be adjusted for each treatment spot. In our gel phantom study, the first lesion was never visible no matter which pathway is used. A rational approach to HIFU treatment would be to have the first treatment spot receive the highest acoustic energy and to gradually decrease the acoustic energy for subsequent treatment spots. A simple algorithm has been proposed and was used to generate uniform lesions for different scanning pathways. Although it seems that the raster scanning requires the least energy for uniform lesion production among the studied scanning pathways, this conclusion may not be extended because the lesion productions depends on many factors, such as the tissue type, HIFU system, and spot spacing. Optimization of specific treatment patterns and HIFU parameters will be the focus of future studies.

References and links

[1] F. Wu, W. Z. Chen, J. Bai, J. Z. Zou, Z. L. Wang, H. Zhu, Z. B. Wang, *Ultrasound Med. Biol. 27(8)*, 1099-1106, (2001).
[2] P. M. Meaney, M. D. Cahill, G. R. ter Haar, *Ultrasound Med. Biol. 26(3)*, 441-450, (2000).
[3] G. R. ter Haar, *Physics Today*, 29-34, (2001).
[4] T. J. Dubinsky, C. Cuevas, M. K. Dighe, O. Kolokythas, J. H. Hwang, *Ultrasound Imaging · Review*, *190*, 191-199, (2008).
[5] M. R. Bailey, V. A. Khokhlova, O. A. Sapozhnikov, S. G. Kargl, and L. A. Crum, *Acoustical Physics 49(4)*, 437-464, (2003).
[6] Y.F. Zhou, L. Zhai, R. Simmons, P. Zhong, *J. Acoust. Soc. Am.*, 120(2), 676-685, (2006).
[7] C. Lafon, V. Zderic, M. L. Noble, J. C. Yuen, P. J. Kaczkowski, O. A. Sapozhnikov, F. Chavrier, L. A. Crum, and S. Vaezy, *Ultrasound Med. Biol. 31(10)*, 1383-1389, (2005).
[8] J. E. Kenney, *Nature Review · Cancer*, *5*, 321-327, (2005).
[9] G. R. ter Haar, *Echocardiography 18(4)*, 317-324, (2001).
[10] S. Vaezy, M. Andrew, P. Kaczkowski, L. Crum, *Annu. Rev. Biomed. Eng. 3*, 375-390, (2001)
[11] V. A. Khokhlova, M. R. Bailey, J. A. Reed, B. W. Cunitz, P. J. Kaczkowski, L. A. Crum, *J. Acoust. Soc. Am. 119(3)*, 1834-1848, (2006).
[12] B.A. Rabkin, V. Zderic, S. Vaezy, *Ultrasound Med. Biol. 31(7)*, 947-956, (2005).

HIFU lesion characterization on liver: acquisition and results

Bruno Durning,[a] Jason Raymond,[b] Charles C. Church,[b]
Robin O. Cleveland,[b] and Eric L. Miller[c]

[a]Department of Electrical and Computer Engineering, Tufts University, Medford, Massachusetts
[b]National Center for Physical Acoustics, University of Mississippi, Oxford, Mississippi
[c]Department of Mechanical Engineering, Boston University, Boston, Massachusetts

Abstract. A key problem in the practical use of high intensity focused ultrasound (HIFU) as a tool for cancer treatment is the non-invasive characterization of the regions of tissue that have been successfully necrosed. Previously, we proposed an approach to image guidance based on the use of echo data obtained from a diagnostic ultrasound transducer and a shape-based inverse scattering approach. Here an experimental apparatus is described to acquire data for *in vitro* phantom experiments and ex vivo experiments with HIFU-induced lesions in porcine liver. The in vitro studies employed tissue-mimicking phantoms with inclusions embedded to simulate HIFU lesions. Using just 5 elements of a 3.5-MHz ultrasound array, the inversion was able to recover the properties of lesions down to a size of 20 mm long by 4 mm in diameter. Experiments were then carried out with fresh excised porcine liver. A 1.1-MHz HIFU transducer was used to create lesions in the liver, and the tissue was then scanned with the ultrasound array. After imaging the tissue was sliced and the true lesion geometry assessed optically. The echo data were then processed to determine the lesion from the data. It was found for lesions with cavitation that the hyperechogenecity from the bubbles made the inversion unable to find the lesion. For the HIFU lesions formed with no cavitation, the lesions had a diameter of less than 3 mm and were too small to be detected with the 5-element array. These results indicate that the shape-based inversion process is promising for detecting purely thermal lesions but that more elements may be needed for detection of HIFU lesions.

Keywords: HIFU detection, inverse problem, model-based.
PACS: 43.60.Lq, 43.60.Uv, 43.80.Jz

INTRODUCTION

The non-invasive nature of HIFU is a attractive feature for cancer treatment but also creates a challenge in that there is no visual feedback on the regions that have been treated. Thus, observing the creation and evolution of lesions during HIFU is a significant barrier to the adoption of the technology. The gold standard in the United States is to use magnetic resonance (MR) to detect temperature elevation and, using a thermal model, to ascertain where lesions form [1]. Ultrasound imaging may appear an attractive modality to detect lesions, however, there is not a robust change in the ultrasound image during HIFU [2] except when cavitation is plentiful – a scenario that many HIFU operators wish to avoid. It has been reported that the acoustic attenuation and sound-speed of tissue change with lesion formation. In particular, attenuation

CP1113, *8th International Symposium on Therapeutic Ultrasound,* edited by E. S. Ebbini
© 2009 American Institute of Physics 978-0-7354-0650-6/09/$25.00

increases 2-8 fold, and the process is irreversible [3]. This has motivated work in trying to detect these changes from standard B-mode data.

The approach investigated here exploits the fact that one does not need to create an image of the soft tissue with a lesion but rather just needs to determine the position and size of the lesion. That is, as described in Ref. [4], the problem can be cast in terms of characterization of a well-defined target rather than image formation.

MATERIAL AND METHODS

The configuration of the data acquisition is as shown in Fig. 1. A HIFU transducer creates an ellipsoid-shaped lesion aligned with its focal axis. An ultrasound imaging array is placed perpendicular to the HIFU beam and multiple transmit-receive data lines between all elements are measured, a form of backscatter tomography. This gives a 2D view of the tissue, and by translating the array a 3D data set is acquired.

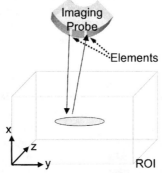

FIGURE 1. Configuration of the HIFU induced lesion and the imaging array.

Inversion Scheme

Each backscattered data line is transformed into the frequency domain as the data to be matched by the inversion algorithm. The forward model used for the inversion, for the case of an object that has changes in sound speed and attenuation, can be cast in the following form:

$$\upsilon_R(\omega, E_{Tx}, E_{Rx}) = \int_{r \in V} K_c(\omega, r, E_{Tx}, E_{Rx}) c_P(r) + K_\alpha(\omega, r, E_{Tx}, E_{Rx}) \alpha_P(r) \, dr \quad (1)$$

where c_p is the perturbation in the sound speed, α_p the perturbation in the attenuation and the kernels for the sound speed can be expressed as:

$$K_c(\omega, r, E_{Tx}, E_{Rx}) = e_{pe}(\omega) \Re\left(k_b(\omega)\right) g(\omega, r, E_{Tx}) g(\omega, r, E_{Rx}) \,. \quad (2)$$

with a similar result holding for K_α. In (2), e_{pe} is the pulse-echo transfer function of the elements, k_b the background wavenumber and $g(.)$ the spatial transfer functions of either the transmitter or receiver. For the details associated with these equations the reader is directed to Ref. [4].

In the inversion scheme c_p and α_p are only non-zero within an ellipsoidal volume where the parameters of the ellipse, position, lengths and rotations are free variables to be determined. Equations (1) and (2) are then used to determine the modeled data v_R for the given ellipsoidal parameters. A cost function is defined as the normalized squared error between the real and the imaginary components of the measured data u_R and the modeled data v_R. Here the cost function was minimized using the LSQNONLIN function from Matlab (The Mathworks, Natick, MA), in order to find the optimal properties of the ellipsoid.

Experimental Methods

For the *in vitro* assessment, a "lesion" was carved from polyurethane (Rencast 6410) which has high acoustic attenuation [5]. Graphite powder was added to give it scattering properties equivalent to tissue. The lesion was held in the middle of a mold using nylon thread, and then an agar-based tissue-mimicking phantom [6] was poured into the mold and allowed to set in order to create the background medium. Both the lesion and the phantom had graphite powder included in their recipe in order to provide equivalent ultrasonic scattering properties. The attenuation coefficients were 0.9 dB/cm and 8.9 dB/cm, with sound speeds of 1525 m/s and 1530 m/s, for the background tissue and lesion, respectively. The higher attenuation and sound speed of the lesion were representative of what one might expect for a HIFU lesion.

The ultrasonic data were taken using a 3.5-MHz probe (Model 8665, BK Medical, Wilmington, MA). The probe was connected to an Analogic Ultrasound Engine (AN2300, Analogic Corp, Peabody, MA) and un-beamformed data recorded where a pulse was transmitted on one element and received on a different element. The raw RF echo data were saved for later processing. For the results reported here, data were acquired using just five elements of the probe. The selected elements were not consecutive, and the effective pitch between the elements was 2.5 mm. Five frequency components were employed evenly distributed from 3 MHz to 4 MHz.

For the experiments involving lesions in tissue, we employed fresh porcine liver. The tissue was placed in PBS and degassed with a vacuum pressure of about 80% for 30 minutes. It was then placed in the tank to be treated. A baseline inversion data set was acquired after which the sample was treated with HIFU. The HIFU source was a 1.1-MHz (ModelH-102, Sonic Concepts, Bothell, WA) with a diameter of 69.94 mm and focal length 62.64 mm. The source was driven with an electrical input power of 20 – 40 W. Pressure measurements in water yielded Isptp = 740-1480 W/cm^2. After HIFU treatment a second image set was taken to determine the ability of the inversion algorithm to detect the lesion. Then the liver was cut into slices approximately 1 mm thick and the lesion photographed from which the true lesion size could be assessed.

RESULTS

Figure 2 shows the phantom lesion and the corresponding B-mode image. The lesion did not appear in B-mode, but the shadow cast due to its high attenuation is observed. The rectangular box shows the region of interest (ROI) where the inversion was performed, and the ellipse shows the result after running the inversion algorithm. This was done for three ellipsoids of different sizes with the results shown in Table 1. It can be seen that the inversion did a good job of capturing the medium and large lesion, but the smaller lesion with a diameter around 3.4 mm was not accurately represented. For the number of elements and frequencies employed here this may be a limit on the resolution of the inversion.

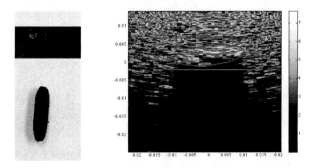

FIGURE 2. Left: Photograph of lesion. Right: B-mode image (axes in metres). The ROI and result from the inversion are overlaid. Note that the inversion did not employ the B-mode data.

TABLE 1. Results (in mm) for the two diameters and the length of the lesions are measured ("True") and as estimated from the inversion ("Result"). For the medium and large lesions the difference was less than 0.5 mm where as for the small lesion it was up to 5 mm.

	Small		Medium		Large	
	True	Result	True	Result	True	Result
Diameter	2.9	4.0	4.8	4.6	5.6	6.1
Diameter	3.8	4.8	5.4	5.8	6.8	6.1
Length	20.5	15	20.6	20.3	19.2	19.4

Figure 3(a) shows a B-mode image of porcine tissue after HIFU treatment and the result from the inversion algorithm (blue circle). In this case the lesion estimated by the inversion was 4.2 mm x 18 mm and that measured in "post mortem" was 4.2 mm x 18 mm. The result though is misleading as the sample was not degassed and cavitation occurred. As the signal induced by cavitation is not incorporated into the algorithm, it was just chance that the inversion returned the correct values. Indeed, the result of the inversion was not robust to changes in the initial guess provided to the algorithm concerning the parameters of the ellipsoid We note that the region of cavitation (echogenenicity) observed on the B-mode image was larger than the measured lesion indicating that cavitation is not necessarily a reliable indicator of lesion position.

Subsequently the tissue was degassed for ~30 minutes before HIFU treatment. In this case the resulting lesion was formed and no cavitation was detected. Figure 3(b) is an optical image from the "post-mortem" assessment showing a lesion of 3 mm diameter. The inversion algorithm was unable to reconstruct this lesion – presumably because it is smaller than the nominal resolution limit found in the *in vitro* study.

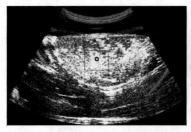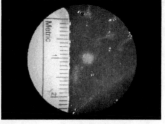

FIGURE 3. Left: B-mode image of tissue phantom. Right: Photograph of lesion.

DISCUSSION AND CONCLUSIONS

An inversion method for detecting ellipsoidal inclusions in tissue has been developed. The *in vitro* validation studies indicate that, for the number of elements and frequencies employed here, it can reliably detect lesions down to diameters of 4 mm. In tissue the algorithm was not able to operate correctly for lesions in which cavitation was present. For the cavitation-free lesions created here, the size was too small to be detected by the inversion. We envision that employing more elements and more frequency components should allow smaller lesions to be detected.

ACKNOWLEDGMENTS

This work was supported in part by the National Institutes of Health through R21 CA 123523 and by CenSSIS, the Gordon Center for Subsurface Sensing and Imaging Systems, under the Engineering Research Centers Program of the National Science Foundation (Award Number EEC-9986821).

REFERENCES

1. Hynynen, K. and N. McDannold, MRI guided and monitored focused ultrasound thermal ablation methods: a review of progress. Int. J. Hyperthermia, 2004. 20: 725-37.
2. Vaezy, S., Shi, X., Martin, R.W., Chi, E., Nelson, R.I., Bailey, M.R., Crum, L.A., "Real-time visualization of high-intensity focused ultrasound treatment using ultrasound imaging," Ultrasound Med. Biol. 27, 33–42 (2001).
3. Techavipoo, U., Varghese, T., Chen, Q., Stiles, T.A., Zagzebski, J.A., Frank, G.R., "Temperature dependence of ultrasonic propagation speed and attenuation in excised canine liver tissue measured using transmitted and reflected pulses," J. Acoust. Soc. Am. 116, 2859–2865 (2004)
4. Ulker Karbeyaz, B., Miller, E.L. and Cleveland, R.O., "Shape Based Ultrasound Tomography for Detection of HIFU Lesions," 123: 2994-2956 J. Acoust. Soc. Am. (2008).
5. Wallace, K.D., T.M. Krueger, C.W. Lloyd, M.R. Holland, and J.G. Miller, Comparison of the (linear) 2f field transmitted with a fully realized two-dimensional effective apodization and the (nonlinear) 2f harmonic field. IEEE Ultrasonics Symposium, 2005: 1203-1206.
6. Huang, J., R.G. Holt, R.O. Cleveland, and R.A. Roy, Experimental Validation of a Tractable Numerical Model for HIFU-Induced Heating in Flow-Through Tissue Phantoms. J. Acoust. Soc. Am., 2004. 116:2451-2458

Preclinical Evaluation of the Accuracy of HIFU Treatments Using a Tumor-Mimic Model. Results of Animal Experiments

D. Melodelima[a], W.A. N'Djin[a], H. Parmentier[a], M. Rivoire[a,b] and J.Y. Chapelon[a]

[a] Inserm, U556, Lyon, F-69003, France ; Université de Lyon, Lyon, F-69003, France
[b] Centre Léon Bérard, Lyon, F-69008, France

Abstract. Presented in this paper is a tumor-mimic model that allows the evaluation at a preclinical stage of the targeting accuracy of HIFU treatments in the liver. The tumor-mimics were made by injecting a warm mixture of agarose, cellulose, and glycerol that polymerizes immediately in hepatic tissue and forms a 1 cm discrete lesion that is detectable by ultrasound imaging and gross pathology. Three studies were conducted: (i) in vitro experiments were conducted to study acoustical proprieties of the tumor-mimics, (ii) animal experiments were conducted in ten pigs to evaluate the tolerance of the tumor-mimics at mid-term (30 days), (iii) ultrasound-guided HIFU ablation has been performed in ten pigs with tumor-mimics to demonstrate that it is possible to treat a predetermined zone accurately. The attenuation of tumor-mimics was 0.39 dB.cm-1 at 1 MHz, the ultrasound propagation velocity was 1523 m.s-1, and the acoustic impedance was 1.8 MRayls. The pigs tolerated tumor-mimics and treatment well over the experimental period. Tumor-mimics were visible with high contrast on ultrasound images. In addition, it has been demonstrated by using the tumor-mimic as a reference target, that tissue destruction induced by HIFU and observed on gross pathology corresponded to the targeted area on the ultrasound images. The average difference between the predetermined location of the HIFU ablation and the actual coagulated area was 16%. These tumor-mimics are identifiable by ultrasound imaging, they do not modify the geometry of HIFU lesions and thus constitutes a viable mimic of tumors indicated for HIFU therapy.

Keywords: Ultrasound, HIFU, liver, metastases, tumor-mimic, imaging.
PACS: 43.80.Sh

INTRODUCTION

To date, the therapeutic efficacy of High Intensity Focused Ultrasound (HIFU) treatments on tumors has been studied on inoculated tumor models of small animals like the rat or the rabbit[1,2]. These models make it possible to perform survival studies but extrapolating results to human is sometimes difficult, especially in terms of volume treated and tolerance. Currently, the pig is an ideal animal model for studying HIFU applied to the treatment of hepatic tumors because of its size and physiology similar to humans. However, there is no established liver tumor model in pigs and HIFU studies are generally performed on healthy pigs. In addition, it was demonstrated that negative margins all around a tumor decrease the recurrence rate[3].

CP1113, *8th International Symposium on Therapeutic Ultrasound,* edited by E. S. Ebbini
© 2009 American Institute of Physics 978-0-7354-0650-6/09/$25.00

The aim of this study was to use a target that is detectable by ultrasound imaging and by gross pathology to evaluate, at the preclinical stage, the spatial accuracy with which a HIFU liver-specific medical device can create a coagulated zone. We propose to use an injectable sonographic tumor-mimic describe in a study on radiofrequency ablation[4]. These tumor-mimics could be excellent tools for assessing whether the position of the induced necrosis actually corresponds to the theoretical position of the HIFU ablation. To date, this model has never been studied acoustically neither over long-term periods. Three studies were conducted. First, several acoustic proprieties of tumor-mimics were studied. Second, tumor-mimics were injected in vivo in 10 pig livers and a radiological, clinical, histological and biological monitoring of the pigs was performed to assess long-term (30 days) tolerance and feasibility. Third, HIFU exposures were performed *in vivo* to determine the feasibility of treating a targeted zone with negative treatment margins.

MATERIAL AND METHODS

Acoustical parameters of tumor-mimics

This approach aims for checking that the mimic-model is suitable to carry out in vivo studies in pig livers by comparing mimic-model acoustical parameters. Tumor-mimics were prepared as described in. A 5 MHz plane transducer and a 0.4 mm needle hydrophone (PZT-Z44-0400, SEA) were used for transmission measurements. The acoustical parameters studied were attenuation, ultrasound celerity and acoustical impedance. The overall measurements were performed at room temperature. Absolute pressure attenuation values of the tumor-mimic and of a sample of pig liver was determined in a frequency band of 1 to 7.5 MHz with a step of 0.5 MHz.

Tolerance of tumor-mimics

This study was performed on ten pigs. Animals with an average weight of 23.2 ± 2.7 kg (19.6-27.3 kg) were used. Premedication was performed using an intramuscular injection of ketamine (15 mg/kg) before anaesthesia which was achieved using a 15 mL intravenous injection of Propofol. Oxygenation was supplied from an assisted ventilation system at a rate of 10 L/min. Anaesthesia was maintained using an intravenous injection of Propofol (20 mL/h) and Sufentanil (5 mL/h) in a continuous perfusion of physiological salt solution. A 25 cm median laparotomy was performed. Each pig has received a mean of 3.9 ± 0.3 (range 3-5) injections of tumor-mimics. This mixture is liquid at 65 °C and solid at 37 °C. The tumor-mimic is injected under ultrasound imaging control using a 12 MHz linear ultrasound imaging probe. Liver movements caused by breathing were eliminated by maintaining pigs under apnea during the injection (1ml for each tumor-mimic). After being injected, tumor-mimic hardens in the liver within one minute producing a hyperechoic discrete lesion. Animals were euthanized at D0 (2 pigs), D4 (4 pigs), D8 (2 pigs), D15 (1 pig) and D30 (1 pig) after the injections. Animals were euthanized under general anesthesia by a single intravenous 0.3 ml/kg injection containing embutramide, mebezonium and tetracaine. Tumor-mimics were removed and sectioned transversally. Histological analysis was performed using routine hematoxylin and eosin methods.

Evaluating accuracy of HIFU preclinical studies

This study was performed on ten pigs. Animals with an average weight of 23.2 ± 2.7 kg (19.6 - 27.3) were used and anaesthetized as described previously. Thermal ablations were produced using an intraoperative toroidial HIFU device with integrated ultrasound imaging probe that has been previously described[5]. HIFU ablations were performed after injection of 4 tumor-mimics per animal. To surround the tumor-mimic with negative margins, 9 juxtaposed HIFU lesions were performed. These lesions were created by juxtaposing single lesions by hand (three rows of three singles lesions with a displacement of 1 cm between each single lesion were created). When the treatment was completed, all the lesions were observed and measured on sonograms. After the end of the procedure, the liver was removed and sliced to inspect ultrasound effects visually. All of the animal procedures were done after local institutional review board approval. These experiments conformed to the requirements of the local Office of Animal Experimentation and were in accordance with the legal conditions of the National Commission on Animal Experimentation.

RESULTS

Acoustic parameters of tumor-mimics

Into the band frequency 1-7.5 MHz, the average attenuation of tumor-mimics was nonlinear and was interpolated by a power function. The log-log slope was 1.63 and the attenuation at 1 MHz was 0.41 dB.cm^{-1} (Figure 1). The average speed of sound in the model was measured at 1522 ± 1 m.s^{-1} (1522 - 1524). The acoustical impedance in the model was 1.84 ± 0.01 MRays (1.84 - 1.88).

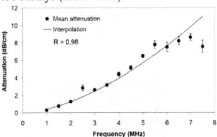

FIGURE 1. Acoustical attenuation in the model between 1-7.5 MHz

Tolerance of tumor-mimics

Thirty-nine out of 44 injections (88%) were successful. Five injections have failed due to injections into blood vessels and one in a biliary duct. One injection was not visible on sonograms. One pig died on D0 following a vena cave hemorrhage due to excessive traction on the liver not related to the injection. 80% of the tumor-mimics were homogenous and ellipsoidal. Pigs recovered from the procedures within two hours after termination of anaesthesia, and resumed eating and normal behavior.

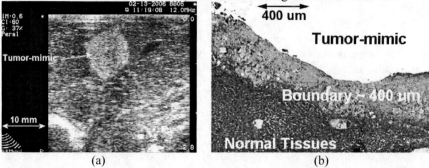

(a)   (b)

FIGURE 2. (a) Tumor-mimic observed on sonogram using a 12 MHz probe the day of injection. (b) Boundary between tumor-mimic and normal tissue observed histologically the day of injection.

Ultrasound imaging (Fig. 2a) and macroscopic analysis show no evidence of changes in the geometry of the tumor-mimics throughout the 30 days of the study. The mean values on D0 for major, longitudinal and minor diameters of tumor-mimics for 1 cc injections measured on sonograms were 13.9 ± 1.8 mm (8.1 - 22.0), 9.8 ± 1.4 mm (5.7 - 15.0) and 6.3 ± 1.1 mm (2.9 - 9.5) respectively. Differences between ultrasound and macroscopic measurements of large, medium and small diameters were respectively 15.5 ± 7.5% (0.0 - 59.0), 19.1 ± 7.2% (0.0 - 48.7%) and 18.0 ± 5.3% (0.0 - 50.0). Histological analysis revealed no changes in healthy hepatic tissue within a 500 μm radius around the injected tumor-mimic (Fig. 2b).

Evaluating accuracy of HIFU preclinical studies

27 HIFU lesions centered on tumor-mimics were produced (Fig. 3). The average longitudinal ablated diameter was 23.0 ± 3.1 mm (14.0 - 32.0) and the average transversal ablated diameter was 40.3 ± 6.4 mm (19.0 - 58.0).

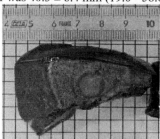

FIGURE 3. Nine juxtaposed HIFU exposures centered in the tumor-mimic with negative margins.

94% of the margins were negative. The margins around the mimic-model were measured in the 3 dimensions respectively at 14.7 ± 5.5 mm (1.0 - 39.0), 5.7 ± 2.3 mm (0.0 - 12.0) and 6.4 ± 3.2 mm (0.0 - 18.0).

DISCUSSION

Acoustic parameters in the tumor-mimics were closed to those in *in vivo* liver tissues and allow use of this model in animals. The first in vivo study confirmed the feasibility and the tolerance of injections. The tumor-mimic formed a discrete lesion in hepatic tissues at least for 30 days. Tumor-mimics dimensions were correlated between sonogram and macroscopic samples. Furthermore, the results of blood analyses performed throughout the study showed that tumor-mimics were tolerated by the animals and, therefore, could be used as a reference target for evaluating the accuracy of preclinical HIFU treatments without creating complications.

Ultrasound guidance makes it possible to juxtapose HIFU lesions on the tumor with negative margins and with homogeneous ablation. During treatment the tumor-mimic remains a fixed reference point on the ultrasound image during the course of HIFU juxtapositions and constitutes an effective target tool. Thus, at the preclinical level the tumor-mimic model allows to confirm that the ultrasound exposure procedure ensures treatment that is adapted in terms of localization and margins.

ACKNOWLEDGMENTS

The authors wish to thank the staff of the institute for experimental surgery for their aid in the animal study. This work was supported by funding from the Cancéropôle Lyon Auvergne Rhône Alpes (PDC 2006.4.8), from the Cancéropôle Grand Ouest (CDTU 2004-01) and from the French Agency for Research on Cancer (ARC 4023). We also wish to thank the Anipath Laboratory and the Pr Scoazec for carrying out the histology study.

REFERENCES

1. Chen L et al. *Ultrasound Med Biol* **25**, 847-856 (1999)
2. Prat F et al. *Hepatology* **21**, 832-836 (1995)
3. McLoughlin JM et al. *Cancer Control* **13**, 32-41 (2006)
4. Scott DJ et al. *J Gastrointest Surg*.**4**, 620-625 (2000)
4. Melodelima D. et al. *Appl. Phys. Letters* **91**, 193901 (2007).

Regrowth of myomas after magnetic resonance-guided focused ultrasound surgery (MRgFUS): Can a repeat procedure improve the clinical outcome?

Kaoru Funaki, M.D. and Hidenobu Fukunishi, M.D.

Department of Gynecology, Shinsuma general hospital, 4-1-6, Isonare-cho, Suma-ku, Kobe, 654-0047,
Japan
TEL; +81-78-735-0001, FAX; +81-78-735-5685
E-mail; kfunakik-shinsuma@yahoo.co.jp

Objective: To estimate the efficacy of repeated magnetic resonance–guided focused ultrasound surgery (MRgFUS) for myomas in cases of established clinical failure. **Significance**: We previously reported that high-intensity myomas (type 3), evaluated by pretreatment T2-weighted magnetic resonance imaging, are less effectively treated by MRgFUS than low- and intermediate-intensity myomas (type 1 and type 2, respectively). These findings indicate that certain myomas resist ablation by focused ultrasound energy. **Results**: Ten of 111 patients who were followed up for at least 6 months after MRgFUS had regrowths and required a repeat procedure. Cases with myomas that required a second treatment because of a large volume or multiple myomas were excluded from the study. The 10 cases considered in this study included 2 with type 1, 4 with type 2, and 4 with type 3 myomas. Five patients were treated again approximately 6 months later, and 5 were retreated between 16 and 33 months after the first MRgFUS. The nonperfused ratio of the treated myomas immediately after the second MRgFUS was greater than that observed after the first MRgFUS. Two patients underwent myomectomy because of persistent hypermenorrhea, and one patient because of a rectal tumor. The volume of most of the myomas, which did not decrease 6 months after the first MRgFUS, noticeably decreased after the second MRgFUS. **Conclusion**: Repeat MRgFUS can improve the treatment outcome for some myomas that resist focused ultrasound energy.

Keywords: myoma, focused ultrasound, MRgFUS, recurrence

PACS: 43.80.+p

INTRODUCTION

Magnetic resonance–guided focused ultrasound surgery (MRgFUS) is one of the treatments for uterine myoma with minimally adverse events. However, some myomas resist ultrasound energy and alternative surgery is required after MRgFUS.

We previously reported that high-intensity (type 3) myomas of pretreatment T2-weighted magnetic resonance images are difficult to treat with MRgFUS. Compared with low-intensity (type 1) and/or intermediate-intensity (type 2) myomas, type 3 myomas have a smaller nonperfused volume immediately after MRgFUS and a smaller volume reduction ratio 6 months after the initial treatment. In addition, type 3 myomas require a second alternative surgery than do type 1 and 2 myomas.

In cases of established clinical failure, we sometimes treat the same myoma twice, not all of which are type 3 myomas. In this study, we intended to estimate the efficacy of repeat MRgFUS for recurrent myomas.

MATERIALS & METHODS

We performed MRgFUS for symptomatic uterine myomas, beginning in June 2004, after receiving an approval from the local ethics committee. Written informed consent was obtained from all patients. Patients who would otherwise have been offered conventional surgery were considered eligible for the study. We treated myomas according to the ExAblate2000™ system software (InSightec Ltd., Tirat Carmel, Israel); the technical details of which were published previously.

Ten of 111 patients who were followed up for at least 6 months after MRgFUS had to be treated again for recurrence of the same myoma. The mean (± standard deviation) follow-up period was 33.1 ± 11.8 months. Cases that initially required a second treatment because of their large volume or multiple myomas were excluded from the study. The 10 cases considered in this study included 2 with type 1, 4 with type 2, and 4 with type 3 myomas.

Three cases underwent gonadotropin-releasing hormone analogue (GnRHa) therapy prior to the first treatment. The results are detailed below and are presented in Table 1.

TABLE 1. The profiles of patients

case	age	GnRHa pre-treatment	Treatment interval (months)	type	1st MRgFUS Myoma volume (cm³)	1st MRgFUS Nonperfused ratio (%)	2nd MRgFUS Myoma volume (cm³)	2nd MRgFUS Nonperfused ratio (%)
a	40	−	22	2	113.0	19.5	336.0	41.3
b	35	−	33	2	344.0	67.2	438.1	57.0
c	40	−	8	3	301.4	33.9	442.3	55.9
d	43	−	25	1	102.8	79.1	118.7	92.7
e	40	−	6	3	173.9	9.3	185.0	48.4
f	39	−	31	2	237.0	44.7	246.1	53.4
g	39	−	16	1	138.8	60.4	106.5	92.0
h	42	+	5	2	184.0	40.2	433.3	UNK
i	44	+	7	3	110.0	43.6	107.3	64.0
j	44	+	9	3	201.2	34.6	488.6	60.0

UNK ; unknown
Mean nonperfused ratio immediately after 1st MRgFUS = 43.3 ± 21.2 (mean ± SD)[*]
Mean nonperfused ratio immediately after 2nd MRgFUS = 62.8 ± 18.0[*]
[*] $p = 0.0037$ (paired T-test)

RESULTS

Five patients were treated again approximately 6 months after (between 5 and 9 months) and five patients were retreated between 16 and 33 months after the first MRgFUS. The nonperfused ratio of the treated myomas immediately after the second MRgFUS (62.8 ± 18.0) was greater (p < 0.01) than that observed after the first MRgFUS (43.3 ± 21.2) (Table 1).

Two patients underwent myomectomy because of persistent hypermenorrhea, and one patient because of a rectal tumor. In most cases, the volume of the re-ablated myomas decreased noticeably after the second MRgFUS (Figure 1). The signal intensities of the treated myomas tended to decrease after MRgFUS (Table 2).

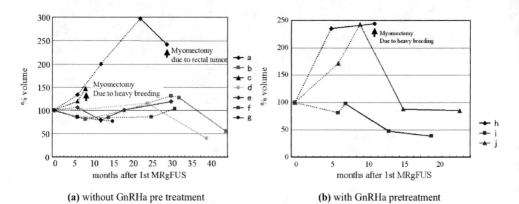

(a) without GnRHa pre treatment   **(b)** with GnRHa pretreatment

Dotted line = post 1st MRgFUS, Solid line = post 2nd MRgFUS

FIGURE1. Volume change ratio

TABLE 2. The signal intensity of the treated myomas on T2-weighted MRIs

case	pretreatment	Post 1st MRgFUS	Post 2nd MRgFUS
a	3.31	2.32 (0.70)	2.51 (0.76)
b	3.47	1.53 (0.44)	1.84 (0.53)
c	4.49	2.59 (0.58)	2.34 (0.52)
d	0.86	1.25 (1.46)	-
e	2.55	-	2.03 (0.80)
f	-	1.50	-
g	0.91	1.56 (1.71)	-
h	2.49	2.43 (0.98)	2.08 (0.83)
i	2.99	1.75 (0.59)	1.74 (0.58)
j	-	2.69	2.17

Proportions of the signal intensity compared to pretreatment are in parentheses.

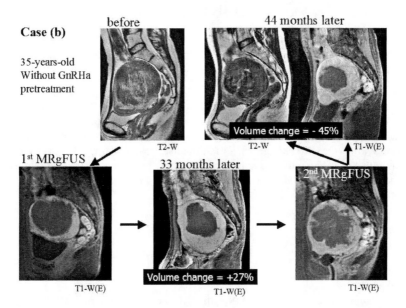

FIGURE 2. Case (b)

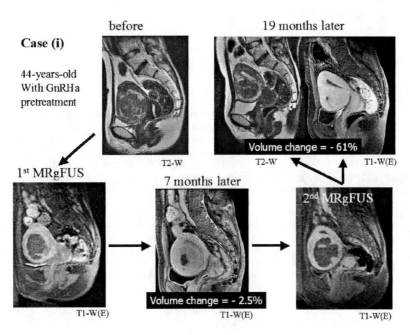

FIGURE 3. Case (i)

COMMENT

We reported here, the outcomes of 10 cases who underwent a second MRgFUS because of the recurrence of their subjective symptoms.

The results are promising. We speculated that retreated myomas became dry from ablation, and the signal intensities on T2-weighted magnetic resonance images decreased after MRgFUS. In general, a high signal intensity on T2-weighted magnetic resonance images indicates water-rich tissue, which resists heat energy. Therefore, the retreated myomas could easily ablate and had a larger nonperfused ratio than the myomas after the first MRgFUS. Additionally, treatment may have changed the proliferative capacity of the myoma. Another possible reason for the larger nonperfused ratio after the second treatment was the improved skill of the operators.

CONCLUSION

1. The nonperfused ratio immediately after the second MRgFUS was larger than that after the first MRgFUS.

2. The volume of most of the retreated myomas decreased after the second MRgFUS.

3. Repeat MRgFUS can improve the treatment outcome of myomas that resist focused ultrasound energy.

REFERENCES

1. Funaki K, Fukunishi H, Funaki T, Sawada K, Kaji Y, Maruo T. Magnetic resonance-guided focused ultrasound surgery for uterine fibroids: Relationship between the therapeutic effects and signal intensity of pre-existing T2-weighted MR images. *Am J Obstet Gynecol.* **196**:184.e1-6 (2007).
2. Funaki K, Fukunishi H. "The early effects of MRgFUS in treating uterine fibroids," In *Therapeutic Ultrasound: 5th International symposium on therapeutic ultrasound,* edited by Clement GT, McDannold NJ, Hynynen K, AIP Conference Proceedings, NewYork, 2006, pp.513-517.
3. Funaki K, Funaki T, Fukunishi H, "The Volume Reduction Ratio of Uterine Fibroid Treated With MRgFUS," In *Therapeutic Ultrasound: 6th International symposium on therapeutic ultrasound,* edited by Constantin-C. Coussios, Gail ter Haar, AIP Conference Proceedings, NewYork, 2007, pp.436-441.
4. Fukunishi H, Funaki K, Ikuma K, Kaji Y, Sugimura K, Kitazawa R, Kitazawa S. Unsuspeccted uterine leiomyosarcoma: magnetic resonance imaging findings before and after focused ultrasound surgery. *Int J Gynecol Cancer.* **17**:724-728 (2007).
5. Funaki K, Sawada K, Maeda F, Nagai S. Subjective effect of magnetic resonance-guided focused ultrasound surgery for uterine fibroids. *J Obstet Gynaecol Res.* **33**:834-839 (2007).
6. Funaki K, Fukunishi H, Funaki T, Kawakami C. Mid-term outcome of Magnetic Resonance-guided Focused Ultrasound Surgery (MRgFUS) for uterine fibroids: from six to twelve months after volume reduction. *J Minim Invasive Gynecol.* **14**:616-621 (2007).
7. Fukunishi H. Treatment of Uterine Leiomyoma with Magnetic Resonance-guided Focused Ultrasound Surgery (MRgFUS). *Nippon Sanka Fujinka Gakkai Zasshi.* **59**:1693-1702 (2007).

Histological Evaluation of Prostate Tissue Response to Image-Guided Transurethral Thermal Therapy After a 48h Recovery Period

Aaron Boyes[a], Kee Tang[a], Rajiv Chopra[a,b], and Michael Bronskill[a,b]

[a]Sunnybrook Health Sciences Centre, 2075 Bayview Ave., Toronto, ON, Canada, M4N 3M5
[b]Department of Medical Biophysics, University of Toronto

Abstract. Image-guided transurethral ultrasound thermal therapy shows strong potential for sparing of critical adjacent structures during prostate cancer treatment. Preclinical experiments were conducted to provide further information on the extent of the treatment margin. Four experiments were carried out in a canine model to investigate the pathology of this margin during the early stages of recovery and were compared to previous results obtained immediately post-treatment. Sedated animals were placed in a 1.5T clinical MRI, and the heating device was positioned accurately within the prostatic urethra with image guidance. Using an MRI-compatible system, the ultrasound device was rotated 365° treating a prescribed volume contained within the gland. Quantitative temperature maps were acquired throughout the treatment, providing feedback information for device control. Animals were allowed to recover and, after 48h, an imaging protocol including T2 and contrast enhanced (CE) MRI was repeated before the animals were sacrificed. Prostate sections were stained with H&E. Careful slice alignment methods during histological procedures and image registration were employed to ensure good correspondence between MR images and microscopy. Although T2 MRI revealed no lesion acutely, a hypo-intense region was clearly visible 2 days post-treatment. The lesion volume defined by CE-MRI increased appreciably during this time. Whole-mount H&E sections showed that the margin between coagulated and normal-appearing cells narrowed during recovery, typically to a width of under 1mm compared to 3mm acutely. These results illustrate the high level of precision achievable with transurethral thermal therapy and suggest methods to monitor the physiological response non-invasively.

Keywords: Prostate; Ultrasound Therapy; Thermal Damage; Histology; Image Registration
PACS: 87.19.lf, 87.19.xj, 87.50.cm, 87.50.ct

INTRODUCTION

Minimally invasive transurethral ultrasound thermal therapy offers strong potential for accurate treatment of localized prostate cancer. A system that enables heating of a prescribed region within the prostate gland using MRI thermometry for feedback control has been developed and validated in a canine model [1]. From these acute studies, we were able to analyze and describe the pathology of thermal lesions produced by this technology following treatments in canine prostate tissue [2]. Histological assessment provides a detailed description of thermal damage *in vivo*, and confirmation of the extent of coagulation predicted by MRI temperature maps [3]. To explore the response to thermal therapy further, this paper focuses on a preliminary set of experiments designed to investigate changes in the thermal lesion during the early stages of recovery as well as the ability of post-treatment MRI to assess thermal damage in the prostate and its potential use as an imaging surrogate. Imaging surrogates for pathology would be valuable clinically, as they would provide a non-

CP1113, 8th International Symposium on Therapeutic Ultrasound, edited by E. S. Ebbini
© 2009 American Institute of Physics 978-0-7354-0650-6/09/$25.00

invasive means to characterize results in multiple follow-up sessions after thermal therapy [4].

METHODS

Four experiments were performed in a canine model with a prototype transurethral thermal therapy system [1] on a 1.5T clinical MR imager (Signa, GE Healthcare). The ultrasound device housed a single planar transducer (15 x 3.5mm) operating at 9.1MHz and up to 7.5W acoustic power. MRI thermometry information was used for guidance and control to enable heating of the targeted region (Fig. 1). Approval for these experiments was obtained from the institutional Animal Care Committee.

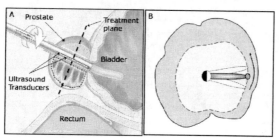

FIGURE 1. A) Diagram illustrating the positioning of the ultrasound device within the prostatic urethra. B) Schematic representation of an MR image at the treatment plane, depicting a target boundary (dashed line), and the collimated ultrasound beam produced by the device. Rotation of the beam sweeps out a continuous prescribed pattern of coagulation within prostate tissue.

Post-treatment imaging was performed at 1h and 48h after treatment. The imaging protocol consisted of acquiring a contrast enhanced (CE) and T2-weighted (T2) MRI. Contours of the prostate boundary on CE images were used to estimate prostate volumes at the acute and chronic time-points. After completion of the imaging protocol at 48h, the animals were sacrificed and prostates were excised for pathological assessment.

Histological Analysis and Image Registration

Transverse, whole-mount hematoxylin and eosin (H&E) sections were obtained as described previously [3]. After 1-2 weeks of formalin fixation, the prostate was sliced into 5mm blocks. Finer sectioning with a microtome produced whole mount prostate slides oriented perpendicular to the urethra, and centered on the plane used for all imaging.

Manually segmented regions of thermal damage on the MR images were registered to images of the histological sections, enabling quantitative comparison of these datasets. The images were warped using a thin plate spline algorithm [5] based on identifiable anatomical landmarks such as the prostate outer boundary, midline, and urethra.

RESULTS

MR imaging has the potential to be used for monitoring of tissue damage at various time-points following thermal therapy [4,6-9]. In this study, CE and T2-weighted images were acquired at 1h and 48h time points following the canine experiments (Fig. 2). As soon as 1h after thermal therapy, a region of reduced signal intensity was apparent on the CE images. In all experiments, this region expanded over the course of the 2 day recovery period. Bright regions throughout the prostate, and particularly surrounding the thermal coagulation, indicated the accumulation of interstitial hemorrhage and edema. Consistent with this, swelling in the gland over the recovery period caused an increase in prostate volume of between 2 and 6cm^3 in these four canines.

Acutely, T2-weighted imaging did not distinguish treated from normal prostate tissue. However, after the recovery period, T2-weighted MRI revealed thermal damage in a pattern very similar to that observed on the CE image.

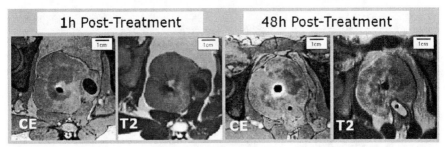

FIGURE 2. Contrast Enhanced (CE) and T2-weighted (T2) images acquired 1 hour and 48 hours after ultrasound delivery to a sub-volume of the gland. MR imaging parameters: CE; 3D FGRE, TE=2.2ms, TR=7ms, FA=13°, FOV=160mm, 256x256, NEX=2. T2; FSE-XL, TE=64ms, TR=1600ms, FA=30°, FOV=200mm, 256x256, NEX=1.

We have previously described regions of acute thermal damage in the prostate [3] (Fig. 3A). In a 2-3mm wide margin at the edge of the ablated region, cell fates were not predictable based on morphological criteria. Closer to the heat source, non-viable tissues appeared either necrotic or thermally fixed. Outside the margin, structural integrity of the basement membrane, and preservation of tissue structure suggested that the tissue was likely to recover.

In prostates excised after 48h, this margin essentially disappeared, and the boundary of tissue necrosis was sharply delineated from apparently recovering prostate tissue (Fig. 3B). At the periphery of the gland, there was accumulation of interstitial edema. Towards the center of the prostate, thermally fixed tissue appeared to have faded over the recovery period, becoming more eosinphillic in comparison to the acute case. Open voids in the tissue sections suggested that sloughing of necrotic tissue was underway at this stage of the tissue reaction.

Hemorrhage could be observed acutely, consisting of patches of hemostasis on microscopy (Fig. 3A), and a red band in gross appearance. The outer boundary of hemorrhagic tissue has been correlated with the boundary of necrosis at the acute time-point [3], and this relationship was clearly visible on H&E in the chronic case. Over the 2 day recovery period, interstitial hemorrhage became much more extensive, spreading throughout the necrotic zone to its periphery.

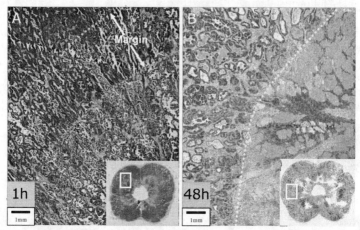

FIGURE 3. Hematoxylin and Eosin stained prostate sections, with enlarged area indicated at the lesion boundary. A) Acute appearance of the thermal damage margin. B) Section of the same prostate shown in Figure 2, excised after the 2 day recovery period.

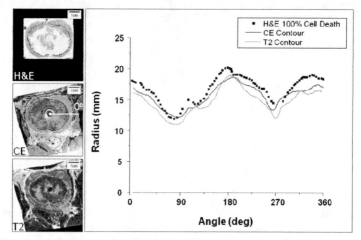

FIGURE 4. Correlation between features of thermal damage on registered H&E, CE and T2 images. Radial distances from the urethra center are plotted against treatment angle. Segmented images are shown at left, with starting position and direction of rotation marked on the CE image.

The CE and T2 images at the 48h stage were registered to whole-mount H&E sections. In two of the four experiments, there was very close correlation between the necrotic region on H&E and the coagulated region visualized on T2 and CE images (Fig. 4). In these experiments the average distances separating the H&E boundary from those on the MR images were 1.3mm (CE) and 1.8mm (T2). In the remaining two cases, good correspondence was observed over partial sectors of the treatment. In these two prostates, the average distance between histological and MRI assessments of thermal damage ranged from 2 to 4mm.

DISCUSSION AND CONCLUSIONS

As early as 48h after treatment with transurethral ultrasound thermal therapy, the severity of thermal tissue damage is well defined on histology. At this stage of recovery, there is little uncertainty in the extent of irreversible thermal damage produced in the prostate.

MRI is a valuable tool for prediction of the results of thermal therapy *in vivo*. In contrast to results obtained in porcine liver [6,9], acute T2 appearance did not distinguish treated from normal prostate tissue. However, at 48h post-treatment, CE and T2 MR images accurately revealed the detailed pattern of thermal damage. The registration procedure was complicated by swelling in the prostate. Still, the results suggest that imaging could be used to describe the extent of thermal ablation quantitatively.

These results indicate that a sharp demarcation between coagulation and sparing of prostate tissue is produced using transurethral thermal therapy. Combined with non-invasive methods for monitoring during and after therapy, this technology offers strong potential for the accurate treatment of localized prostate cancer, with reduced negative outcomes relative to current clinical standards.

ACKNOWLEDGMENTS

We gratefully acknowledge Laibao Sun and Dr. Linda Sugar (Sunnybrook HSC) for assistance in preparation and analysis of the histological slides, as well as the following funding agencies who have supported this work: The Terry Fox Foundation, Ontario Research and Development Challenge Fund, Ontario Institute of Cancer Research, and the Canadian Institutes of Health Research.

REFERENCES

1. R. Chopra *et al.*, "MRI-compatible transurethral ultrasound system for the treatment of localized prostate cancer using rotational control," Med.Phys. 35 (4), 1346-1357 (2008).
2. Sharon L. Thomsen, In: edited by Thomas P. Ryan and Terence Z. Wong (SPIE, 1999) pp. 82-95.
3. A. Boyes *et al.*, "Prostate tissue analysis immediately following magnetic resonance imaging guided transurethral ultrasound thermal therapy," J.Urol. 178 (3 Pt 1), 1080-1085 (2007).
4. K. Hynynen *et al.*, "MR imaging-guided focused ultrasound surgery of fibroadenomas in the breast: a feasibility study," Radiology 219 (1), 176-185 (2001).
5. F. L. Bookstein, "Principal warps: thin-plate splines and the decomposition of deformations," Pattern Analysis and Machine Intelligence, IEEE Transactions on 11 (6), 567-585 (1989).
6. M. S. Breen *et al.*, "Radiofrequency thermal ablation: correlation of hyperacute MR lesion images with tissue response," J.Magn.Reson.Imaging 20 (3), 475-486 (2004).
7. R. S. Lazebnik *et al.*, "Radio-frequency-induced thermal lesions: subacute magnetic resonance appearance and histological correlation," J.Magn.Reson.Imaging 18 (4), 487-495 (2003).
8. I. A. Morocz *et al.*, "Brain edema development after MRI-guided focused ultrasound treatment," J.Magn.Reson.Imaging 8 (1), 136-142 (1998).
9. K. K. Vigen *et al.*, "In vivo porcine liver radiofrequency ablation with simultaneous MR temperature imaging," J.Magn.Reson.Imaging 23 (4), 578-584 (2006).

In Vivo Animal Studies

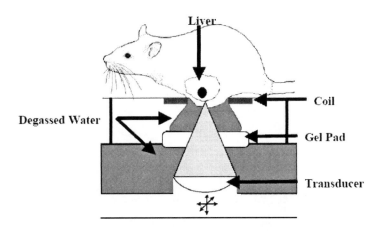

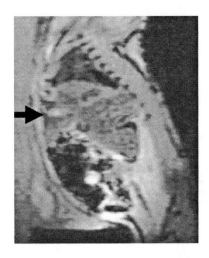
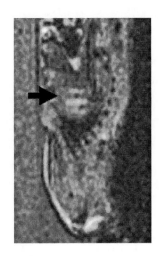

Focused Ultrasound Surgery Control Using Local Harmonic Motion: VX2 Tumor Study

Laura Curiel[a,b], Rajiv Chopra[a], David Goertz[a] and Kullervo Hynynen[a]

[a]*Sunnybrook Health Sciences Centre, 2075 Bayview Ave, Toronto, ON, M5N 3M5, Canada*
[b]*Thunder Bay Regional Research Institute, 980 Oliver Rd, Thunder Bay, ON, P7B 6V4*

Abstract. The objective of this study was to develop a real-time method for controlling focused ultrasound surgery using ultrasound imaging. The approach uses measurements of localized harmonic motion (LHM) in order to perform controlled FUS exposures by detecting changes in the elastic properties of tissues during coagulation. Methods: Nine New Zealand rabbits with VX2 tumors implanted in the thigh were used for this study. LHM was generated within the tumors by periodic induction of radiation force using a FUS transducer (80-mm focal length, 100-mm diameter, 20-mm central hole, 1.485-MHz). Tissue motion was tracked by collecting and cross-correlating RF signals during the motion using a separate diagnostic transducer (3-kHz PRF, 5-MHz). After locating the tumor in MR images, a series of sonications were performed to treat the tumors using a reduction in LHM amplitude to control the exposure. Results: LHM was successfully used to control the sonications. A LHM amplitude threshold value was determined at which changes were considered significant and then the exposure was started and stopped when the LHM amplitude dropped below the threshold. The appearance of a lesion was then verified by MRI. The feasibility of LHM measurements to control FUS exposure was validated.

Keywords: Focused Ultrasound Surgery, HIFU, Harmonic Motion, Tissue Elasticity.
PACS: 87.50.yk

INTRODUCTION

Magnetic Resonance offers an accurate but high cost control for focused ultrasound surgery (FUS). The use of more affordable modalities like ultrasound is attractive to target tissues and control the exposure. However, the treatments currently using ultrasound control rely on previously determined treatment parameters [1-3] making clinical outcome variable because of changing tissue properties [4, 5].

Imaging of elastic properties of tissues is an ideal technique to control FUS exposure since thermal ablation changes elastic characteristics. Different approaches have been proposed in this direction [6-11]. Localized harmonic motion (LHM) has been recently reported as a method to visualize thermal lesions *in vitro* and *in vivo* [12-13]. A FUS transducer is used to induce a time-varying force causing tissues oscillation at the modulation frequency. Motion is then estimated using cross-correlation of RF signals from a separate diagnostic ultrasound beam [12].

In the present study we propose the use of Local Harmonic Motion measurements to control and monitor FUS tumor treatments by using the induced harmonic motion amplitude as a parameter to determine when the tissues reach coagulation and the FUS exposure should be stopped.

CP1113, *8th International Symposium on Therapeutic Ultrasound*, edited by E. S. Ebbini
© 2009 American Institute of Physics 978-0-7354-0650-6/09/$25.00

METHODS

Transducer Set-up

The same FUS transducer (1.485 MHz, 100-mm diameter, 80-mm focal length, 20-mm diameter central hole) was used to induce the harmonic motion and to create the thermal ablation. Tissues movements were tracked by a separate diagnostic transducer (single element, 5 MHz, 47-mm focal length, 20-mm, Imasonic, France) placed at the central hole of the FUS transducer with their focal volumes aligned.

Animal Experiments

Experiments were conducted after approval from the local Institutional Animal Care Committee. Nine New Zealand White male rabbits were injected with VX2 cells in both thighs and treated one week later. They were anesthetized with a mixture of ketamine and xylazine, had both thighs depilated, and were placed on top of a water tank with the thigh in front of the transducer assembly. The animal was covered with a heating blanket and its temperature was monitored using a rectal probe.

The rabbit thigh was imaged on the MRI scanner (Signa SP, GE Healthcare, USA) to locate the tumor using T1-weighted imaging (FSE, 256x256, TE/TR=9.03/500, FOV=16cm, Slice=2mm, ETL=4, 3NEX) with contrast agent injection (gadolinium, 0.2ml/kg). After the FUS exposures were performed on the animal, it was sacrificed using Pentobarbital Sodium (2ml/4.5kg), the muscle was then exposed and the tumor was located, excised and immersed in 10% buffered formalin solution.

Histological analysis was performed to evaluate the tissue reaction to thermal exposure and the apparition of coagulation within the targeted tumor (H&E stain).

Control of FUS Exposures

The transducer assembly was mounted on a MR-compatible system which allowed positioning of the FUS relative to the MR images. Multiple controlled FUS exposures were performed within each tumor. In Figure 1 the procedure flow for the controlled exposures is shown: before the exposure, harmonic motion was induced and the

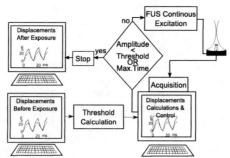

FIGURE 1. Controlled exposures flow chart.

amplitude was obtained 10 times; a threshold was then defined as the mean value of these measurements minus two times the standard deviation; the excitation was then applied continuously obtaining LHM measurements every 1.2 s and the exposure was stopped if the amplitude at the focus dropped below the threshold or if a maximum time was reached; after 1-minute cooling, ten LHM measurements were performed.

During the continuous ultrasound exposure MR thermometry with a fast gradient echo sequence using the Proton Resonant Frequency shift method was performed in a plane transverse to the ultrasound beam at the focal location (FGRE, 256x128, TE/TR=17.3/34.9, FOV=16cm, Slice=3mm, Img. time=4.6 s, 1NEX, temperature dependence of the proton-resonant frequency shift 0.00909 ppm/°C). After exposure the apparition of coagulation was verified by MRI using T2-weighted MR imaging (FSE, 256x256, TE/TR=69.10/2000, FOV=16cm, Slice=2.5mm, ETL=4, 1NEX) [14].

RESULTS

Controlled Exposures

It was considered that the FUS exposure was successfully controlled when the exposure was stopped after the amplitude was lower than the threshold and coagulation was confirmed by the T2-weighted MR images, or when the exposure was never stopped before the maximum time and no coagulation was observed. The overall results are shown in Figure 2. The control was successful for 74 sonications over the 108 (68.5%). For 48.1% of the cases the system successfully stopped after reaching the threshold with coagulation confirmed and for 20.4% the system stopped because the maximum time was reached and no coagulation was observed.

For the 34 sonications (31.5%) where the control was not successful two different situations were observed: the system never stopped but the MR images did show coagulation (14.8%), or the system stopped but no coagulation was observed (16.7%). Analysis of the unsuccessful sonications showed that for 24 sonications (22.2%), noise or severe changes in the RF signal explained an over or underestimation of the motion making the system continue or stop prematurely the exposure. For the remaining cases (9.3%) no noise or changes in RF signal were observed.

An example of the LHM amplitudes measured during three controlled exposures is shown in Figure 3. In (a) and (b) the motion amplitude dropped below the threshold

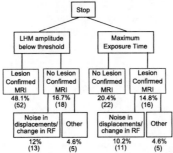

FIGURE 2. Different situations observed after the system stopped.

and the system stopped with a coagulation confirmed in the MR images. In (c) the system stopped when the maximum exposure time (50 s) was reached without measurements below the threshold and no coagulation observed in the MR images.

The thermal doses for the cases where coagulation was observed were consistently higher than the minimum value reported for rabbit muscle [15]. However, values were consistently higher; indicating that the thermal dose needed to achieve coagulation in tumor cells was higher than for muscle.

Amplitude Before and After Exposure

For all the locations where thermal coagulation was confirmed by MRI, the measured amplitude of the induced harmonic motion after thermal coagulation was between 9% (p=0.04) and 57% (p<0.0001) lower than the amplitude before exposure.

Figure 4 shows an example of tissue displacement at the focus before and after FUS exposure and the corresponding MR images (T2-weighted, FSE, 256x256, TE/TR=58.02/2000, FOV=16cm, Slice=2mm, ETL=4, 1NEX) for cases in Figure 3.

Histological analysis of all slices confirmed the presence of tumor at the targeted area and that cell damage was present for all the cases where coagulation was observed in the MR images.

DISCUSSION

This goal of the study was to use local harmonic motion (LHM) induced with ultrasound to control focused ultrasound exposure. It was possible to perform LHM measurements before and after thermal coagulation as well as during exposure.

The method here proposed to control an exposure relies on the definition of a LHM amplitude threshold below which the system stops the energy deposition. This threshold value was chosen accordingly to previously reported data [13]. Different threshold values can be still explored to improve the control.

Sources of error for the technique can come from changes in the RF signal causing de-correlation: out-of-plane movements, expansion/compression of tissues or changes in the nature of tissues that alter the echo. By acquiring at high PRF de-correlation can be minimized and short measuring times make the technique less sensitive to large and slow movements. However, if the technique was to be used in fast-moving organs, this movement could be an issue.

Thermal dose values for which coagulation was obtained were higher than 60 equivalent minutes at 43°C consistently with reported values for rabbit muscle [15].

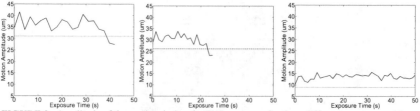

FIGURE 3. Amplitude of the motion during the FUS exposure for three different exposures with an average acoustic power of: (a) 10 W, (b) 17 W and (c) 8 W. Dotted lines represent threshold.

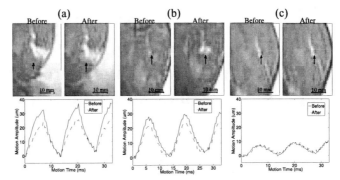

FIGURE 4. MR images before/after exposure (top) and local harmonic motion (bottom) at the focus and for the three different locations for which the FUS exposure control is shown in Figure 3.

However, we obtained thermal doses as high as 180 equivalent minutes at 43°C for which no tissue damage was observed and thermal dose values appear to be higher than the reported values. This could be explained by a higher perfusion in tumors or by an MRI temperature coefficient higher than for the muscle.

Future work needs to be conducted to verify that when the noise is not an issue, the system has a higher reliability. Finally, the use of LHM technique to map and locate tumor and coagulation after FUS exposures would improve the monitoring of treatment by locating the target and treated area.

ACKNOWLEDGMENTS

Work supported by CRC, NIH R21/R33 CA102884-01 and Terry Fox foundation.

REFERENCES

1. J. Y. Chapelon, M. Ribault, F. Vernier, R. Souchon, A. Gelet. *Eur J Ultrasound* **9**, 31-38 (1999).
2. T. Uchida, N. T. Sanghvi, T. A. Gardner, et al. *Urology* **59**, 394-398 (2002).
3. L. Curiel, F. Chavrier, B. Gignoux, S. Pichardo, S. Chesnais, J. Y. Chapelon. *Med Biol Eng Comput* **42**, 44-54 (2004).
4. B. E. Billard, K. Hynynen, R. B. Roemer. *Ultrasound Med Biol* **16**, 409-420 (1990).
5. K. Hynynen, D. DeYoung, M. Kundrat, E. Moros. *Int J Hyperthermia* **5**, 485-497 (1989).
6. B. J. Fahey, K. R. Nightingale, S. A. McAleavey, M. L. Palmeri, P. D. Wolf, G. E. Trahey. *IEEE Trans Ultrason Ferroelectr Freq Control* **52**, 631-641 (2005).
7. T. Karjalainen, J. S. Thierman, K. Hynynen. *Proc IEEE Ultrason Symp* **2**, 1397-1400 (1999).
8. A. Alizad, L. E. Wold, J. F. Greenleaf, M. Fatemi. *IEEE Trans Med Imaging* **23**, 1087-1093 (2004).
9. L. Curiel, R. Souchon, O. Rouviere, A. Gelet, J. Y. Chapelon. *Ultrasound Med Biol* **31**, 1461-1468 (2005).
10. Y. Le Y, K. Glaser, O. Rouviere, R. Ehman, J. P. Felmlee. *Magn Reson Med* **55**, 700-705 (2006).
11. F. L. Lizzi, R. Muratore, C. X. Deng, et al. *Ultrasound Med Biol* **29**, 1593-1605 (2003).
12. E. E. Konofagou, K. Hynynen. *Ultrasound Med Biol* **29**, 1405-1413 (2003).
13. L. Curiel L, R. Chopra, K. Hynynen. *Ultrasound Med Biol* in press (2008).
14. A. H. Chung, F. A. Jolesz, K. Hynynen. *Med Phys* 26, 2017-2026 (1999).
15. N. J. McDannold, R. L. King, F. A. Jolesz, K. Hynynen. *Radiology* 216, 517-523 (2000).

Acoustic Droplet Vaporization, Cavitation, and Therapeutic Properties of Copolymer-Stabilized Perfluorocarbon Nanoemulsions

Kweon-Ho Nam[a], Douglas A. Christensen[a], Anne M. Kennedy[b], and Natalya Rapoport[a]

[a]*Department of Bioengineering, University of Utah, Salt Lake City, UT 84112, USA*
[b]*Department of Clinical Radiology, Health Science Center, University of Utah, Salt Lake City, UT 84112, USA*

Abstract. Acoustic and therapeutic properties of Doxorubicin (DOX) and paclitaxel (PTX)-loaded perfluorocarbon nanoemulsions have been investigated in a mouse model of ovarian cancer. The nanoemulsions were stabilized by two biodegradable amphiphilic block copolymers that differed in the structure of the hydrophobic block. Acoustic droplet vaporization (ADV) and cavitation parameters were measured as a function of ultrasound frequency, pressure, duty cycles, and temperature. The optimal parameters that induced ADV and inertial cavitation of the formed microbubbles were used *in vivo* in the experiments on the ultrasound-mediated chemotherapy of ovarian cancer. A combination tumor treatment by intravenous injections of drug-loaded perfluoropentane nanoemulsions and tumor-directed 1-MHz ultrasound resulted in a dramatic decrease of ovarian or breast carcinoma tumor volume and sometimes complete tumor resolution. However, tumors often recurred three to six weeks after the treatment indicating that some cancer cells survived the treatment. The recurrent tumors proved more aggressive and resistant to the repeated therapy than initial tumors suggesting selection for the resistant cells during the first treatment.

Keywords: Cancer Therapy, Targeted Drug Delivery, Nanobubbles, Perfluoropentane, Ultrasound.
PACS: 87.50.yt, 87.63.dh.

INTRODUCTION

During the last decade, a number of novel modalities for a targeted tumor therapy have been suggested. These modalities are based on developing stimuli-responsive nanoparticles that release their drug load in response to environmental or physical stimuli, such as pH, hyperthermia, light, or ultrasound. In our previous work, we have developed the nanoemulsions that converted into nano- and microbubbles *in situ* upon injection or under the action of therapeutic ultrasound [1], [2]. These systems combined passive tumor-targeting capacity with ultrasound responsiveness and could be used for combining ultrasonography with ultrasound-mediated chemotherapy. Here we describe acoustic properties of these systems.

The nanoparticles we have developed are composed of nano- or micro-scale echogenic emulsions that convert into nano- and/or microbubbles *in situ* upon injection and tumor sonication. A set of their properties includes drug carrying, tumor-

CP1113, *8th International Symposium on Therapeutic Ultrasound*, edited by E. S. Ebbini
© 2009 American Institute of Physics 978-0-7354-0650-6/09/$25.00

targeting, enhancing intracellular drug delivery, and enhancing the ultrasound contrast of the tumor. The cores of the nanoemulsion droplets or nanobubbles were formed by organic perfluoro- compounds; in this work, perfluoropentane (PFP) was used; the PFP was encased in the walls formed by the biodegradable amphiphilic block copolymer, poly(ethylene oxide)-co-poly(L-lactide) (PEG-PLLA) or poly(ethylene oxide-co-polycaprolactone (PEG-PCL).

Due to the impedance difference from the surrounding medium, not only perfluorocarbon bubbles but also droplets have echogenic properties; however bubbles manifest higher echogenicity than droplets, which allows using ultrasound imaging to monitor acoustic droplet vaporization (i.e. the ADV effect that was discovered and investigated in a series of works by Kripfgans, Fowlkes *et al.* for a different type of perfluorocarbon emulsions [3], [4]). Besides producing high ultrasound contrast, bubbles serve as potent enhancers of ultrasound-mediated drug delivery. Therefore nanodroplet vaporization *in situ* to generate bubbles is highly desirable for both ultrasonography and drug delivery. The PFP has a boiling temperature of 29 °C thus producing nanoemulsions at room temperature. The ADV effects in PFP nanoemulsions stabilized by PEG-PLLA and PEG-PCL are described below. Another issue addressed in the paper is related to the ADV effect and bubble cavitation in highly viscous gel systems used as tissue models. This information is relevant to acoustic effects produced in tumor interstitium after bubble extravasation. The information on the acoustic properties of these novel formulations obtained in this study was used for optimizing *in vivo* tumor imaging and therapy.

MATERIALS AND METHODS

Block copolymers. Block copolymers used in this study were bought from Polymer Source (Quebec, Canada). The PEG-PLLA copolymer had a total molecular weight of 9,700. The PEG-PCL copolymer had a total molecular weight of 4,600 D.

Micellar solutions and drug loading. Micellar solutions of the block copolymers were prepared by a solvent exchange technique as described in details previously [1]; DOX loading into the micelles was performed at the micelle preparation stage. Genexol-PM was bought from Samyang Corp. (Daejeon, South Korea) and dissolved in PEG-PLLA micellar solution.

Preparation of nanoemulsions. An aliquot of PFP was pipetted into a corresponding micellar solution and sonicated by 20-kHz ultrasound in ice-cold water.

Nanoparticle size distribution. Size distribution of nanoparticles was measured by dynamic light scattering at an angle of 165° using Delsa Nano S instrument (Beckman Coulter, Osaka, Japan) equipped with a 658 nm laser and a temperature controller. Size distribution was analyzed using Non-Negative Least Squares (NNLS) method.

Sonication. Unfocused 1- or 3-MHz ultrasound was generated by an Omnisound 3000 instrument (Accelerated Care Plus Inc, Sparks, NV) equipped with a 5 cm^2 transducer head.

Cavitation activity. Cavitation activity was assessed by measuring subharmonic, harmonic, and broadband noise amplitudes in a scattered beam. The microbubble formulation inserted in a Samco polyethylene transfer pipette (5 mm internal diameter, 0.3 mm wall thickness, Fisher Scientific, Pittsburg, PA) was positioned at a distance of 0.5 cm from the transducer that was housed in an open glass tank containing filtered distilled degassed water. To minimize possible standing wave formation, a 2.5 cm thick rubber liner was mounted opposite the transducer. Ultrasound pressure was measured using a needle hydrophone (HNR-1000, Onda, Sunnyvale, CA) with a 20 dB preamplifier (AH-1100, Onda, Sunnyvale, CA). The hydrophone was placed perpendicular to the beam direction at a distance of 3 cm from the sample.

Monitoring acoustic droplet vaporization by visual observation and ultrasound imaging. Formation of the microbubbles from the nanodroplets under the action of ultrasound was monitored visually and by ultrasound imaging using a 7.5-MHz scanner (Scanner 250, Pie Medical, Maastricht, The Netherlands).

Cells and tumor models. Ovarian cancer A2780 cells were obtained from American Type Culture Collection (Manassas, VA). The cells were cultured and inoculated to nu/nu mice as described previously [1].

RESULTS AND DISCUSSION

Acoustic droplet vaporization

These experiments were performed for two types of the droplet stabilizing copolymers (PEG-PLLA and PEG-PCL) and two types of matrices (liquid (PBS) and gel (0.2% agarose or a bovine plasma clot) for 1-MHz or 3-MHz ultrasound. Some experiments were performed using low-frequency CW 90-kHz ultrasound generated in the ultrasound bath (SC-100, Sonicor Instrument Co., Copiague, NY) with intensity close to that of 1-MHz ultrasound (peak-to-peak pressure of 0.7 MPa). Ultrasound intensities that (a) induced the formation of the first visible bubbles; and (b) induced droplet-to-bubble transition in the whole volume of the sample were recorded.

For both emulsion types, the first visible bubbles were always formed on the distal wall of the container at low ultrasound intensities thus suggesting their nucleation in the surface crevices. In liquid systems, the onset of the droplet-to-bubble transition in the whole volume of the sample was accompanied by intensive bubble coalescence into the large bubbles that were raised to the sample surface thus mimicking sample boiling. In what follows, we call this phenomenon "global ADV". The threshold of the global ADV was noticeably higher than that for the formation of first bubbles on the wall surface.

Effect of the type of droplet-stabilizing copolymer. For the droplets stabilized by a PEG-PCL copolymer, the ADV threshold was lower than that for the bubbles of the same composition stabilized by a PEG-PLLA copolymer; as an example, at room temperature and under 1-MHz ultrasound with a 20% duty cycle (1.2 ms pulse duration and 4.8 ms inter-pulse interval), the global ADV threshold for the 1% PFP/0.25% PEG-PCL system was 0.57 MPa compared to 0.85 MPa for the droplets of the same composition stabilized by PEG-PLLA.

Effect of the duty cycle. The ADV threshold strongly depended on the ultrasound duty cycle and was significantly higher for pulsed ultrasound as compared to CW ultrasound. In PFP/PEG-PCL system, five-fold higher nominal ultrasound energy was required for initiating the global ADV effect by 1-MHz ultrasound of 20% duty cycle than by CW ultrasound; moreover, in PFP/PEG-PLLA systems, pulsed ultrasound with 20% duty cycle did not induce global ADV effect while CW ultrasound did.

Effect of temperature. For both types of the emulsions, the ADV threshold was lower at 37 °C compared to room temperature. As an example, for 1% PFP/0.25% PEG-PCL system sonicated for 1 min by 1-MHz ultrasound with 20% duty cycle, ADV threshold dropped from 0.68 MPa at room temperature to 0.44 MPa at 37 °C.

Effect of ultrasound frequency. For both types of the emulsions, the ADV threshold was higher for 3-MHz compared to 1-MHz ultrasound.

Effect of gel matrices. While liquid systems can mimic bubble behavior in blood vessels, much more viscous environment surrounds the bubbles extravasated into the extracellular matrix in tumor tissue. Introduction of the nanodroplets into a gel matrix substantially hampered global formation of large bubbles. Visual observations and ultrasound imaging indicated the formation of isolated large bubbles (FIGURE 1(a), sonication by CW 1-MHz ultrasound at 1.18 MPa peak-to-peak pressure for 1 minute); for comparison, in PBS suspensions, an intensive global "boiling" was observed almost immediately at a pressure as low as 0.3 MPa. However the absence of the global formation of large bubbles does not signify the absence of the droplet-to-bubble transition. As indicated by the generation of harmonics and broadband noise (see below), ultrasound did induce droplet-to-bubble transition in gel matrices; however, gel precluded intensive bubble coalescence in the sample volume. FIGURE 1(a) suggests that the isolated bubbles formed under ultrasound initiated droplet-to-bubble transition in their immediate vicinity and grew by coalescence with these bubbles. This effect was much stronger at lower ultrasound frequencies; an example for gel sonication by 90-kHz ultrasound at 0.7 MPa is shown in FIGURE 1(b). For the optimal intratumoral drug delivery and imaging, it appears reasonable to modulate megahertz frequency range (which is required for ultrasound focusing) by a hundred kilohertz frequency range in therapeutic ultrasound.

Bubble Cavitation

For the effective drug delivery, the formation and cavitation of the nano/microbubbles from the nanoemulsions are extremely beneficial because the oscillation and cavitation of the bubbles trigger the release of the encapsulated drug and also perturb cell membranes thus enhancing the intracellular drug uptake. In the present study, the cavitation effects have been explored for unfocused ultrasound at a frequency of 1 MHz. The appearance and amplitudes of harmonic frequencies and broad band noise were monitored in Fast Fourier Transform emission spectra. The representative data on the relative subharmonic peak amplitudes are shown in FIGURE 2(a) for the PFP/PEG-PCL emulsion in PBS and in FIGURE 2(b) for the droplets inserted in the agarose gel. The threshold of the stable bubble cavitation (about 0.5 MPa) is clearly seen in FIGURE 2(a) (but not in FIGURE 2(b) because the gel comprised some preexisting bubbles). To characterize inertial cavitation, we measured mean relative amplitude of a broadband noise in the frequency intervals that avoided fundamental, harmonic, and superharmonic frequencies. The data obtained clearly indicated that inertial cavitation of the bubbles proceeded in both liquid and gel systems at the ultrasound pressure of 1.18 MPa that was chosen for *in vivo* experiments. The promising results of *in vivo* studies are shown in FIGURE 3. Ovarian carcinoma tumors were grown in the left and right flank of a mouse; PTX-loaded PEG-PLLA nanoemulsions were injected systemically; only one (the right) tumor was sonicated. The unsonicated tumor grew with the same rate as control indicating a strong retention of the drug in the bubbles while the sonicated tumor was resolved after four treatments.

Very promising chemotherapy results were also obtained with DOX-loaded PEG-PCL nanoemulsion

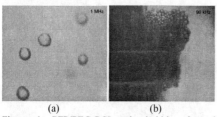

(a)   (b)

Figure 1. PFP/PEG-PCL microbubbles formed from the nanodroplets inserted in the bovine plasma clots under ultrasound of 1 MHz (a) or 90 kHz (b).

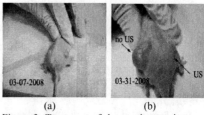

(a)   (b)

Figure 3. Treatment of the ovarian carcinoma by PEG-PLLA nanobubble-encapsulated paclitaxel; (a) – before treatment; (b) – three weeks after treatment.

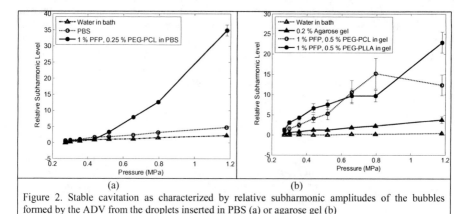

(a)   (b)

Figure 2. Stable cavitation as characterized by relative subharmonic amplitudes of the bubbles formed by the ADV from the droplets inserted in PBS (a) or agarose gel (b)

ACKNOWLEDGMENTS

This work was supported by the NIH R01 EB1033 Grant to N. Rapoport.

REFERENCES

1. N. Rapoport, Z. Gao, and A. M. Kennedy, *J. Natl. Cancer Inst.* **99**, 1095-1106 (2007).
2. Z. Gao, A. M. Kennedy, D. A. Christensen, and N. Rapoport, *Ultrasonics* **48**, 260-270 (2008).
3. O. D. Kripfgans, J. B. Fowlkes, *et al.*, *Ultrasound Med. Biol.*, **26**, 1177-1189 (2000).
4. A. H. Lo *et al*, *IEEE Trans. Ultrasons. Ferroelect. Freq. Contr.*, **54**, 933-946 (2007).

Histotripsy of the Prostate for the Treatment of BPH: Chronic Results From a Canine Model

Timothy L Hall[a], Chris R Hempel[a], Alison M Lake[a], Kathy Kieran[a], Kim Ives[c], J Brian Fowlkes[b,c], Charles A Cain[c], and William W Roberts[a,c]

[a]University of Michigan Department of Urology, Ann Arbor, MI, USA.
[b]University of Michigan Department of Radiology, Ann Arbor, MI, USA.
[c]University of Michigan Department of Biomedical Engineering, Ann Arbor, MI, USA.

Abstract. Histotripsy was evaluated as a non-invasive BPH treatment. The prostates of 21 canine subjects were targeted with one of three histotripsy doses. Prostates were harvested immediately, 7 days, or 28 days after treatment and assessed for changes. Lower treatment doses were found to produced scattered cellular disruption and hemorrhage that was sometimes reversible. Higher doses perforated the urethra and produced cavities in the glandular prostate that healed to leave an enlarged urinary channel.

Keywords: Ultrasound therapy, histotripsy, BPH, prostate.
PACS: 43.80.

INTRODUCTION

Benign prostate hyperplasia (BPH) is a condition of an enlarged prostate occurring in older men. As the prostate grows, confinement by the surrounding capsule causes compression of the urethra and leads to symptoms of urinary hesitancy, frequent urination, and general discomfort as well as increased risk of urinary tract infections. In 2000, primary diagnosis of BPH accounted for 4.5 million physician visits.[1] Milder cases are sometimes resolved with long term use of medications. Minimally invasive interventions using HIFU or RF ablation have yielded poor results for treatment of more severe cases.[2] The standard for treatment is a surgery called trans-urethral resection of the prostate (TURP) using a knife and electrocautery or photovaporization. In this procedure, the center of the prostate is removed to enlarge the urinary channel. TURP is highly effective and provides immediate relief of symptoms, but carries a significant morbidity risk.[3]

Histotripsy is a method of ultrasound therapy where repeated intense bursts of ultrasound at a low duty cycle cause direct mechanical disruption of tissue through cavitation mechanisms. Using a highly focused sound field, these effects can be confined to a precise volume. The accumulated cellular disruptions from a large number of bursts can reduce the targeted tissue to a liquid state.[4]

The overall goal of this work was to investigate histotripsy as a non-invasive treatment for BPH. By rendering the center of the prostate to a liquid state, histotripsy was hypothesized to be capable of providing immediate relief of symptoms as the ablated tissue could be flushed from the urinary channel. This study had the following

CP1113, *8th International Symposium on Therapeutic Ultrasound,* edited by E. S. Ebbini
© 2009 American Institute of Physics 978-0-7354-0650-6/09/$25.00

aims: 1) demonstrate accurate targeting of the prostate non-invasively and initiation of histotripsy therapy, 2) successful removal of urethral and glandular prostate tissue, 3) identify effective ablative doses for urethral and glandular prostate tissue, 4) assess the safety, acute, and chronic effects of histotripsy ablation.

METHODS

21 mixed breed adult canine subjects were used in this study. Subjects were selected to have a prostate volume of at least 10 cm^3 (median = 23.2 cm^3). Subjects were anesthetized with acepromazine (0.1 mg/kg) and thiopental (3.5 to 5.5 mg/kg intravenously) and then intubated. Anesthesia was maintained throughout the remaining procedures with inhaled 1-2% isoflurane.

Subjects were placed supine, the lower abdomen shaved, and ultrasound coupling gel was applied. The penis was gently clamped with a modified towel clamp and pulled to the right side. A stainless steel bowl with a cutout was placed over the abdomen. Into the bowl was placed a thin plastic bag which was then filled with degassed water.

Therapeutic ultrasound was delivered with a piezoceramic composite array transducer (Imasonic) trans-abdominally. The transducer was an annulus shape with an outer diameter of 14 cm, inner diameter of 6 cm and geometric focal length (radius of curvature) of 10 cm. All the array elements were excited in phase such that the steering capability was not used. The transducer was mounted to a 3-axis positioning system with the focus scanned mechanically. An endocavitary ultrasound imaging probe (E8C, GE Medical Systems) was aligned in the center of the transducer for preliminary targeting.

Exciting the therapy system briefly in the water bolus above the subject produced a bubble cloud that was marked on the image from the E8C. This focal point was then positioned in the desired location within the prostate. Subsequent treatment in the prostate was monitored with a trans-rectal probe (I739, GE Medical Systems) which provided markedly superior image quality but was not physically registered with the therapy transducer.

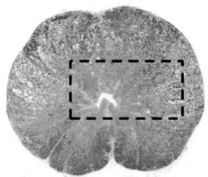

FIGURE 1. Representation of the targeted volume (dashed box) in the prostate. Fibrous tissue (urethra and scattered bands) appear pink whereas glandular tissue is stained purple.

38 treatment volumes were targeted usually 2 per prostate with one volume towards the apex and the other placed towards the base. Only one volume was placed in some of the smallest prostates to avoid problems discriminating the treatments. Each volume consisted of a grid of 1 mm spaced focal locations to cover approximately 2 cm^3. The volumes were placed to intersect both the urethra and a portion of glandular tissue (figure 1). Treatment consisted of repeated 3 cycle pulses of 750 kHz ultrasound with a peak negative pressure amplitude of 20 MPa. The total therapy dose delivered to each volume was either 56000, 160000, or 540000 pulses. The pulse repetition frequency was 300 Hz yielding treatment times of 3, 9, and 30 minutes respectively.

Following treatment, 6 subjects (acute) were euthanized immediately and the prostate removed and processed for histology. 7 subjects were recovered from anesthesia and kept for 7 days before prostate removal and 8 subjects were kept for 28 days. Non-acute subjects were catheterized for 1-3 days to prevent urinary obstruction.

Blood samples were collected for standard analysis before treatment, 24 hours after, and at prostate harvest. Urine samples were collected after treatment and cultured to detect infection. Pain was assessed each day starting from before the procedure using a standard behavioral assessment method.

Harvested prostates were fixed for 5-7 days in formalin and then grossly sectioned in 5 mm slabs. The slabs were paraffin embedded and sectioned in 1 mm increments to yield a complete sectioning of the prostate in 1 mm increments. All slides were stained with Hematoxylin and Eosin (H&E).

RESULTS

The treatment was well tolerated by all subjects. Daily pain score assessments showed a small deviation from baseline which normalized within 24 hours of catheter removal. One subject developed a minor forearm injury unrelated to treatment.

Blood analysis showed minor elevations in white blood count, serum creatine kinase and liver enzymes post-operatively. These values all normalized by the time of harvest (7 or 28 days). The increase in liver enzymes was consistent with a normal response to anesthesia. All urine cultures demonstrated no growth. Mild post-operative hematuria was present and resolved in a few days.

Histotripsy was successfully initiated in all 38 target volumes shown by a bubble cloud observed on ultrasound imaging in the targeted location. All 38 volumes were also identified histologically. Tissue effects in acute subjects ranged from scattered points of hemorrhage and cell disruption to cavities filled with a completely acellular liquid. Chronic subject effects ranged from scattered fibrosis to large cavities. These are described in detail below with respect to applied dose.

13 volumes were targeted with a 56k dose (figure 2). In acute subjects, the volumes displayed scattered focal sites of disruption and hemorrhage 10 – 100 microns in diameter. Both urethral tissue and glandular tissue showed damaged, however, no macroscopic cavities were formed and none of the urethras were perforated. Prostates harvested 7 days after treatment showed additional necrosis compared with acutes in the glandular tissue. Fibrosis and the beginning of tissue reorganization were present. 2 of 5 volumes displayed macroscopic cavities within the glandular tissue occupying only a portion of the full treatment volume. 3 of 5 urethras continued to show some

scattered hemorrhage, one showed no damage, and one showed a perforation. The four volumes in prostates harvest 28 days after treatment showed only scattered areas of fibrosis in glandular tissue. No macroscopic cavities were formed. All urethras showed no damage.

Acute   7 days   28 days

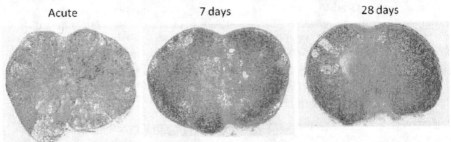

FIGURE 2. Representative slides of cross sections of targeted volumes exposed to a 56k dose.

12 volumes were targeted with a 160k dose (figure 3). In acute subjects, contiguous regions of hemorrhage and cellular disruption were found in glandular tissue. The urethra was substantially destroyed or perforated in two volumes and only damaged in two other volumes. For three volumes from prostates harvested 7 days after treatment, a macroscopic cavity was formed in communication with a perforated urethra. One volume displayed a damaged but not perforated urethra and only scattered disruption to glandular tissue. All four volumes harvested 28 days after treatment showed perforated urethras in communication with a large drained cavity in the glandular prostate tissue. A urothelium lining had reformed on the cavity and urethra. The lobes of the prostate targeted by the treatment volume were noticeably smaller than the opposite sides suggesting some loss of prostate volume and partial collapse of the cavities created.

Acute   7 days   28 days

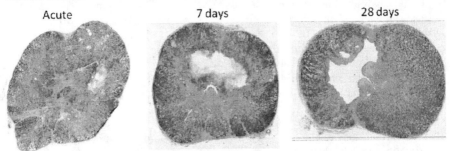

FIGURE 3. Representative slides of cross sections of targeted volumes exposed to a 160k dose.

13 volumes were targeted with a 540k dose (figure 4). 5 volumes in prostates harvested acutely showed contiguous regions of hemorrhage and cell disruption. 2 of the 5 volumes had visibly perforated or absent urethras. All 8 volumes from prostates harvested 7 days or 28 days after treatment had perforated or absent urethras contiguous with cavities in the glandular tissue. Shrinkage of the targeted lobe was noted. A urothelium lining was present on the 28 day cavities.

132

Acute   7 days   28 days

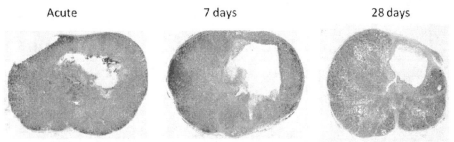

FIGURE 4. Representative slides of cross sections of targeted volumes exposed to a 540k dose.

To summarize, trans-abdominal histotripsy was successful at debulking glandular prostate tissue in the canine. The urethra could be perforated allowing disrupted tissue to be drained. Treatment was well tolerated by all subjects.

REFERENCES

1. J.T. Wei, E. Calhoun and S.J. Jacobsen, "Urologic diseases in America project: benign prostatic hyperplasia", *J Urol* 173 (2005), pp. 1256–1261.
2. H.S. Tunuguntla and C.P. Evans, "Minimally invasive therapies for benign prostatic hyperplasia", *World J Urol* 20 (2002), pp. 197–206.
3. W.K. Mebust, H.L. Holtgrewe and A.T. Cockett et al., "Transurethral prostatectomy: immediate and postoperative complications—a cooperative study of 13 participating institutions evaluating 3,885 patients", *J Urol* 141 (1989), pp. 243–247.
4. W.W. Roberts, T.L. Hall and K. Ives et al., Pulsed cavitational ultrasound: a noninvasive technology for controlled tissue ablation (histotripsy) in the rabbit kidney, *J Urol* 175 (2006), pp. 734–738.

Feasibility of MRI-guided Focused Ultrasound as Organ-Sparing Treatment for Testicular Cancer

Robert Staruch[a], Laura Curiel[b], Rajiv Chopra[a,b] and Kullervo Hynynen[a,b]

[a]Department of Medical Biophysics, University of Toronto
[b]Imaging Research, Sunnybrook Health Sciences Centre
2075 Bayview Avenue, Toronto, Ontario, Canada M4N 3M5

Abstract. High cure rates for testicular cancer have prompted interest in organ-sparing surgery for patients with bilateral disease or single testis. Focused ultrasound (FUS) ablation could offer a noninvasive approach to organ-sparing surgery. The objective of this study was to determine the feasibility of using MR thermometry to guide organ-sparing focused ultrasound surgery in the testis. The testes of anesthetized rabbits were sonicated in several discrete locations using a single-element focused transducer operating at 2.787MHz. Focal heating was visualized with MR thermometry, using a measured PRF thermal coefficient of -0.0089 ± 0.0003 ppm/°C. Sonications at 3.5-14 acoustic watts applied for 30 seconds produced maximum temperature elevations of 10-80°C, with coagulation verified by histology. Coagulation of precise volumes in the testicle is feasible with MRI-guided focused ultrasound. Variability in peak temperature for given sonication parameters suggests the need for online temperature feedback control.

Keywords: Focused ultrasound, MRI, thermometry, proton resonance frequency shift, testis.
PACS: 87.50.yk, 87.50.yt, 87.61.-c.

INTRODUCTION

Testicular cancer is the most common malignancy in young men, affecting 1 in 10000 men between 15 and 34 [1]. With surgical removal of the testis, long term survival approaches 100%, but for the 5% of patients with bilateral disease, removal of both organs causes infertility. This group faces lifelong testosterone deficiency leading to osteoporosis, abnormal muscle and fat distributions, and mood disorders. Androgen replacement therapy is ineffective in one third of cases [2]. To preserve quality of life for these young patients, less invasive approaches are being investigated.

Marberger *et al* [3,4] have investigated the use of high intensity focused ultrasound (HIFU) to ablate testicular lesions, and published results for seven patients who had metachronous bilateral disease [4]. Using a clinical HIFU system designed for prostate ablation, multiple sonications were performed to thermally coagulate an US-targeted volume. With adjuvant radiotherapy, they showed excellent cure rates and sustained hormone function, but could only verify lesion production in the one patient who refused RT and had a new germ cell tumor arise adjacent to the HIFU lesion.

Temperature elevations for identical sonication parameters vary widely *in vivo* due to spatial and temporal variations in tissue absorption and perfusion. MR thermometry

CP1113, *8th International Symposium on Therapeutic Ultrasound*, edited by E. S. Ebbini
© 2009 American Institute of Physics 978-0-7354-0650-6/09/$25.00

can not only quantify heating in the testis, but can also be used to perform feedback control during sonication to overcome inhomogeneities and achieve a desired spatial heating pattern. The objective of this study was to determine the feasibility of using MR thermometry to guide organ-sparing focused ultrasound surgery in the testis.

METHODS

To determine the feasibility of using MR thermometry to guide focused ultrasound organ-sparing surgery in the testis, focused ultrasound heating was performed *in vivo* in rabbit testicles over a range of ultrasound exposures. During sonication, the spatial temperature distribution was measured with MRI [5] and the locations of measured temperature elevations were later compared with histology.

Spatial temperature distributions were calculated from MR phase images using the proton resonance frequency shift method [5]. A spatial resolution of approximately 1 x 1 x 3 mm and temporal resolution of 5 seconds were achieved in coronal images using a spoiled gradient echo sequence (FSPGR, TE: 10 ms, TR: 38.6 ms, 30° flip angle, 8-16 cm FOV, 3 mm slice, 128x128, NEX: 1). To our knowledge, a measurement of the PRF shift coefficient for the testis has not been reported in the literature. To calibrate, freshly excised rat testes were immersed in a 6 mM solution of $MnCl_2$ pre-heated to 60°C. As they cooled in the MRI, temperature was measured every 30 seconds in all samples with fiber-optic temperature probes (Luxtron 3100, Luxtron Corp., Santa Clara, CA). Measurements coincided with FSPGR image acquisition (8 cm FOV, NEX: 6). Complex phase subtractions were calculated offline, and the mean phase shifts in a 200 pixel ROI were correlated with the fiber-optic measurements.

Sonications were performed in five New Zealand White rabbits (3.4-3.6 kg) with a single-element transducer (2.787 MHz, 5 cm aperture, 10 cm radius) using an MRI-compatible positioning system (Figure 1a) in a clinical 3T imager (Signa, GE Healthcare). Acoustic coupling is provided by a flexible plastic sleeve of degassed water. Transducer focus was localized by the water jet produced at low power.

The rabbit, anesthetized with 50 mg/kg ketamine and 5 mg/kg xylazine followed by maintenance with 2% isoflurane, had its testicles and surrounding area carefully depilated (Veet, Reckitt Benckiser North America, Inc., Parsippany, NJ) and locally anesthetized. The animal was positioned prone on the apparatus, with depilated testes centered in the top aperture, allowed to rest at the water surface (Figure 1b).

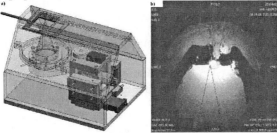

FIGURE 1. a) Schematic of MRI-compatible transducer positioning system showing transducer's acoustic field sonicating up through an aperture in the top plate of the apparatus. b) Axial image showing the position of the transducer with respect to the rabbit testis and the ultrasound focus.

Discrete locations in the testis were sonicated continuously for 30 seconds at 3.5-14 acoustic watts during acquisition of phase images for thermometry. By remotely repositioning the transducer between sonications, up to four individual thermal lesions were created in each testis, spaced about 1 cm apart.

Animals were sacrificed immediately after experiments. Testes were excised and fixed in 10% buffered formalin. Histological sections sliced coronally at 5 μm every 250 μm were stained with hematoxylin and eosin. The size and locations of observed lesions were compared with measured temperature distributions.

RESULTS

Figure 2 shows the correlation between phase difference and temperature elevation measured in the excised rat testes. A least-squares fit to these values yielded a linear dependence in the phase difference on temperature of -4.11 ± 0.14 °/°C (mean ± SD), which corresponds to a PRF temperature coefficient of α = -0.0089 ± 0.0003 ppm/°C, similar to results published for other tissues [5,6]. This value of α was used for *in vivo* thermometry in rabbit testes during MRgFUS.

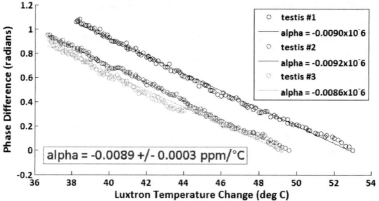

FIGURE 2. PRF shift calibration for three freshly excised rat testes. Correlation between phase difference and fiber-optic temperature measurements displayed in ppm/°C.

Figures 3(a)-(d) show measured temperature elevations in the testis of a rabbit during a 30 second sonication at 8.75 W. Figure 3(e) shows the corresponding peak temperature elevations measured in a 10 pixel region of interest at the focus.

Figure 4 shows peak temperature elevations measured with MR thermometry for 19 sonications in 5 animals at 3.5-14 acoustic watts. Peak temperature elevations ranged from 5-80°C. Image SNR at peak temperature elevation varied from approximately 60 to 200, with corresponding temperature uncertainties of ±0.5 to ±1.5°C.

H&E staining showed clearly demarcated lesions with a ring of interstitial edema surrounding a region of cells destroyed by coagulation necrosis. An example for a sonication of 12 acoustic watts for 30 seconds is shown in Figure 5.

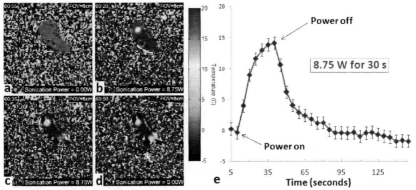

FIGURE 3. Spatial temperature distribution during ultrasound heating of rabbit testicle. a)-d) Coronal temperature maps through the focal plane during and after sonication. e) Peak temperature elevation at the ultrasound focus during testicular MRgFUS treatment.

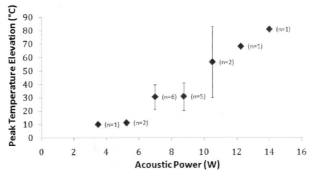

FIGURE 4. Peak temperature elevations measured with MR thermometry for nineteen 30s sonications at 3.5-14 acoustic watts in the testes of five rabbits.

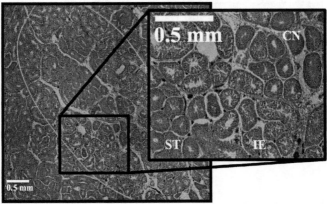

FIGURE 5. Histologically identified HIFU lesion (outlined) after 30 second sonication at 12 W. Lesion boundary shows regions of normal seminiferous tubules (ST), interstitial edema (IE), and coagulation necrosis (CN). H&E x 40.

137

DISCUSSION

The study demonstrates the feasibility of MRI-guided focused ultrasound of the testis. MR thermometry using the proton resonance frequency shift was shown to be a feasible method for online guidance of FUS thermotherapy, providing temperature distributions through a plane of interest with spatial, temporal, and temperature resolutions of less than 1 mm, 5 seconds, and ± 1.0°C. Large variations (up to 30°C) in the peak temperatures using identical sonication parameters were observed. These variations, caused by tissue and perfusion inhomogeneities, make online dosimetry an important part of focused ultrasound exposures. Further experiments to identify the appropriate thermal dose for ablation of testicular parenchyma, and to implement online temperature feedback control are warranted.

ACKNOWLEDGMENTS

Funding provided in part by an NSERC Alexander Graham Bell Canada Graduate Scholarship. Hardware and software support for the MR-compatible positioning system were provided by Anthony Chau and Sushil Kumar. Animal expertise was provided by Alexandra Garces. Freshly excised rat testes were graciously provided by Michelle Ladouceur-Wodzak.

REFERENCES

1. S. Krege *et al*, "European consensus conference on diagnosis and treatment of germ cell cancer: a report of the second meeting of the European germ cell cancer consensus group (EGCCCG): Part I," *Eur. Urol.* **53**, 478-496 (2008).
2. S. D. Fossa *et al*, "Androgen replacement and quality of life in patients treated for bilateral testicular cancer," *Eur. J. Cancer* **35**(8): 1220-1225 (1999).
3. S. Madersbacher *et al*, "Transcutaneous high-intensity focused ultrasound and irradiation: an organ-preserving treatment of cancer in a solitary testis," *Eur. Urol.* **33**: 195-201 (1998).
4. C. Kratzik *et al*, "Transcutaneous high-intensity focused ultrasonography can cure testicular cancer in solitary testis," *Urology* **67**(6): 1269-1273 (2005).
5. Y. Ishihara *et al*, "A precise and fast temperature mapping using water proton chemical shift," *MRM* **34**, 814-823 (1995).
6. R. D. Peters *et al*, "Ex vivo tissue-type independence in proton-resonance frequency shift MR thermometry," *MRM* **40**, 454-459 (1998).

Thermal Ablation by High-Intensity-Focused Ultrasound Using a Toroid Transducer Increases the Coagulated Volume and Allows Coagulation Near Portal and Hepatic veins in Pigs

D. Melodelima[a], W.A. N'Djin[a], H. Parmentier[a], M. Rivoire[a,b] and J.Y. Chapelon[a]

[a] Inserm, U556, Lyon, F-69003, France ; Université de Lyon, Lyon, F-69003, France
[b]Centre Léon Bérard, Lyon, F-69008, France

Abstract. A new geometry of HIFU transducer is described to enlarge the coagulated volume. The geometry of the transducer was not spherical. The surface of the transducer was built based on a toroid geometry. The transducer was generated by the revolution of a circle about an axis lying in its plane. Eight emitters operating at a frequency of 3 MHz were diced out of a single toroid piezocomposite element. Each of the eight emitters was divided into 32 transducers. The focal zone is conical and located at 70 mm from the transducer. A 7.5 MHz ultrasound imaging probe is placed in the centre of the device for guiding the treatment. Our long-term objective is to develop a device that can be used during surgery. In vivo trials have been performed on 13 pigs to demonstrate this new principle and to evaluate the vascular tolerance of the treatment. This new geometry combined with consecutive activation of the eight emitters around the toroid allows achieving a mean thermal ablation of 7.0 ± 2.5 cm3 in 40 seconds. All lesions were visible with high contrast on sonograms. The correlation between the size of lesions observed on sonograms and during gross examination was 92%. This allows the user to easily enlarge the coagulated volume by juxtaposing single lesions. The pigs tolerate the treatment well over the experimental period even when coagulation was produced through portal and/or hepatic veins.

Keywords: Ultrasound, HIFU, liver, metastases, tumor, imaging.
PACS: 43.80.Sh

INTRODUCTION

Colorectal cancer is among the highest most common causes of cancer death in the western world, ranking second in Europe and third in United States[1]. Nearly half the patients will develop liver metastases at some point during the course of the disease, with 15–25% having metastases at the time of diagnosis. Hepatic resection is the gold standard in the treatment of colorectal liver metastases and currently is the only treatment that can, to date, ensure long-term survival in 25 - 40% of the patients[2]. Patients are eligible for hepatic resection if complete resection of colorectal metastases is possible with tumor free margins. Additionally, the remaining functional hepatic

CP1113, *8th International Symposium on Therapeutic Ultrasound*, edited by E. S. Ebbini
© 2009 American Institute of Physics 978-0-7354-0650-6/09/$25.00

volume must be sufficient to ensure adequate postoperative liver function. Only 20% of patients with liver metastases are suitable for resection.

Focused beams of High Intensity Focused Ultrasound (HIFU) treatments produce sufficiently strong heating in the focal zone to coagulate cells, even at distances relatively far from the transducer. This method allows for the creation of well-defined conformal treatments. Excellent results have been obtained both experimentally and clinically in inducing homogeneous and reproducible tumor destruction[3].

Here we report that a HIFU transducer with toroid geometry can rapidly induce large coagulation necroses. The device was divided into eight elements to produce a conical focal zone located 70 mm from the transducer, allowing for deep and large thermal ablation. An ultrasound imaging probe located in the centre of the device provides image guidance for the treatment. The medical device presented in this study could be used in conjunction with resection. Therefore the approach selected is surgical laparotomy and consequently makes it possible to reach all regions of the liver without penetrating the hepatic capsule. Furthermore, an open procedure enables the protection of organs in the vicinity while eliminating the risk of secondary lesions. Using a porcine model, the feasibility and efficiency of this new HIFU therapy was examined.

MATERIAL AND METHODS

The geometry of the transducer was toroidial which allows creating conical shaped focal zone. From a geometrical point of view a toroid is a surface of revolution obtained by rotating a closed plane curve about an axis lying in its plane. The emitting surface has a diameter of 70 mm and a radius of curvature of 70 mm. The transducer was divided radially into eight piezocomposite emitters and produces a conical focal zone located 70 mm from the transducer. Each of the eight emitters is divided radially and into concentric rings to create 32 transducers so the location and intensity of the pressure field created can be controlled electronically by modulating the amplitude and phase applied to each transducer. Each individual transducer is 0.13-mm^2 and operates at a frequency of 3 MHz. As a result, each of the eight emitters focuses on a distinct 1/8 of ring and contributes to the formation of a single HIFU lesion. In this configuration, the acoustic energy was distributed over a larger volume. During the creation of a single lesion, each of the eight emitters was activated one at a time for 5 seconds while the 7 other emitters are inactive. There is no pause during changeover, which makes it possible to use the heat deposited by the previous exposures. According to this treatment principle, the total HIFU exposure time to produce a single lesion that is 2 cm in diameter by 2.5 cm on its major axis is 8×5 seconds or 40 seconds. A 7.5 MHz ultrasound imaging probe (Vermon, Tours, France) was placed in the centre of the device and connected to a BK HAWK 2102 EXL scanner (B-K Medical, Herlev, Denmark) to guide the treatment.

Trials were conducted on 13 pigs, 12-14 weeks old, with an average weight of 31.3 ± 4.2 kg (min. 23 – max. 37 kg). Twenty-four hours before and after HIFU, the food intake of the animal was restricted with free access to water. Premedication was performed 30 minutes before anesthesia using an intramuscular injection of ketamine at a rate of 20 mg/kg. A 6.5 French venous catheter was placed in an auricular vein.

Induction was made by an intravenous injection of propofol. Ventilation was ensured at 10 l/min and at a frequency of 18 to 20 respiratory movements per minute with a 70% air/oxygen mixture. Anesthesia was maintained by a 1% propofol pressure infuser at a dose of 20 mg/kg/h, and sufentanil at a dose of 5 to 10 μg/kg/h. A 25 cm median laparotomy was performed from the xyphoïd process after classical surgical asepsis. Treatments were performed under sterile conditions. The HIFU device was held by hand and placed in acoustic contact with the liver using a sterile ultrasound coupling fluid which is contained in a sterile polyurethane envelope. The transducer-driving equipment was similar to that reported previously[4]. The total exposure time for a single lesion was 40 seconds. Larger lesions were created by juxtaposing single lesions (two rows of three singles lesions with a displacement of 1 cm between each single lesion were created). When the treatment was completed, all the lesions were observed and measured in sonograms.

Animals were revived using infrared lamps, and clinically monitored before being taken back to the animal quarters. Post-operative analgesia was administered by a fentanyl patch at a 100-μg dosage every three days. The pigs were euthanized under general anesthesia by a single intravenous 0.3 ml/kg injection containing embutramide, mebezonium and tetracaine (T61®, Intervet, Beaucouze, France). Total hepatectomy took place one hour (3 pigs), 4 days (4 pigs), 7 days (2 pigs), 15 days (2 pigs) and 30 days (2 pigs) after treatment. The hepatectomies were carried out on different dates to study local and general treatment tolerance and the evolution of the sizes of the lesions over a period of time. The lesions were cut along the exposure axis. Each lesion was then sliced into thin sections of 5 mm thick to determine whether thermal damages were homogeneous. Representative portions of treated tissue were then immersed in 10% formalin for fixation and set in paraffin. Staining was done with hematoxylin-phloxine-saffron (HPS).

All of the animal procedures were done after local institutional review board approval. These experiments conformed to the requirements of the local Office of Animal Experimentation and were in accordance with the legal conditions of the National Commission on Animal Experimentation.

RESULTS

In total, 67 single lesions were created (13 observed at D0, 34 at D4, 8 at D7, 6 at D15 and 6 at D30). An average of 5.8 ± 1.7 (min. 5 – max. 9) lesions were created in each liver. Single lesions were homogeneous with a mean diameter of the single lesions was 19.3 ± 4.0 mm (min. 12.0 – max. 29.0 mm). Analysis of single lesions showed, on 32 specimens, that necrosis could circumscribe completely vessels up to 5 mm in diameter (Figure 1a). Bile stains were equally noted in many lesions indicating a rupture of minor intrahepatic bile duct. The sizes of the lesions did not change over time as shown in Figure 1b. The diameter of the lesions observed at D0 was not significantly different as compared with the diameter at D4 (p=0.55), D7 (p=0.85), D15 (p=0.13) or D30 (p=0.11). A slight decrease was observed at D15 and D30 since the fibrous tissue response around the coagulated region was not taken into account in the measurement of the diameter. Fifteen large lesions were produced (two observed at

D0, two at D4, five at D7, four at D15 and two at D30). The sonication time, defined as the time from the first to the last sonication was on average 21 ± 8 minutes (min. 9 – max. 42). The mean diameter of the multiple lesions was 33.5 ± 13.5 mm (min. 14.0 – max. 60.0)

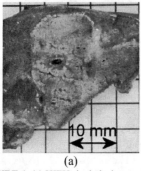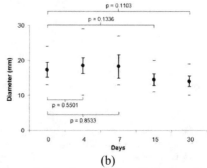

(a)   (b)

FIGURE 1. (a) HIFU single lesion produced in 40 seconds through a vessel 5 mm in diameter. (b) Evolution of the diameter of HIFU single lesions over 30 days. There is no significant difference between the lesions observed one hour after treatment and those observed 4 days, 7 days, 15 days and 30 days after treatment.

HIFU lesions in the liver were seen as a hypoechoic region with a central hyperechoic zone (Figure 2). A correlation was noted between the sizes of lesions measured macroscopically and the sizes of the same lesions measured by ultrasound ($R2 = 0.90$). The mean difference between the ultrasound and gross pathological diameters was 2.4 ± 2.1 mm (0 – 11.4).

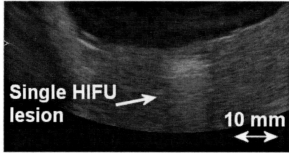

FIGURE 2. Single HIFU lesion observed on sonograms using the integrated ultrasound imaging probe.

The local and biological tolerances of the treatment were excellent. The pigs remained hemodynamically stable during the procedure. They recovered from the procedure within two hours after termination of anesthesia, and quickly resumed eating and normal behavior. The mean weight gain was 14 kg in one month for the 2 pigs studied until D30.

Using standard hematoxylin and eosin staining, histological evaluation of formalin fixed paraffin-embedded sections of excised HIFU ablation in liver tissues revealed evidence of tissue necrosis and cell death from D0. Complete and homogeneous coagulation necrosis in the entire treated region was confirmed from D15. A conjunctive fibrous cap appeared at the periphery of the lesions at D15 and D30. Tissue damage was confined to regions that had been given HIFU exposure. Within these treated regions, there was no evidence of intact cells. The ablated region was not reduced around blood vessels of less than 5 mm in diameter. There was no intervening healthy tissue surrounding vessels that were lower than or equal to 5 mm in diameter.

DISCUSSION

Using the transducer geometry presented in this paper each emitter is excited alternatively and consecutively, but the heat deposition is continuous in the focal zone. This principle allows for the creation of a broad heating pattern over short period of time, since each exposure benefits from the heat produced by previous sonications. In addition, this method allows for lower ultrasound energy in surrounding tissues since each of the eight emitters is excited only once to produce a lesion of 2 centimeters in diameter. Therefore, this toroid geometry of HIFU transducers is a promising technique for large thermal ablations and may be particularly useful for the treatment of liver metastases of colorectal cancer. The use of such a device can increase the number of patients eligible for hepatic resection by treating large metastases or metastases that are inaccessible to surgery or other local ablative technologies. Necroses induced by HIFU treatment circumscribe vessels with a maximum diameter of 5 mm. Thus, treatment near large vascular structures is conceivable.

ACKNOWLEDGMENTS

The authors wish to thank the staff of the institute for experimental surgery for their aid in the animal study. This work was supported by funding from the Cancéropôle Lyon Auvergne Rhône Alpes (PDC 2006.4.8), from the Cancéropôle Grand Ouest (CDTU 2004-01) and from the French Agency for Research on Cancer (ARC 4023). We also wish to thank the Anipath Laboratory and the Pr Scoazec for carrying out the histology study.

REFERENCES

1. Jemal A. et al. *CA Cancer J Clin* **55**, 10-30 (2005).
2. Antoniou A. et al. *Surgery* **141**, 9-18 (2007).
3. Kennedy J. E. *Nat Rev Cancer* **5**, 321-327 (2005).
4. Melodelima D. et al. *Med Phys* **33**,2926-2934 (2006).

A toroidial-shaped HIFU transducer for assisting hepatic resection: a complementary tool for surgery

N'Djin WA[a], Melodelima D[a], Schenone F[b], Rivoire M[b], Chapelon JY[a]

[a]Inserm, U556, Lyon, F-69003, France ; Université de Lyon, Lyon, F-69003, France.
[b]Institute of Experimental Surgery –Centre Léon Bérard, Lyon, F-69008, France ;
Université de Lyon, Lyon, F-69003, France.
apoutou.ndjin@.inserm.fr

Abstract. A toroidial-shaped HIFU medical device with integrated ultrasound imaging was developed for the treatment of colorectal liver metastasis. The HIFU toroidïal-shaped transducer contained 256-elements (working frequency: 3 MHz) and allows creating a single conical lesion of 7 cm^3 in 40 seconds (I_{focal} = 1700 $W.cm^{-2}$). Volumes of treatment can then be significantly increase by juxtaposing single lesions. Presented here is the use of this device in an animal model as a complementary tool to improve surgical resection in the liver. A zone of coagulative necrosis before transecting the liver was performed using this device in order to minimize blood loss and dissection time during hepatectomy. Resection assisted by HIFU (RA-HIFU) was compared with classical dissections with clamping (RC) and without clamping (Control). For each technique 14 partial liver resections were performed in seven pigs. Blood loss per dissection surface area was the main outcome parameter. Blood loss during liver transection was significantly lower in RA-HIFU (7.4 ± 3.3 $ml.cm^{-2}$) than in RC (34%) and Control (47%). The duration of transection in RA-HIFU (13 ± 3 min) was significantly shorter than in RC (44%) and Control (28%). Precoagulation also resulted in the use of significantly fewer clips; the number of clips used per square centimetre was 50% lower in RA-HIFU (0.8 ± 0.2 cm^{-2}) than in the other groups.

Keywords: HIFU; Liver; precoagulation; dissection; Blood losses; ultrasound

PACS: 01.30.Cc

INTRODUCTION

Colorectal cancer represents 940 000 new cases per year in the world. For 50 to 70% of these cases, patients develop metastases in the liver (LMCC) [1-2]. To date, the gold standard treatment of LMCC is the surgical resection but only concern 20 % patients. When resection is possible, the 5-years survival rate is 40% whereas for unresectable patients, this rate is null. However, non negligible difficulties could be encountered during the procedure of resection, due to the risk of extensive bleeding in many patients, leading to operative complications and the requirement of blood transfusions. Conventional resection techniques include vessel ligation and cauterization (bipolar electrocautery, radiofrequency, water dissector, ultrasound dissector). Some of these techniques implies hepatic trauma induced when probes penetrates the liver. Resection during clamping of the hepatic pedicle is in use since

CP1113, 8th International Symposium on Therapeutic Ultrasound, edited by E. S. Ebbini
© 2009 American Institute of Physics 978-0-7354-0650-6/09/$25.00

this procedure allows decreasing the volume of blood losses [3-4-5] but is associated with some morbidity (ischemia). In this paper, we propose to use the haemostatic properties of HIFU to reduce blood losses and assist resection without clamping. However, standard HIFU treatments are not well-suited as they are limited by the small size of the grain of rice shaped lesion and the long time necessary to enlarge the necroses by juxtaposition of multiple treatments. A previous study used a reflector to enlarge the typical region of necroses and assist resection [6]. In our study, a toroidial HIFU medical device developed for the treatment of LMCC is presented as a tool for assisting liver resection [7].

MATERIAL

The toroidial shaped HIFU transducer operates at a frequency of 3 MHz (focal distance: 70 mm) and enables the creation of a large single HIFU lesion (7 cm^3) in 40 seconds (acoustic power: 50-60 W, I_{focal} = 1700 W.cm^{-2}). This medical device is used manually during an open procedure. HIFU lesions appear on sonogram as a conical area in the liver tissues (hypoechoic on the center and hyperechoic on the boundary up to day 14 [8]. An integrated ultrasound imaging probe working at 7.5 MHz allows controlling the position of the HIFU treatment in real time on sonogram. Then, multiple single HIFU lesions can be juxtaposed accurately to enlarge the final necroses in the liver [9].

METHODS

Animal experiments were performed under an approved research protocol. These experiments conformed to the requirements of the local office of animal experimentation and were in accordance with the legal conditions of the French National Commission on Animal Experimentation. In a mid term preclinical study, the resection assisted by HIFU (RA-HIFU) was compared with classical resections with clamping (RC) and without clamping (Control) in pig liver. 21 pigs were treated and divided into 3 groups of 7 pigs. A 25-cm median laparotomy was performed from the xiphoid process. In the RA-HIFU group, the HIFU probe was used during an open procedure to precoagulate the liver before resection. The wall of necroses was created by juxtaposing manually multiple single conical HIFU lesions on the line of resection. HIFU exposures were stopped when operators considered by controlling on sonogram and macroscopically on palpation, that the barrier of lesions was homogeneous throughout the lobe. In the RC group, intermittent clamping (10/5 minutes) of the hepatic pedicle (Pringle manoeuvre) were performed using a Rummel tourniquet. During period of revascularisation, resection procedure was suspended to prevent haemorrhage associated to the dissection. In the 3 groups, each animal underwent two resections in their right central and left central lobes. Ultrasound controls, biological and clinical follows up were carried out up to 14 days (D14) after the treatment. At D14, after the euthanasia, macroscopic and histological analyses of the slice of resection were performed on the remaining parenchyma. The interest of RA-HIFU was studied regarding the vascular control during the resection, the time of procedure and the local and biological tolerance of the treatment.

RESULTS

The day of the treatment (D0), the average weight of the pigs was 29.1 ± 1.4 kg (min. 24.5 max. 34.2 kg). In group RA-HIFU, the walls of HIFU lesions were created in 22 ± 5 minutes (min. 10 max. 36 minutes) and were homogeneous (Fig.1). The resection rate was 11.2 ± 1.4 % (min. 6.1 max. 16.4 %). The average thickness of resected lobes was 2.5 ± 0.2 cm (min. 1.6 max. 3.4 cm) and the length of the resection line was 8.4 ± 0.8 cm (min. 6.0 max. 11.7 cm). The surface of the slice of resection had an area of $17.4 ± 3.5$ cm^2 (min. 8.7 max. 49.7 cm^2).

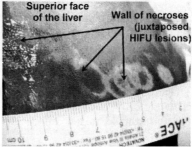

FIGURE 1. Wall of necroses in pig liver on the line of transaction before hepatectomy

Vascular control

The number of surgical clips used during resection to control vessels was 50 % lower in RA-HIFU ($0.8 ± 0.2$ cm^{-2} (min. 0.4 max. 1.5 cm^{-2})) compared with RC ($1,6 ± 0,2$ cm^{-2} (min. 0,8 max. 2,5 cm^{-2})) and Control ($1,8 ± 0,4$ cm^{-2} (min. 0,8 max. 3,2 cm^{-2})). Blood losses were also decreased in RA-HIFU ($7,4 ± 3,3$ ml.cm^{-2} (min. 1,7 max. 21,7 ml.cm^{-2})) since they were 34% lower compared with RC ($11,2 ± 2,2$ ml.cm^{-2} (min. 3,7 max. 17,9 ml.cm^{-2})) and 47% lower compared with Control ($14,0 ± 3,4$ ml.cm^{-2} (min. 7,8 max. 30,0 ml.cm^{-2})) (Fig.2).

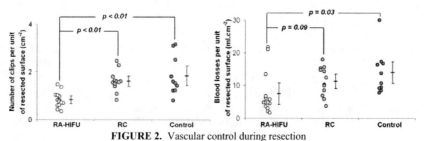

FIGURE 2. Vascular control during resection

Time of procedure

The procedure of resection was composed of HIFU exposures (only in the group RA-HIFU), 1 transection of a lobe, possible vessel ligations and a final homeostasis with electrical bistouries. In these conditions, the time of procedure was 24% and 29% higher in RA-HIFU (31 ± 6 minutes (min. 20 max. 62 minutes)), which contain additional HIFU sequences, compared respectively with RC (25 ± 4 minutes (min. 12 max. 42 minutes)) and Control (24 ± 3 minutes (min. 10 max. 34 minutes)). However, when focusing on the phase of transection, the time dedicated to this stage was 44% and 28% lower in RA-HIFU (13 ± 3 minutes (min. 7 max. 30 minutes)) compared with RC (23 ± 4 minutes (min. 12 max. 39 minutes)) and Control (18 ± 3 minutes (min. 10 max. 27 minutes)).

Biological and clinical follows up

20 on 21 pigs recovered uneventfully and quickly resumed eating and normal behavior up to D14. One pig died at D0 during the awakening phase in Control group. Ultrasound imaging control showed well defined sections of resection and in most cases, no abscess was detected (only one case was noticed of a sub capsular hematoma, 53×29 mm closed to the section in RC group). Macroscopic and histological analyses at D14 described normal cicatrisation of the remaining parenchyma with the presence of inflammatory reactions and the formation of fibrosis.

DISCUSSION

RA-HIFU requires controlling fewer vessels since the number of surgical clips was significantly lower (50%) compared with classical resections. After having created a wall of precoagulation on the line of resection in 20 minutes, vessels up to 5 mm in diameter were occluded and can be located and controlled faster in necrotized tissues than in normal tissues. This method makes possible to carry out continuous resections without having to synchronize the procedure with intermittent periods of revascularization. The total time of procedure in RA-HIFU group is longer but does not exceed 29% and is due to the preliminary period of HIFU exposures for precoagulating liver tissues. However, this parameter was considered acceptable since the stage of liver resection is performed faster (up to 44%) and easier using RA-HIFU. In addition, RA-HIFU improves vascular control and blood losses encountered during resection were significantly decreased compared with standard resections with clamping (34%) and without clamping (47%). Then, RA-HIFU limits risks of complication due to significant bleeding. Morbidity usually associated with clamping (ischemia) is eliminated during the RA-HIFU procedure. In previous studies, liver HIFU treatments performed with this medical device were already shown to be well tolerated at mid term in pig *in vivo* [8]. In this new study, RA-HIFU method benefits from this tolerance and general conditions of pigs were good up to two weeks.

In conclusion, this medical device dedicated for the treatment of LMCC allows assisting and improving standard liver resection at a preclinical stage. RA-HIFU method holds promise for future clinical applications in resection of LMCC associated with safe and efficient hemorrhage control.

ACKNOWLEDGEMENTS

The authors wish to thank the staff of the laboratory for experimental surgery for their aid in the animal study. This work was supported by funding from the Cancéropôle Lyon Auvergne Rhône Alpes (PDC 2006.4.8), from the Cancéropôle Grand Ouest (CDTU 2004-01) and from the French Agency for Research on Cancer (ARC 4023).

REFERENCES

1. Pohlen et al. Morbidity and mortality of elderly patients after surgery of liver metastases. Gastroent 2003;124(4):A737
2. Wildi et al. Intraoperative sonography in patients with colorectal cancer and resectable liver metastases on preoperature FDG-PET-CT. J Clin Ultrasound 2008;36:20-26
3. Hogart Pringle. Note on the arrest of hepatic hemorrhage due to trauma. Ann Surg 1908;48(4):541-549
4. Huguet et al. Tolerance of the human liver to prolonged normothermic ischemia: a biological study of 20 patients submitted to extensive hepatectomy. Arch Surg 1978;113:1448-1451
5. Petrowsky et al. A prospective, randomized, controlled trial comparing intermittent portal clamping versus ischemic preconditioning with continuous clamping for major liver resection. Ann Surg 2006;244(6):921-930
6. Zderic et al. Resection of abdominal solid organs using high-intensity focused ultrasound. Ultrasound Med Biol 2007;33(8):1251-1258
7. Melodelima et al. Ultrasound surgery with a toroïd transducer allows the treatment of large volumes over short periods of time. Appl Phys Lett 2007;91:193901
8. Melodelima et al. High Intensity Focused Ultrasound ablation for the treatment of colorectal liver metastases during an open procedure. Study on the pig. Ann Surg 2008; in press
9. N'Djin et al. Utility of a tumor-mimic model for the evaluation of the accuracy of HIFU treatments. Results of in vitro experiments in the liver. Ultrasound Med Biol 2008;34:in press

The Feasibility of HIFU Liver Ablation Through the Ribcage and Cartilage in a Rodent Model

Randy King, Viola Rieke, Kim Butts Pauly

Department of Radiology, Lucas MRI Center, Stanford University, 1201 Welch Road, Stanford, CA 94305-5488.
Department of Bioengineering, Lucas MRI Center, Stanford University, 1201 Welch Road, Stanford, CA 94305-5488.

Abstract. We examined the feasibility of the rat model for the study of HIFU treatment of liver cancer. Significance: HIFU is being developed for the minimally invasive treatment of primary and metastatic liver cancer. In patients, obstruction of the ultrasound by the ribs poses a significant problem, and current studies are under way which investigate the efficacy of focusing around or sonicating between the ribs. Such techniques show promise for patient treatments, but are not feasible when using rodent models. Results: Six recently euthanized (within the hour) Sprague-Dewey rats were used. The hair over the anterior surface was removed. Sonications were performed with the InSightec ExAblate system at 0.95 MHz, 1.1 MHz, and 1.35MHz through the rib cage. Temperature rise was monitored with MRI-based thermometry. Lesions were created in the livers of 5/6 rats. In the five rats, energy levels between 572-1194 Joules produced lesions every time. With energies greater than 1393 Joules, skin damaged was observed which prevented the ultrasound from propagating to the liver on subsequent sonications, accounting for the one study that failed to produce lesions. No thermal damage was observed at the skin with sonications that resulted in liver lesions, and no significant heating was observed at or near the skin in the MRI temperature maps. Conclusions: It is possible to ignore the effect of ribs and sternum in rodents and create lesions within the rat liver. This technique opens the door to using hepatocellular carcinoma rodent models in HIFU studies.

INTRODUCTION

Primary and secondary hepatic tumors are very common worldwide [1]. Unfortunately, surgical resection is considered the only potentially curative option. While authorities agree that surgery remains the treatment of choice for patients with respectable hepatic tumors, few patients are surgical candidates [1]. Therapeutic ultrasound, specifically high intensity focused ultrasound (HIFU), has become increasingly prominent among the range of treatments for localized tumors. This technique is used clinically for the treatment of prostate, liver and uterine fibroids [2,3,4,5,6]. To study hepatocellular carcinoma an appropriate animal model must be established. Recently, the pig has been suggested as being the ideal model for studying HIFU applied to the treatment of hepatic tumors because of the animal's size and physiology is close to that of humans [7]. The pig may be a good model when replicating the size of the human is important, e.g. when examining volume treated and tolerance, but there is no established porcine liver tumor model. Rodent models are preferred to larger animals because of the cost associated with survival studies, convenience of experimental setup, and available tumor cell lines. We propose that the rat could be a viable model for HIFU therapy.

CP1113, *8th International Symposium on Therapeutic Ultrasound,* edited by E. S. Ebbini
© 2009 American Institute of Physics 978-0-7354-0650-6/09/$25.00

In previous FUS studies the rat liver has been exteriorized to allow access to the tissue [8,9]. To be a useful model, the effects of the ribcage, including the bone and cartilage, on the ultrasound beam must be able to be ignored without exteriorizing the liver. Sonication around the ribcage in such a small animal is impractical. In the following study we show that it is possible to sonicate through the ribcage of the rat and create thermal lesions localized to the liver with no skin burns. By limiting motion of the rat, treatment monitoring using MR thermal imaging is possible.

Materials and Methods

All the experiments in this study were done with the InSightec (Haifa, Israel) MR guided focused ultrasound system, ExAblate 2000. The animals used in this study were Sprague-Dewey rats placed feet first in prone position on the therapy table inside the MRI (3 Tesla, GE Signa) using a standard GE (Milwaukee, WS) 3-inch surface coil attached under the rat so that the abdomen is suspended through the coil into a water bath This water bath is used to achieve acoustic coupling between the animal and the transducer (Fig. 1). *In situ* rats (n=6) were used within 1hr of sacrificing. *In vivo* rats (n=3) were anesthetized using 1.5%-2.0% isoflourine, 2 L/min Oxygen while their heart rate and oxygen saturation were monitored The abdomen of the rats were shaved to remove most of the hair; the remaining hair was removed with a chemical depilatory (Nair, Church and Dwight Co., Lakewood, NJ). For the hepatocellular carcinoma tumor model (n=1) 1 x 10^6 McA-RH 7777 Morris hepatoma cells were injected in PBS into the middle lobe of the liver of the rat. Sonications on *in situ* rats were performed using frequencies 0.95 MHz-1.35 MHz and energy levels of 572-1194 Joules. *In vivo* rats were limited to 1.35 MHz, but the energy levels used remained the same as the *in situ* cases.

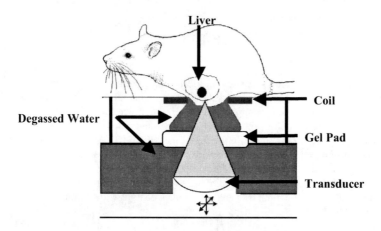

FIGURE 1. Schematic of experimental setup

Results

In the in situ studies, we found it was possible to create thermal lesions localized to the liver of rats by sonicating directly through the ribcage. No thermal burns were observed by visual inspection at energy levels below 1393 Joules on the skin on in the underlying tissue between the liver and the ribcage. Skin lesions were observed at energies levels above 1393 Joules. This was used as the threshold for the in vivo experiments, during which thermal lesions were created in the liver of the rat while no skin burns were observed (Fig. 2)

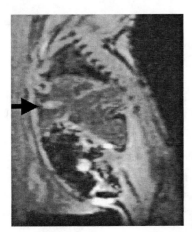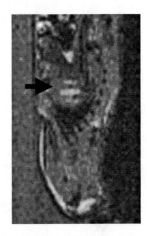

FIGURE 2. T1 weighted MR images of thermal lesions created *in vivo* in rat livers

Respiratory and bowel motion, as well as flow artifact from the cardiovascular system of the rat were minimized in several ways. The suspension of the abdomen through the MRI coil reduced the motion of the liver from its respiration. By keeping the phase encode direction of the MR system in the R/L direction, flow artifact from the heart and cardiovascular system is limited to the area superior to the liver. Finally, bowel motion was greatly reduced by fasting the animals for twelve hours before the experiment. Using all these techniques we were able to limit the motion and obtain MR temperature profiles during treatment (Fig. 3).

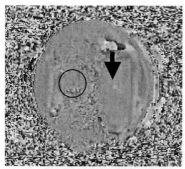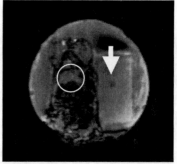

FIGURE 3. MR temperature profile during sonication (lef) and MR magnitude image (right) during the same sonication. The circled liver shows minimal physiological motion. Also shown is a heating spot in a phantom adjacent to the animal (arrows).

The in vivo studies demonstrated the ability to deliver the ultrasound through the ribs, while still creating a focus in the liver with intensities high enough to ablate tissue, but not damaging the skin or interlaying tissue. We have also shown the ability to monitor the HIFU treatment with MRI temperature mapping by limiting motion actifacts in the rat. With these techniques, treatment of a hepatocellular carcinoma tumor implanted into the liver of the rat is possible. Thermal ablation of the implanted tumor with the HIFU system was performed and MR temperature maps were obtained during the treatment. Maximum temperature rises, as well as thermal dose were monitored to determine when areas had been ablated (Fig. 4). These areas of thermal ablation matched thermal lesions localized to the tumor, which were visually observed during necropsy.

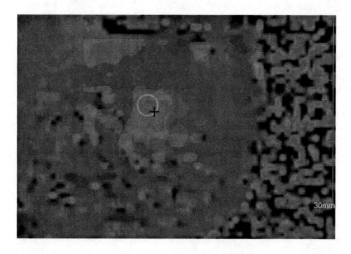

FIGURE 4. MR temperature profile during HIFU ablation of a rat HCC performed in vivo. The crosshairs indicate a peak temperature of 88°C with an average of the surrounding pixels of 77°C.

Conclusions and Future Work

In this study we have shown that the rat can be a feasible model for HIFU liver treatments, including hepatocellular carcinoma. It is possible to ignore the effect of the ribs and the sternum in rats and create *in vivo* thermal lesions localized to the liver of the rat. By limiting motion artifacts this ablative treatment can be performed while acquiring MRI temperature data. The resulting temperature maps can be used to monitor the HIFU treatment. Protocols for rat HCC treatments still need to be developed in terms of optimized power, frequency, and duration, as well as imaging parameters for better location and visualization of the tumors, but this technique opens the door to using HCC rat models in HIFU studies. Such models are needed for the advancement of patient treatments.

References

1. G.D. Dodd, M.C. Soulen, R.A. Kane, et al, Radiographics, 2000; 20; PP 9-27.
2. H. Madersbacher, M. Stohrer, R. Richter, et al, Cancer Res, 1995, Aug 1; 55; PP3346-51.
3. J.Y. Chapelon, M. Ribault, M. Vernier, R. Souchon, A. Gelet, Eur J Ultrasound, 1999, Mar; 9; PP 31-38.
4. R.O. Illing, J.E. Kennedy, F. Wu, et al, Br J Cancer, 2005;Oct; 93; PP 890-895
5. F. WU, Z.B. Wang, W.Z. Chen, et al, Ann Surg Oncol, 2004; Dec; 12; PP 1061-1069.
6. C.M. Tempany, E.A. Stewart, N. McDannold, et al, Radiology, 2003; Mar; 3; PP 897-905.
7. W.A. N'djin, D. Melodelima, H. Parmentier, Ultrasound in Med Biol, 2008; 34; article in press
8. L. Chen, GR. ter Harr, D. Robinson, et al, Ultrasound in Med Biol, 1999; 5; PP 847- 856.
9. L. Chen, GR. ter Harr, C.R. Hill, S.A. Eccles, G. Box, Ultrasound in Med Biol, 1998; 24; PP 1475- 1488.

Investigating Sonothrombolysis with High Frequency Ultrasound

Cameron Wright[*,†], Kullervo Hynynen[*,†], and David Goertz[*,†]

[*]Department of Medical Biophysics, University of Toronto, Canada
[†]Imaging Research, Sunnybrook Health Sciences Centre,
2075 Bayview Ave, Toronto ON, M4N 3M5, Canada

Abstract. Despite a significant body of work establishing the feasibility of ultrasound mediated thrombolysis in vitro, in vivo, and in clinical settings, there remains considerable uncertainty about the specific mechanisms involved in this process. This motivates further work to elucidate these mechanisms, which will be central to optimizing safe and effective operating conditions, and to guide the development of novel approaches and instrumentation. In this study, we investigate the use of high frequency ultrasound as a means of gaining mechanistic insight into sonothrombolysis. A high frequency ultrasound (20-50 MHz) instrument is employed which provides the ability to conduct volumetric clot imaging as well as pulsed-wave Doppler to monitor hemodynamics within vessels and clots. With modifications, it is enabled to perform the acquisition of RF data to assess the displacement of clots and vessel walls subjected to therapeutic pulses. Additional modifications were made to perform nonlinear imaging of micron to submicron sized bubbles, which are of interest in enhancing clot lysis. Experiments were performed on in vitro clots, and in vivo using a rabbit femoral artery clot model initiated by the injection of thrombin. Therapeutic pulses are provided by a single element spherically focused air backed transducer with transmit frequencies of 1.68 MHz. Clear visualization of the clots, displacements, and presence or absence of flow within these vessels is shown to be feasible, indicating the potential of this approach as a tool for providing insight into sonothrombolysis.

Keywords: Ultrasound, Thrombolysis, Microbubble
PACS: 43.80.Sh, 87.50.yg, 87.50.yt

INTRODUCTION

Ultrasound potentiated thrombolysis has been shown to have considerable potential for applications in stroke, cardiology and peripheral artery disease [1,2]. There has been a substantial body of research examining this process from a mechanistic perspective [3,4,5] and a range of factors have been identified or proposed to play roles in this process, including acoustic streaming, cavitation, and radiation pressure induced displacements. There still remains however significant uncertainty about mechanistic details, and their relative importance under different operating conditions. This motivates further work to elucidate and characterize these effects, particularly with a view to optimizing safe and effective operating conditions and to guide the development of novel approaches and instrumentation. The objective in this study was to investigate the use of high frequency ultrasound (20-50 MHz) as a tool to investigate sonothrombolysis. Specifically we attempted to a) image clots

CP1113, 8th International Symposium on Therapeutic Ultrasound, edited by E. S. Ebbini
© 2009 American Institute of Physics 978-0-7354-0650-6/09/$25.00

volumetrically and perform hemodynamic monitoring during sonothrombolysis treatment b) image microbubbles (micron to submicron) within and surrounding clots and c) measure and map displacements of clots subjected to therapeutic pulses of ultrasound.

METHODS

Ultrasound Imaging

Imaging was performed at 30 MHz using a commercial high frequency imaging system (VisualSonics Inc.), which offers high spatial resolution (~60-80 microns) and the ability to perform 3D volumetric scans and pulsed-wave Doppler. We note that in [6], such a system was employed to examine 2D Bscan sections through a rabbit ear thrombus. In the present study volumetric images were acquired pre- and post-sonothrombolysis treatment along the femoral vessels. The commercial imaging system was modified to perform 30-15 MHz subharmonic contrast imaging [7] to enable the visualization of microbubbles within and surrounding clots.

Imaging was done on a rabbit femoral artery clot, formed in the manner described in [8]. Tissue was resected from New Zealand White rabbits to expose the artery. Thrombin was injected proximal to the first branch point initiating ~ 1cm clot.

High intensity focused ultrasound (HIFU) in the absence of pharmacological agents was used to lyse clots. The therapy transducer was annular (10 cm diameter, 8 cm focus, 1.68 MHz) and was employed from below. Image-guidance was provided by a combination of a coaxial 9 MHz imaging array transducer situated within the therapy annulus. Treatment was performed at 1 mm spacings along the clot, exposing for 60 seconds at each location (1 Hz PRF, 10 ms pulse, 80 acoustic W).

Displacements

Modifications to the imaging setup were made to enable the use of high frequency ultrasound spatial mapping of displacements in clots. By interleaving imaging and therapeutic pulses (1 Hz PRF, 1 ms pulse, 1-3 acoustic W) successive RF imaging lines could be processed using a 2D autocorrelator [9] to measure displacements as a function of time along one line of sight. Rabbit whole blood was withdrawn from femoral artery. Clots were left at room temperature for 3h then stored at 5° C for minimum 3 days. Clots were situated in an agar phantom during exposure.

RESULTS

Figure 1(a) and (b) demonstrates the use of pulsed-wave Doppler to assess flow characteristics within the in vivo clot, in this case confirming that flow has been shut down entirely by the occlusion. Figure 2 shows a 3D volumetric image of the femoral artery and veins acquired in the vicinity of the clot (proximal to 1st bifurcation point) after the HIFU treatment session. From this volumetric data, patterns of clot erosion can be visualized. Example pre- and post-treatment longitudinal views of a femoral clot are shown in Figure 3(a) and (b), for a case where pulsed-wave Doppler monitoring indicated that flow restoration had not been achieved. Residual thrombus was found to be proximal to the bifurcation point, indicating an incomplete treatment.

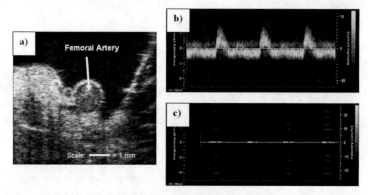

Figure 1. (a) 30 MHz B-scan post thrombus formation. 30 MHz PW Doppler before (b) and after (c) thrombus formation.

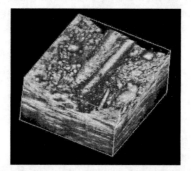

Figure 2. 30 MHz 3D volumetric image of femoral vessels (step sizes of 1mm).

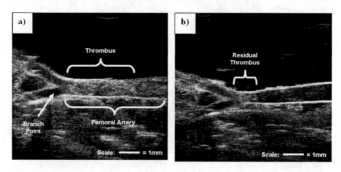

Figure 3. Longitudinal cross section of femoral artery before (a) and after (b) HIFU thrombolysis treatment.

Example B-scan and subharmonic contrast images are shown in Figure 4(a) and (b) respectively (same scale and location). The contrast images show that agent is in the vein, but has not penetrated within the clot at this level (~4 mm distal to the clot surface).

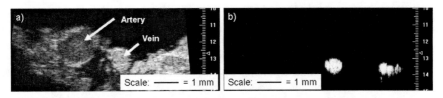

Figure 4: a) 30 MHz B-mode image of femoral artery and vein after HIFU treatment. b) Subharmonic image of femoral vessels in same location after injection of Definity microbubbles.

Example displacement results for a 2.5 watt pulse are shown in Figure 5(a) and (b). The spatial distribution of displacements as a function of depth along the imaging beam are visualized, with the peak corresponding to the point of intersection with the therapy beam (14 mm).

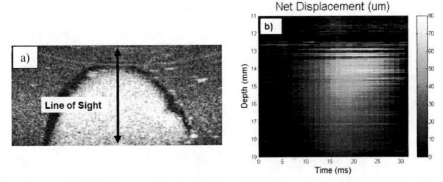

Figure 5. (a) 20 MHz B-mode of clot situated in agar for displacement measurement. (b) Net displacement (μm) of clot embedded in agar subjected to therapeutic ultrasound along one line of sight as a function of time

DISCUSSION AND CONCLUSIONS

This study has investigated the use of high frequency ultrasound as a tool for gaining mechanistic insight into sonothrombolysis. Using a rabbit femoral artery thrombus model, high frequency imaging showed clear visualization of the presence or absence of blood flow in the femoral artery with PW Doppler. This technique enables one to ensure the clot has been successfully formed within the artery and additionally, provides the ability to monitor flow recanalization through the vessel before and after treatment to determine treatment outcome.

High frequency imaging also provided clear visualization of the lysis pattern with 3D volumetric imaging of a rabbit femoral artery thrombus. This technique allows one to quantify volumetric and morphological changes of clots pre- and post- treatment providing valuable insight into how the thrombus breaks up based on different sonication parameters.

The ability to visualize microbubbles within and surrounding clots would provide valuable information for microbubble mediated sonothrombolysis treatments. Such information has previously been reported in [10] at lower frequencies, and we anticipate that the improved spatial resolution of high frequency ultrasound, in conjunction with volumetric morphologic data will be of increased utility in examining the thrombolytic process.

It has been previously suggested that clot displacements due to radiation forces may play a role in clot lysis, but this effect appears not to have been measured to date. The results of this study have shown the feasibility of measuring the spatial distribution of clot displacements with high frequency ultrasound. The quantification of the spatial distribution of thrombus motion at various sonication levels may help provide insight into the significance of this mechanism on overall clot lysis.

REFERENCES

1. Alexandrov et al. "Ultrasound-Enhanced Systemic Thrombolysis for Acute Ischemic Stroke". N Engl J Med 2004;351:2170-8.
2. Pffaffenberger et al. "Ultrasound Thrombolysis". Thromb Haemost. 2005 Jul;94(1):26-36. Review.
3. Francis et al. "Binding of Tissue Plasminogen Activator to Fibrin: Effect of Ultrasound". Blood. Vol. 91, No 6, 1998.
4. Holland et al. "Correlation of Cavitation with Ultrasound Enhancement of Thrombolysis". Ultrasound in Medicine and Biology., Vol. 32, No 8, 2006.
5. Frenkel et al. "Pulsed High-Intensity Focused Ultrasound Enhances Thrombolysis in an in Vitro Model". Radiology: Volume 239: Number 1-April 2006.
6. Stone et al. "Pulsed-high intensity focused ultrasound enhanced tPA mediated thrombolysis in a novel in vivo clot model, a pilot study". Thromb Res. 2007;121(2):193-202. Epub 2007 May 4.
7. Goertz et al. "High Frequency Nonlinear B-Scan imaging of Microbubble Contrast Agents". Trans IEEE UFFC, 2005.
8. Helft et al. "Comparative time course of thrombolysis induced by intravenous boluses and infusion of staphylokinase and tissue plasminogen activator in a rabbit arterial thrombosis model". Blood Coagul Fibrinolysis. 1998 Jul;9(5):411.
9. Loupas et al. "An Axial Velocity Estimator for Ultrasound Blood Flow Imaging, Based on a Full Evaluation of the Doppler Equation by Means of a Two-Dimensional Autocorrelation Approach". IEEE UFFC, 1995.
10. Porter et al. "Treatment of Deeply Located Acute Intravascular Thrombi with Therapeutic Ultrasound Guided by Diagnostic Ultrasound and Intravenous Microbubbles". J Ultrasound Med. 2006 Sep;25(9):1161-8.

MR Monitoring of the Near-Field HIFU Heating

Charles Mougenot[a,b], Max O. Köhler[c], Julia Enholm[c], Bruno Quesson[b],
Ari Partanen[c], Chrit T.W. Moonen[b], Gösta J. Ehnholm[c,d]

[a] Philips Systèmes Médicaux, 33 rue de Verdun, 92156 Suresnes, France
[b]Laboratory for Molecular and Functional Imaging, 146, rue Léo Saignat, 33076 Bordeaux, France
[c]Philips Healthcare, Äyritie 4, 01510 Vantaa, Finland
[d]Philips Research North America, 345 Scarborough Road, Briarcliff Manor, 10510 New York, USA

Abstract. The ablation of tumoral tissue with High Intensity Focused Ultrasound under MRI control has become clinical practice.[1,2] However, the most common adverse effect is skin burns induced in the near-field between the transducer and the focal point.[3] We present a study, based on animal trials, with monitoring and quantification of near field temperature increase in order to prevent skin burns.

Keywords: HIFU, MRI, near field, safety
PACS: 43.80.Sh

OBJECTIVES

HIFU produces accurate thermal ablation with local energy deposition. However, a major risk related to sonication, especially volumetric heating, is possible skin burns and unintended thermal damage of near-field tissue. HIFU is frequently combined with MRI to monitor the temperature increase in the treatment region. An animal trial study was conducted to examine the usefulness of MR for monitoring near-field temperature increase aimed at preventing skin burns.

MATERIAL & METHODS

Animal trials approved by the local ethical committee were performed on a Philips HIFU system and a 1.5T Achieva Philips MRI. Sonications were performed in the thigh muscle of 9 pigs (~50kg) under full anesthesia. Electronic displacement of the focal point along circular trajectories ranging from 4mm to 16mm diameter was used to produce volumetric heating of variable size (2kJ to 8kJ acoustic).

The MR temperature monitoring (based on the PRF method [4]) of the volumetric heating was composed of 6 slices acquired every 2.9s with an EPI sequence (EPI-factor = 11, echo time 20ms). One sagittal slice including the beam axis provided an overview of the heating. Three coronal slices around the focal point provided a quantification of the necrosis size produced. Two coronal slices located in the near field, in between the transducer and the focal point, were used aimed at preventing skin burns.

Because one near field slice was located in between the gel pad and the fat layer interface and the other near field slice was located in between the fat layer and the muscle interface, the fat signal had to be suppressed (water selective 121-binomial excitation). In addition a median filter (5×5 voxels) was used to improve the quality of thermal map before looking for the maximum temperature increase produced in the near field.

RESULTS

Figure 1 shows typical example of MR thermal map obtained at the end of a 12mm diameter volumetric heating within the acoustical near field in between fat layer and muscle. However, the partial volume effect with the fat suppressed tends to reduce the SNR and the temperature accuracy. However, temperature increase observed in the near field is also relative, typically below 10°C.

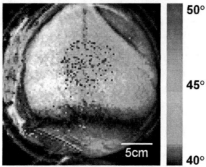

FIGURE 1. MR thermal map of the acoustical near field in between fat layer and muscle at the end of 12mm diameter volumetric heating.

Since an unnecessary high spatial resolution was used, the temperature accuracy was improved by using a spatial filter. Figure 2 illustrates the effect and the temperature accuracy improvement obtained with a median filter of 5×5 voxels applied on the thermal map shown the Fig. 1.

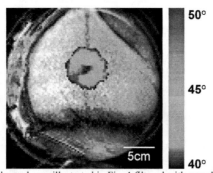

FIGURE 2. MR thermal map illustrated in Fig. 1 filtered with a median of 5×5 voxels.

Based on the filtered near field thermal map a reliable quantification of the maximum temperature increase in the near field was obtained. This maximum temperature increase detected correlated linearly with acoustic energy density. In the 120 sonications performed, 4 of 5 skin burns observed in histological analysis were correctly estimated by MR temperature monitoring without any false positives. Only one skin burn was not detected, probably due the progressive thermal build up induced by successive sonications with insufficient cooling duration as this duration was not yet optimized for this initial trial.

CONCLUSION

Near field MR thermal maps provide accurate and reliable detection of maximum temperature with a median filter even with in the presence of partial volume effects due to fat suppression. The maximum temperature detected in the near field is mainly influenced by energy density, which can therefore be used as a good indicator to reduce the risk of inducing skin burns.

However, this method is limited since the MR thermal maps provide only the relative temperature variation and not the absolute temperature. As a consequence, a slight risk of undetected skin burns remains in the case of insufficient cooling duration and if progressive thermal build up induced by successive sonications is not monitored.

REFERENCES

1. C.M. Tempany, E.A. Stewart, N.J. McDannold, B.J. Quade, F.A. Jolesz, and K.H. Hynynen, *Radiology*, **226**, 897-905 (2003).
2. F.M. Fennessy and C.M. Tempany, *Top Magn Reson Imaging*, **17**, 173-179 (2006)
3. E.A. Stewart, W.M. Gedroyc, C.M. Tempany, B.J. Quade, Y. Inbar, T. Ehrenstein, A. Shushan, J. Hindley, R.D. Goldin, M. David, M. Sklair, and J. Rabinovici, *Am J Obstet Gynecol*, **189**, 48-54 (2003).
4. J. Hindman, *J Chem Phys* **44**, 4582-4592 (1966).

TREATMENT PLANNING AND MODELING

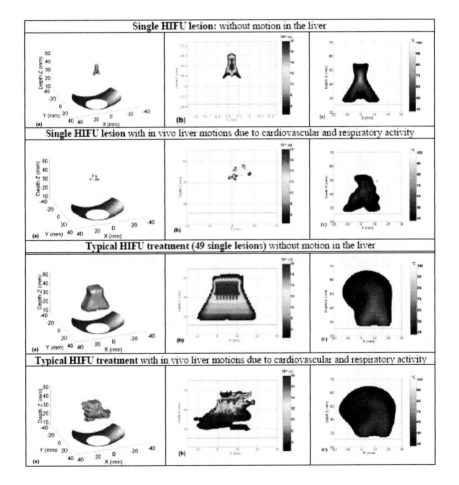

A User-Friendly Software Package for HIFU Simulation

Joshua E. Soneson

Center for Devices and Radiological Health, US Food and Drug Administration, Silver Spring, Maryland 20993
joshua.soneson@fda.hhs.gov

Abstract. A freely-distributed, MATLAB (The Mathworks, Inc., Natick, MA)-based software package for simulating axisymmetric high-intensity focused ultrasound (HIFU) beams and their heating effects is discussed. The package (HIFU_Simulator) consists of a propagation module which solves the Khokhlov-Zabolotskaya-Kuznetsov (KZK) equation and a heating module which solves Pennes' bioheat transfer (BHT) equation. The pressure, intensity, heating rate, temperature, and thermal dose fields are computed, plotted, the output is released to the MATLAB workspace for further user analysis or postprocessing.

Keywords: Software, nonlinear acoustics, numerical methods
PACS: 43.80.Sh, 43.25.Cb

INTRODUCTION

The current state of free software available for simulating medical ultrasound is limited to diagnostic applications. Existing freely-distributed codes include FIELD II[1] and KZKTEXAS[2], both of which were originally designed to simulate diagnostic ultrasound. The former is constrained to linear acoustic systems while the latter computes nonlinear effects but is best suited for short tone bursts. The software package HIFU_Simulator was designed to fill the need for inexpensive (both economically and computationally) modeling of high-power continuous wave (CW) beams and heating effects typical of therapeutic devices.

This article describes the technical aspects of this package, including the numerical methods used to solve the KZK and BHT equations. Instructions for use of HIFU_Simulator is described in the included user's manual[3].

PROPAGATION MODULE

The KZK equation is solved using a split-step method which permits the linear and nonlinear terms to be integrated using different techniques. The linear parts of the equation are solved in the frequency-domain, so for each of the K harmonics included in the calculation, there is a corresponding equation

$$\frac{\partial \hat{p}_k}{\partial z} + \frac{ic_0}{2}\nabla_r^2 \hat{p}_k + \alpha_k \hat{p}_k = 0, \quad k = 1, 2, \ldots, K,$$

(1)

CP1113, *8th International Symposium on Therapeutic Ultrasound*, edited by E. S. Ebbini
2009 American Institute of Physics 978-0-7354-0650-6/09/$25.00

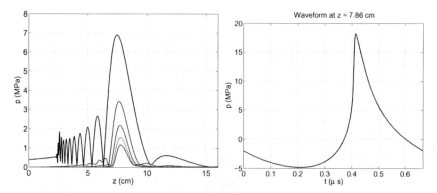

FIGURE 1. Simulation of a 5 cm diameter 8 cm focal length, 1.5 MHz transducer operating at 100 W total acoustic power. The first 5 cm of the propagation path is through water, the remaining 11 cm through generic tissue. Left: axial pressure distribution of the first five harmonics. Right: time-domain waveform at maximum peak positive pressure. In this simulation, a 5 cm diameter transducer with 8 cm focal length

where $\hat{p}_k$ is the complex-valued pressure field of the kth harmonic, z and r are the axial and radial coordinates, c_0 is the small-signal sound speed, $\mathrm{Re}(\alpha_k)$ and $\mathrm{Im}(\alpha_k)$ are the respective absorption and dispersion coefficients, and $\nabla_r^2 = \partial^2/\partial r^2 + r^{-1}\partial/\partial r$ is the axisymmetric transverse Laplacian. The absorption coefficient may vary with frequency according to any power-law relationship and the dispersion coefficent is calculated at runtime using a local approximation of the Kramers-Kronig relations[4]. The boundary condition at the transducer face is a parabolic approximation of a spherically-converging harmonic waveform with a uniform pressure distribution[5]. Equations (1) are discretized in r using second-order finite differences on a uniform grid and integrated using two methods. In the boundary layer at the transducer face, where the solution is highly oscillatory, a second-order, diagonally-implicit Runge Kutta (DIRK) method with stiff decay[6] is used. Traditionally the backward-Euler method and very small integration steps are used to preserve stability in this boundary layer and accuracy beyond it, but the DIRK method used here allows much larger integration steps, provides the required stability, and speeds computation. Once past the boundary layer, the trapezoidal method is used for the remainder of the integration.

For user convenience, the stepsizes Δz and Δr are determined at runtime by estimating the resolution requirements for a corresponding linear beam, but may be modified by the user if more resolution is deemed necessary.

To eliminate artifacts caused by reflection of waves from the unphysical boundaries of the computational domain, a perfectly matched layer[7] absorbing boundary condition is implemented. The perfectly matched layer, located just outside the region of interest, converts propagating waves whose wavenumbers have nonzero r-components into decaying evanescent waves, absorbing them before they corrupt the solution. This technique allows the radial extent of the computational domain to remain small: only 25% greater than the transducer radius, reducing computational overhead.

At each integration step the solution is converted to the time-domain representation using the fast Fourier transform, and the nonlinear part of the KZK equation

$$\frac{\partial p}{\partial z} = \frac{\beta p}{\rho_0 c_0^3} \frac{\partial p}{\partial t},$$

(2)

is solved using the upwind method[8]. Here t is time, β is the coefficient of nonlinearity, and ρ_0 is mass density. At each gridpoint in the computational domain, the amplitude of the solution is determined; if it is negligibly small, the nonlinear step is skipped, reducing computation time. Otherwise, the amplitude is used to determine the number of integration substeps required for the upwind method to remain stable, and the solution is computed. The upwind method is used to integrate a single cycle of the CW beam and periodic boundary conditions are imposed. After integration, the solution is converted back to the frequency-domain representation and the cycle is repeated until the simulation is complete.

One benefit of computing the solution in both time- and frequency-domains is that information is easily accessed from both. In Fig. 1, the left plot shows the axial pressure distribution of the first five harmonics, which is generated from frequency domain data. The right plot shows the time-domain waveform at maximum peak positive pressure.

HIFU_Simulator also has provisions for layered media. If some of the propagation path is through water and the rest through tissue, the code computes the incident beam and the transmitted beam, taking account of the impedence mismatch using the standard formula[9]. The beam reflected from the material interface is not computed.

The spatial distribution of intensity and heating rate are computed at runtime using the plane-wave approximation:

$$I(r,z) = \frac{1}{2\rho_0 c_0} \sum_{k=1}^{K} |\hat{p}_k|, \quad H(r,z) = \frac{1}{\rho_0 c_0} \sum_{k=1}^{K} \text{Re}(\alpha_k)|\hat{p}_k|$$

(3)

Plots of the axial distribution of these quantities are shown in Fig. 2.

HEATING MODULE

To determine the temperature rise T, Pennes' bioheat transfer equation

$$\rho_0 C \frac{\partial T}{\partial t} = \kappa \nabla^2 T + H - wCT$$

(4)

is solved. Here, C is heat capacity, H is heating rate, and w is perfusion rate. A second-order finite difference discretization is used with Dirichlet boundary conditions and the solution is evolved in time using an efficient second-order implicit Runge Kutta method[1]. The appropriate timestep Δt is determined by the code and is based on the user-defined

---

[1] This IRK method is different from the one used for KZK, it trades some stability for efficiency

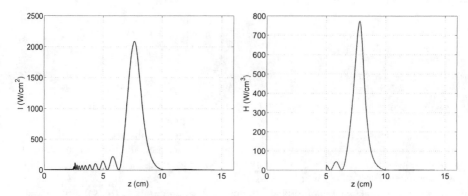

FIGURE 2. Same simulation as Fig. 1. Left: axial intensity distribution. Right: axial heating rate. Note spike in heating rate at $z = 5$ cm due to water/tissue interface.

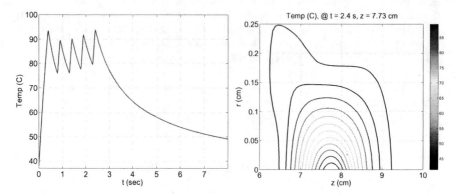

FIGURE 3. Same simulation as Fig. 1. Here the treatment consists of an initial 0.5 s sonication followed by four 0.1 s sonications on a 20% duty factor. Left: peak temperature vs. time. Right: temperature contours at 2.4 s.

sonication protocol. Fig. 3 shows a plot of the peak temperature as a function of time and a contour plot of the thermal field at the instant the peak temperature is achieved.

The thermal dose is computed at runtime using the following formula[10] for cumulative equivalent minutes at 43°C:

$$\text{CEM}_{43}(r,z) = \int_0^{t_f} R^{T(r,z,s)+T_0-43}\,ds, \quad R = \begin{cases} 4 & \text{if } T \le 43°C \\ 2 & \text{if } T > 43°C, \end{cases} \tag{5}$$

where t_f is the duration of the simulation and T_0 is equilibrium temperature (user-defined). A plot of the thermal dose contours for an example HIFU treatment is shown in Fig. 4.

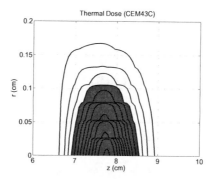

FIGURE 4. Thermal dose contours on a logarithmic scale. The shading indicates the region in which greater than 240 CEM_{43} is acheived. Same treatment as Fig. 3.

CONCLUSION

To close, a few words should be mentioned regarding the limitations of the propagation model used in this package. Since the KZK equation is a parabolic approximation, this constrains the allowable transducer geometry to greater than approximately f/1.4. Also, while the algorithm used is suitable for simulating CW beams, gated pulses containing fewer than approximately 100 acoustical cycles may not be accurately modeled. Finally, this model does not account for cavitation or boiling bubble effects.

ACKNOWLEDGMENTS

The author thanks Matt Myers and Jerry Harris for their support and Subha Maruvada and Diane Nell for testing the α-version of the HIFU_Simulator. This work was partially supported by the Defense Advanced Research Projects Agency through AIG # 224-05-6016.

REFERENCES

1. J. A. Jensen, *J. Acoust. Soc. Am* **89**, 182–191 (1991).
2. Y.-S. Lee and M. F. Hamilton, *J. Acoust. Soc. Am* **97**, 906–917 (1995).
3. J. E. Soneson, in preparation.
4. M. O'Donnell. E. T. Jaynews, and J. G. Miller, *J. Acoust. Soc. Am.* **63**, pp. 696–701 (1981).
5. M. F. Hamilton, "Sound Beams," in *Nonlinear Acoustics*, edited by M. F. Hamilton and D. T. Blackstock, Academic Press, San Diego, 1998, p. 244.
6. U. M. Ascher, and L. R. Petzold, *Computer Methods for Ordinary Differential Equations and Differential-Algebraic Equations*, Society for Industrial and Applied Mathematics, Philidelphia, 1998, p. 106.
7. J. P. Berenger, *J. Comp. Phys.* **114**, 185–200 (1994).
8. R. J. LeVeque, *Numerical Methods for Conservation Laws*, Birkhauser-Verlag, Basel, 1990.
9. L. M. Brekhovskikh, *Waves in Layered Media*, Academic Press, New York, 1960, pp. 15–17.
10. S. A. Sapareto and W. C. Dewey, *Int. J. Radiat. Oncol Biol. Phys.*, **10**, pp. 787–800 (1984).

Optimization of HIFU Treatments for Use in Model Predictive Control

A. Payne[a,b], A. Blankespoor[a], N. Todd[b], U. Vyas[c], D. Christensen[c], D. Parker[b] and R. Roemer[a,b]

[a]University of Utah, Dept of Mechanical Engineering, 50 S. Central Campus Dr., Salt Lake City, UT 84112
[b]Utah Center for Advanced Imaging Research, 729 Arapeen Dr., Salt Lake City, UT 84108
[c]University of Utah, Dept. of Bioengineering, 20 S. 2030 E. Rm. 108, Salt Lake City, UT 84112

Abstract. It is shown that the time needed to deliver a specified thermal dose while satisfying normal tissue safety requirements can be minimized through optimization of the individual HIFU pulse heating and cooling times. Numerical simulations were performed using a finite difference approximation of the 3-D Pennes' bioheat transfer equation. Treatment times decreased with increased maximum power density for all scan paths simulated. The effects of normal tissue temperature constraint location, desired thermal dose and perfusion were found to be significant. The presented simulations demonstrate that HIFU treatment optimization is possible, but on-line adjustments with a model based predictive controller are necessary to minimize the overall treatment time.

Keywords: thermal modeling, optimization, model predictive control, HIFU
PACS: 87.55.de

INTRODUCTION

HIFU treatments are usually performed by ablating individual sub-regions by either mechanical movement of a transducer or by electrically steering a multiple element phased array transducer. A serious problem with ablating sizeable tumors is the thermal buildup in the intervening normal tissue that lies between the tumor and transducer [1]. If enough thermal buildup occurs, the transducer power must be turned off to allow the normal tissue to cool. In practice, several studies have shown that a fixed delay time, or cooling period is needed between pulses to limit near field, normal tissue heating [2-4]. While this is effective in reducing thermal damage in the normal tissue, it creates excessively long treatment times. In response, several studies have been done to try and optimize this difficult 3D thermal problem [5-8].

While all of these studies provide valuable insight, each study applied fixed heating and cooling times, not optimizing each individual pulse within the treatment. In addition, none of the studies rigorously considered the overheating of normal tissue. In this paper, simulations are presented that optimize the heating and cooling times for a multiple sonication HIFU treatment in a homogeneous three dimensional volume. Results are presented for the effects of applied power density, pre-selected scanning paths, perfusion levels and normal tissue constraint locations.

CP1113, 8th International Symposium on Therapeutic Ultrasound, edited by E. S. Ebbini
© 2009 American Institute of Physics 978-0-7354-0650-6/09/$25.00

METHODS

The simulations presented here use a finite difference approximation of the 3D Pennes' BHTE [9],

$$\rho C_t \frac{\partial T}{\partial t} = k\nabla^2 T - WC_b\left(T - T_b\right) + Q_{ap} \qquad (4)$$

Here T is temperature (°C), ρ is the tissue density (kg/m^3), C_t is the specific heat of tissue (J/kg/°C), k is the thermal conductivity of the tissue (W/m/°C), Q_{ap} is the power density deposited by an external applicator (W/m^3), W is the Pennes' perfusion parameter (kg/m^3/s), C_b is the specific heat of blood and T_b is the arterial blood temperature. The geometry of the simulated system is shown in Figure 1.

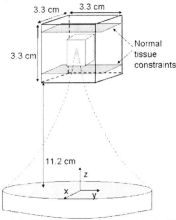

FIGURE 1. Geometric layout of the 3D simulated treatment domain. The origin is located in the center of the transducer's face.

The ultrasound power deposition was modeled from a 256 element phased array transducer using the hybrid angular spectrum method [10], an extension of the traditional angular spectrum method. The transducer operates at a frequency of 1MHz with a radius of curvature of 13cm. A simulated power deposition at the geometric focus is seen in Figure 2.

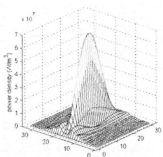

FIGURE 2: Theoretical prediction of the power deposition (100W electrical) of a 256 element phased array. Shown is the central plane at the geometric focus. 1x1x1mm spatial resolution.

A 1.5cm^3 tumor sub-region was treated with 45 sonications. Three paths were tested, a back to front raster, a top to bottom raster, and an alternating path. The goal of the treatment optimization was to find the optimal heating and cooling times at every pulse for a given perfusion rate and applied power density to minimize the overall treatment time. The optimization was accomplished with an iterative procedure with the following constraints; the entire thermal dose (240 CEM43°C) must be delivered in a single pulse, and all normal tissue temperature constraints must remain below the defined normal tissue temperature limit (43°C).

RESULTS

The optimal treatment time for increasing applied power density for the three pre-determined paths is shown in Figure 3. As has been seen in previous results [11], the treatment time decreases with increasing applied power for all paths. However, there is a point of diminishing returns, where there is minimal decrease in treatment time for an increase of power. There is also a strong path dependence, with the alternating path having an approximately 40% reduced treatment time over both raster paths.

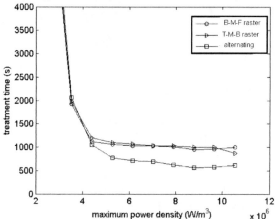

FIGURE 3: Optimized treatment time for three pre-determined paths as a function of maximum power density. The simulated volume had a homogeneous perfusion value of 0.5 kg/m^3/s.

The same simulations are shown in Figure 4, with individual heating and cooling times presented. For all paths, the heating time decreases with increased applied power and the cooling time subsequently increases. However, the alternating path requires less interpulse cooling than the two raster paths, resulting in the shorter total treatment time, as shown in Figure 3. The alternating path increases the distance between pulses, reducing the amount of thermal buildup in the ultrasound near field, requiring less interpulse cooling time.

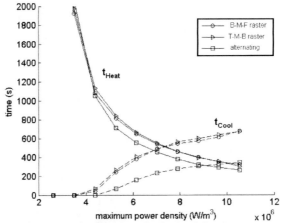

FIGURE 4: Optimized heating and cooling times for the simulation parameters seen in Figure 3.

The effect of normal tissue temperature constraint value ($T_{NTlimit}$) and thermal dose target are seen in Figures 5 and 6, respectively. As expected, a higher $T_{NTlimit}$ significantly reduces total treatment time. In the same regard, lower thermal dose levels require significantly shorter treatment times. These results point to the need for more comprehensive studies to determine the true isoeffect value of thermal dose *in vivo*, for a range of tissue types [12].

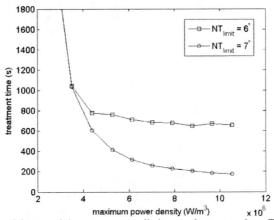

FIGURE 5: Effect of the normal tissue temperature limit on total treatment time. The legend indicates temperature rise above ambient.

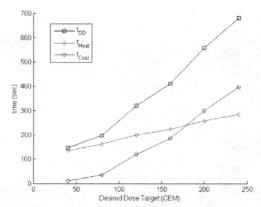

FIGURE 6: Effect of thermal dose target on treatmet time. Results were simulated using the alternating scan path, a homogeneous perfusion value of 0.5 kg/m^3/s and maximum applied power density of 0.88x10^7 W/m^3.

CONCLUSIONS

The results presented show that a multiple pulse HIFU treatment time can be minimized through the optimization of the heating and cooling times of each sonication pulse. Factors which influence treatment time are the power deposition pattern, predetermined scanning path, normal tissue constraint location and desired thermal dose value. In order to implement this optimization scheme experimentally, the use of a model based predictive feedback controller is required.

ACKNOWLEDGMENTS

We gratefully acknowledge the support of NIH-1-R01-CA87785, Siemens Medical Solutions, the Focused Ultrasound Foundation, the University of Utah and the Ben B. and Iris M. Margolis Foundation.

REFERENCES

1. N. McDannold et al., *J Magn Reson Imaging*: **8**, 91-100 (1998).
2. N. McDannold et al., *Radiology*: **211**, 419-426 (1999).
3. C. Damianou and K. Hynynen, *Ultrasound Med Biol*: **19**, 777-787 (1993).
4. X. Fan and K. Hynynen, *Ultrasound Med Biol*: **22**, 471-482 (1996).
5. M. Malinen et al., *Phys Med Biol*: **50**, 34373-90 (2005).
6. W. Lin et al., *Med Phys*: **28**, 2172-2181 (2001).
7. B. Billard et al., *Ultrasound Med Biol*, **16**, 409-420 (1990).
8. H. Wan et al., *IEEE Trans. On Ultrason*: **43**, 1085-1097 (1996).
9. H. Pennes, *Appl Physiol*: **1**, 93-122 (1948).
10. U. Vyas and D. Christensen, "Hybrid angular spectrum method for ultrasound beam propagation" in *International Society for Therapeutic Ultrasound* 2008.
11. A. Payne, *Phys Med Biol*, submitted.
12. M. Dewhirst, *Int J Hyperthermia*: **19**, 267-294 (2003).

Impact of Real Liver Motion on HIFU Treatments: an in-vivo-data-based modeling

N'Djin WA[a], Miller NR[b], Bamber JC[b], Chapelon JY[a], Melodelima D[a]

[a]Inserm, U556, Lyon, F-69003, France ; Université de Lyon, Lyon, F-69003, France.
[b]Royal Marsden NHS trust and Institute of Cancer Research, Sutton, United Kingdom.
Apoutou.ndjin@.inserm.fr

Abstract. Organs motion is a key component in the treatment of abdominal lesions by HIFU, since it may influence the efficacy and treatment time. Previous studies on HIFU treatments showed the effect of motor-controlled translations applied to in vitro liver samples. In vivo organs motions are more complex and could lead to various effects on HIFU treatments. Here we report that a combined method can be used for simulating the effect of real in vivo motion on HIFU lesion in the liver. Sequences of ultrasound images were acquired in vivo during an open procedure on 4 pigs during breathing and apnea using a 12 MHz ultrasound imaging probe. Ultrasound correlation-based methods were used to estimate liver motion using speckle tracking. These in vivo motion data were included in numerical simulations based on Bio Heat Transfer Equation for evaluating the influence of motion on treatments performed with a 3 MHz spherical HIFU transducer. Data acquired during breathing confirmed that liver motions were mainly encountered in the cranial-caudal direction (f=0.2 Hz, magnitude: 13.3 ± 1.1 mm). Liver motions due only to cardiovascular activity were negligible (f=0.96 Hz, magnitude < 0.5 mm). When considering in vivo liver motion, simulated HIFU lesions were significantly modified (size, homogeneity) between control (no motion) and breathing samples. These results allow the estimation of the influence of effective liver motion on HIFU treatments. Additionally this combined method may be used to simulate the effectiveness of solutions suggested for correcting tissue motion during HIFU therapy.

Keywords: Liver; Motion; tracking; Modeling; HIFU; ultrasound

PACS: 01.30.Cc

INTRODUCTION

Significant difficulties generated by organ motions due to the respiratory activity have already been highlighted during clinical studies about HIFU treatments of liver cancers. Breathing during the HIFU procedure may reduces the accuracy of the treatment. When apnea is performed during a HIFU session to eliminate major organ movements, the treatment time may be significantly increased. Previous *in vitro* studies have observed the effect of artificial tissues motions on HIFU standard treatments. However, *in vivo* motions are expected to be more complex and could lead to various effects on HIFU treatments. This study aims to quantify the effect of *in vivo* pig liver motion on the size, shape, homogeneity and location of the ablated region generated during a typical HIFU treatment described in [1].

CP1113, *8th International Symposium on Therapeutic Ultrasound*, edited by E. S. Ebbini
© 2009 American Institute of Physics 978-0-7354-0650-6/09/$25.00

METHODS

Ultrasound images

Animal experiments were performed under an approved research protocol. These experiments conformed to the requirements of the local office of animal experimentation and were in accordance with the legal conditions of the French National Commission on Animal Experimentation. Acquisitions of ultrasound images of pig livers were performed during experiments which involved HIFU exposures during an open procedure [2]. Pigs were anaesthetized and mechanically ventilated. Sequences of ultrasound images of the liver were acquired *in vivo* on 4 healthy pigs with an average weight of 26.7 ± 2.2 kg (range 22.0 -31.2 kg). Freehand acquisitions were performed during periods of breathing and apnea by placing the ultrasound imaging probe into acoustic contact with the superior face of the liver. The ultrasound scanner was a BK® HAWK 2102 EXL, with a 2D linear imaging probe working at a frequency of 12 MHz. The image depth was 45 mm, the ultrasound scanner frame rate was 54 fps and the size of frames was 720×576 pixels.

Quantification of the nature of in vivo liver movements

Ultrasound images were acquired in two orthogonal planes along cranial-caudal and transverse directions. Additionally, acquisitions were performed in the left lateral (LL), left central (LC) and right central (RC) lobes of each pig in order to determine if liver motion magnitudes depended of the position in the liver. The right lateral (RL) lobe was not observed since it was less accessible in the abdomen and did not allow acquiring the two orthogonal planes with the ultrasound imaging probe. In order to determine the relative influence of respiration and cardiovascular activity on liver motions, ultrasound images were acquired in regions containing hepatic veins. First, acquisitions were done during breathing to access the liver movement due to respiration. Second, acquisitions were performed during an apnea to separate the liver movement only due to cardiovascular activity. Special attention was paid to liver tissues on the surrounding of hepatic veins which dilated with blood pressure pulses. Then, an ultrasound correlation-based method was used to estimate liver motion using speckle tracking. 2D motion tracking algorithm was previously described in [3].

Modeling of in vivo liver motions effects on HIFU treatments

Data of liver displacements measured by the 2D motion tracking method were integrated in a 3D numerical modeling of the equivalent time at 43°C ($t_{43°C}$) based on the resolution of the Bio Heat Transfer Equation described in [4]. Simulations were carried out for a truncated spherical transducer (3 MHz, f = 45 mm) described in [1] with a hole at its center for taking into account the presence of an integrated ultrasound imaging probe. The effects of liver motions were studied for a single HIFU lesion (exposure conditions: 5s On / 5s Off) and for a HIFU treatment of 490 seconds (juxtaposition of 49 single HIFU lesions as described in [1]). Simulations were conducted by considering (i) no motion (control), (ii) *in vivo* motion during apnea and (iii) *in vivo* motion during breathing.

RESULTS

Evaluation of in vivo liver movements
(data acquisitions and motion tracking)

Liver motions (with cardiovascular and respiratory activity) are mainly encountered in the cranial-caudal plane. When using ultrasound images recorded during period of breathing, motion tracking method allowed access to the respiratory frequency ($f_{respiratory}$= 0,20 Hz) which is similar to the respiratory frequency imposed by the mechanical respirator ($f_{respirator}$= 0,20 Hz). Considering cranial-caudal planes, magnitude of the liver motion was relatively homogeneous for each pig and in each lobe. The average relative amplitude of liver movements was 13.3 ± 1.1 mm (range 9.0 – 15.5). After speckle tracking of ultrasound images sequences, the mean correlation coefficient between each ultrasound image was calculated for each sequence. For the overall images sequences studied, the average value of correlation coefficients were respectively for cranial-caudal and transverse directions, 0.79 ± 0.01 (range 0.75 – 0.81) and 0.67 ± 0.04 (range 0.58 – 0.79). When using images recorded during periods of apnea, motion tracking method allowed access to the heart beat frequency ($f_{heart\ beat}$= 0.96 Hz) which is similar to the heart beat frequency monitored with ECG (monitoring: 56 beats/minutes, 0.93 Hz). Magnitude of liver motion due to heart beat was considered as negligible (<0.3 mm) compared with liver motion due to breathing.

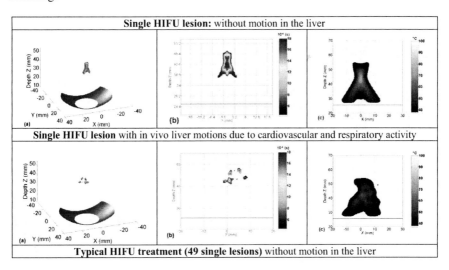

Single HIFU lesion: without motion in the liver

Single HIFU lesion with in vivo liver motions due to cardiovascular and respiratory activity

Typical HIFU treatment (49 single lesions) without motion in the liver

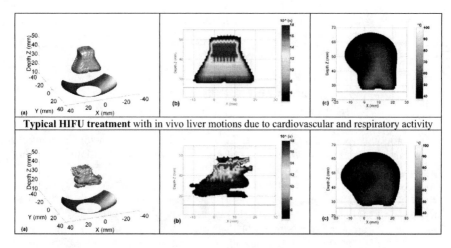

FIGURE 1. In vivo liver motion effects on HIFU treatments

Modeling of in vivo liver motions effects on HIFU treatments

All results show the temperature and the lesion just after the last HIFU exposure (Fig.1): (a) $t_{43°C}$ displayed in 3D with a minimal threshold fixed to 14400 seconds + surface of the HIFU transducer, (b) $t_{43°C}$ displayed in 2D with a minimal threshold fixed to 14400 seconds in the cranial-caudal direction and (c) temperature in the cranial-caudal direction displayed with a minimal threshold fixed to 37°C. The coagulated volume changes significantly when liver motions due to breathing were considered (Tab.1).

TABLE 1. Summary of HIFU Simulated Lesions

	Single lesion		Typical HIFU treatment (49 juxtaposed lesions)	
Motion considered in modeling	No motion	Cardiovascular + respiratory	No motion	Cardiovascular + respiratory
Lesion volume (cm^3)	0.17	0.02 (↘ 88%)	7.91	4.78 (↘ 40%)
Average $t_{43°C}$ in the cranial caudal median plane (10^{15} seconds)	89	6.8	133	7.6
Temperature after HIFU treatment (°C)	70	50 (↘ 29%)	85	55 (↘ 88%)
Homogeneity	Standard	Splitting	Standard	Distortion

DISCUSSION

The presented combined method based on both in vivo and simulated data allows evaluation and quantification of effective *in vivo* liver movements. Acquisitions performed during an open procedure make possible the use of high definition ultrasound imaging probes. Therefore, spatial definition and image acquisition rate are suitable for measuring the heart beat frequency. An open procedure also allows a facilitate access to many parts of the liver and images can be acquired without artifacts due to the rib cage or adjacent organs. The effects of *in vivo* liver motion on HIFU lesions have been highlighted. Significant changes were observed on the homogeneity, size and shape of HIFU lesions when real motion of the liver was taken into account in the simulation. These changes are significant and mainly due to breathing. Some regions of the HIFU lesions are established with the minimal $t_{43°C}$ required for irreversible necroses. By considering liver motion (with breathing), these regions should be considered to have the most important uncertainty, as they are highly dependent on the input parameters and could easily be below the minimal threshold for necrosis. Regarding the different solution for compensating liver motion, a tracking of the motion in real time seems to remain today the more efficient method [5]. However, this technology requires a lot of development and may also require complex and expensive equipment. Gating was another option and several simulations are in progress. But to date, no conclusive results emerge from simulations since HIFU treatments involved when using gating take too much time comparing with standard treatments and do not allow the creation of acceptable and homogeneous lesions. Several other configurations of gating have to be tested. Changing the spatial and temporal step between consecutive single HIFU exposures may also compensate the changes observed in the resulting lesion. It would consist on constant changes to the whole array or different changes for different exposures according to the deformation of the lesion. Then, a new energy distribution fitted to motion effects predictions should be applied in liver tissues to compensate and cover regions previously untreated.

ACKNOWLEDGEMENTS

The authors wish to thank the staff of the laboratory for experimental surgery for their aid in the animal study. This work was supported by funding from the Cancéropôle Lyon Auvergne Rhône Alpes (PDC 2006.4.8) and from the French Agency for Research on Cancer (ARC 4023).

REFERENCES

1. Gignoux B.M.H., Scoasec J.Y., Curiel L., Beziat C., Chapelon J.Y., "HIFU destruction of hepatic parenchyma", Ann. Chir. 2003; 128: 18-25
2. Melodelima D., N'Djin W.A., Parmentier H., Chesnais S., Rivoire M., Chapelon J.Y, "Ultrasound surgery with a toric transducer allows the treatment of large volumes over short periods of time", Applied Physics Letters, 2007, in press
3. Hsu A., Miller N.R., Evans P.M., Bamber J.C., Webb S., "Feasibility of using ultrasound for real-time tracking during radiotherapy", Med. Phys. 2005; 32(6): 1500-1512
4. Chavrier F., Chapelon J.Y., GeletA., Cathignol D., "Modeling of high-intensity focused ultrasound-induced lesions in the presence of cavitation bubbles", J. Acoust. Soc. Am. 2000; 108:432-440
5. Pernot M., Tanter M., Fink M., "3-D real-time motion correction in high-intensity focused ultrasound therapy", Ultrasound Med. Biol. 2004; 30(9): 1239-1249

Theoretical Analysis of the Accuracy and Safety of MRI-Guided Transurethral 3-D Conformal Ultrasound Prostate Therapy

Mathieu Burtnyk, Rajiv Chopra and Michael Bronskill

Sunnybrook Health Sciences Centre, 2075 Bayview Ave, Toronto ON, M4N 3M5, Canada
and Department of Medical Biophysics, University of Toronto, Canada

Abstract. MRI-guided transurethral ultrasound therapy is a promising new approach for the treatment of localized prostate cancer. Several studies have demonstrated the feasibility of producing large regions of thermal coagulation adequate for prostate therapy; however, the quantitative assessment of shaping these regions to complex 3-D human prostate geometries has not been fully explored. This study used numerical simulations and twenty manually-segmented pelvic anatomical models derived from high-quality MR images of prostate cancer patients to evaluate the treatment accuracy and safety of 3-D conformal MRI-guided transurethral ultrasound therapy. The simulations incorporated a rotating multi-element planar dual-frequency ultrasound transducer (seventeen 4x3 mm elements) operating at 4.7/9.7 MHz and 10 W/cm^2 maximum acoustic power. Results using a novel feedback control algorithm which modulated the ultrasound frequency, power and device rate of rotation showed that regions of thermal coagulation could be shaped to predefined prostate volumes within 1.0 mm across the vast majority of these glands. Treatment times were typically 30 min and remained below 60 min for large 60 cc prostates. With a rectal cooling temperature of 15°C, the rectal wall did not exceed 30EM43 in half of the twenty patient models with only a few 1 mm^3 voxels above this threshold in the other cases. At 4.7 MHz, heating of the pelvic bone can become significant when it is located less than 10 mm from the prostate. Numerical simulations show that MRI-guided transurethral ultrasound therapy can thermally coagulate whole prostate glands accurately and safely in 3-D.

Keywords: MRI-guided, 3-D, control, transurethral, thermal therapy, thermometry.
PACS: 87.50.yt, 87.55.Gh, 87.55.N, 87.57.nm, 87.61.-c.

INTRODUCTION

Although prostate cancer is currently the most common cancer in men, incidence rates continue to rise and the disease is migrating towards a younger, low-risk population [1]. While conventional therapies for prostate cancer offer good local disease control, they are associated with high rates of urinary, bowel and sexual complications, often reducing the quality of life of patients significantly [2].

MRI-guided transurethral ultrasound therapy is gaining interest as a minimally-invasive treatment option for men with localized prostate cancer [3, 4]. A device inserted in the urethra gains direct access to the prostate such that the delivered energy does not have to pass through sensitive anatomical structures. An array of multiple

CP1113, 8th International Symposium on Therapeutic Ultrasound, edited by E. S. Ebbini
© 2009 American Institute of Physics 978-0-7354-0650-6/09/$25.00

transducers emits directional (unfocused) ultrasound beams capable of heating prostate tissue to thermal coagulation. Control of the ultrasound parameters and the device rate of rotation can confine the thermal coagulation pattern to the prostate gland and reduce damage to important surrounding anatomy. In order to shape the region of thermal coagulation to conform to the target prostate volume, accurate temporal and spatial temperature measurements are essential for feedback control. Magnetic resonance imaging (MRI) technology can provide such information non-invasively during treatment.

Several studies have demonstrated the feasibility of producing large regions of thermal coagulation adequate for prostate therapy; however, the quantitative assessment of shaping these regions to complex 3-D human prostate geometries, as well as the consequential thermal impact on the surrounding anatomy, have not been fully explored. This study used numerical simulations and twenty pelvic anatomical models to evaluate the treatment accuracy and safety of 3-D conformal MRI-guided transurethral ultrasound therapy.

METHODS

Three-dimensional anatomical models of prostate cancer patients were developed to provide a realistic geometrical framework for the theoretical analysis of treatment accuracy and safety. Twenty patient models were created by manually segmenting the prostate, urethra, rectum and pelvic bone on high resolution MR images of prostate cancer patients. Segmented prostate volumes ranged from 14 to 60 cc.

Computer simulations were used to model transurethral ultrasound prostate therapy with a rotating linear array of dual-frequency planar rectangular transducers and feedback temperature measurements. An array of seventeen 4x3 mm transducer elements was modeled to span the length of the prostates in the set of patient models and to provide high treatment resolution along the applicator. An approximation to the Rayleigh-Sommerfeld integral was used to calculate high spatial resolution ultrasound fields (0.25 mm isotropic) generated by these small virtual transducer elements. The frequencies were set to 4.7 and 9.7 MHz to provide the range of depth of heating required to treat the segmented prostate volumes [5]. An explicit finite-difference solution to the Bioheat Transfer Equation (BHTE) was used to model tissue temperature dynamics considering heat conduction, blood perfusion and ultrasound energy deposition at a temporal and spatial resolution of 1 s and 1 mm^3 respectively. The simulated tissue volumes were soft tissue, cortical bone and bone marrow.

A feedback control algorithm adjusted the treatment delivery by modulating the transducer rotation rate and the ultrasound power and frequency of each transducer element based on multiple temperature measurements at the prostate boundary. The goal of the feedback control algorithm was to shape the region of thermal coagulation in 3-D to the MRI-segmented prostate geometry, by raising the temperature along the entire surface of the prostate to 52°C, representative of thermal coagulation. The control parameters were updated after each temperature measurement (1 s) and determined according to the following equations:

$$\omega = \min_{i=1..n}\{\omega_i\},$$

$$\omega_i = \begin{cases} \omega_{min} \leq \dfrac{k_\omega(r_i)}{\Delta Tr_i} \leq \omega_{max}(r_i), & \Delta Tr_i > 0 \\ \omega_{max}(r_i), & \Delta Tr_i \leq 0 \end{cases}$$

$$p_i = \begin{cases} p_{min} + k_p(r_i)\cdot \Delta Tr_i \leq p_{max}, & \Delta Tr_i > 0 \\ 0, & \Delta Tr_i \leq 0 \end{cases}$$

$$f_i = \begin{cases} f_{high}, & r_i < 13.5\,mm \\ f_{low}, & r_i \geq 13.5\,mm \end{cases}$$

where ω is the device rate of rotation ($^\circ$ min^{-1}), $k_\omega(r_i)$ is the rotational gain constant, r_i is the distance from the transducer to the prostate (mm), p_i is the individual element acoustic power (W_a), p_{max} is the maximum power (10 W_a/cm^2), $k_p(r_i)$ is the power gain constant, f_i is the ultrasound frequency (MHz), f_{high} and f_{low} are the high and low ultrasound frequencies of the dual-frequency elements.

RESULTS AND DISCUSSION

Treatment accuracy was quantified using the treatment difference distance, which was defined as the radial distance between the boundary of thermal coagulation (52°C isosurface) and the target prostate boundary. For all twenty patient models, the mean and standard deviation of the treatment difference remained less than 0.3 and 1.0 mm, respectively. For comparison, the total volume of the treatment difference was less than 50% of the volume of a constant 1 mm overt-treatment margin. Typical results are shown in Figure 1 where the treatment difference is plotted over the surface of three representative target prostate geometries. Similar results with high treatment accuracy were achieved for all 20 patient models.

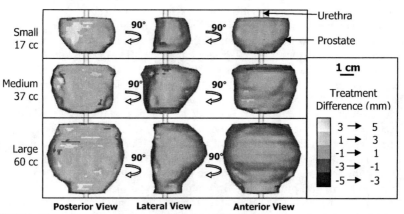

FIGURE 1. Three views of typical treatment results of MRI-guided transurethral ultrasound therapy for small 17 cc, medium 37 cc and large 60 cc prostates. The region of thermal coagulation was within 1 mm of the prostate over most of these volumes.

Figure 2 shows the treatment time for transurethral ultrasound prostate therapy which, as expected, increased with prostate volume. Treatment times are typically about 30 min, ranging up to 60 min for large 60 cc prostates. Also shown in Figure 2 are the mean values reported in selected literature on clinical transrectal HIFU.

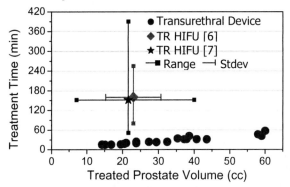

FIGURE 2. Treatment times for transurethral ultrasound therapy increase with prostate volume. The mean and range for treatment times reported for transrectal (TR) HIFU are shown for comparison.

Heating of the rectum is of particular concern because it is in very close proximity to the posterior portion of the prostate, where the majority of cancers are found [8]. Consequential heating of the rectal wall was evaluated by calculating the volume of rectal tissue that accumulated a thermal dose greater than 30 EM43, a very conservative threshold for potential damage [9]. The mean and range of this value are plotted versus the temperature of the water flowing through the rectal cooling device in Figure 3a. As the rectal cooling temperature decreases, so does the volume of potentially damaged rectal tissue. With a rectal cooling temperature of 15°C, the rectal wall did not exceed 30EM43 in half of the twenty patient models with only a few 1 mm³ voxels above this threshold in the other cases.

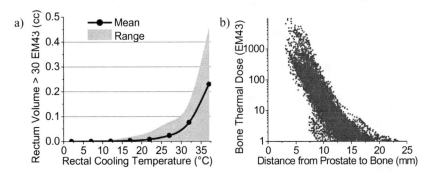

FIGURE 3. Evaluating the consequential heating to: a) the rectal wall and b) the pelvic bone, during transurethral ultrasound prostate therapy. a) Significant heating of the rectum can be avoided using a rectal cooling device. b) Heating of the pelvic bone can become significant when it is located less than 10 mm from the prostate (at 4.7 MHz).

The pelvic bone is not located as close to the prostate as the rectum, but its high ultrasound absorption makes it susceptible to thermal damage during transurethral ultrasound therapy. Heating of the pelvic bone was evaluated by calculating the thermal dose in each voxel of cortical bone which was directly facing the prostate. Figure 3b shows that the thermal dose increased rapidly as the separation distance between the prostate and the bone decreased. The simulations indicated that, at 4.7 MHz, heating of the pelvic bone can become significant when it is located less than 10 mm from the prostate. Treatment strategies are being investigated, for example using a higher frequency, to reduce the amount of pelvic bone heating at those locations.

CONCLUSIONS

Numerical simulations show that MRI-guided transurethral ultrasound therapy devices using a rotating planar array of dual-frequency transducers can create volumes of thermal coagulation that conform accurately in 3-D to complex but realistic prostate geometries of differing shapes and sizes.

The amount of consequential heating to the rectum and pelvic bone is highly dependent on a patient's specific anatomical geometry (seen in the range of the data in Figure 3). As transurethral ultrasound therapy moves to the clinic, patient-specific modeling and pre-treatment planning will help determine the parameters and energy delivery strategies that optimize the risk/benefit ratio on an individual patient basis.

ACKNOWLEDGMENTS

Support for this study was provided by the Terry Fox Foundation, the Ontario Research and Development Challenge Fund, the Ontario Institute of Cancer Research and the Canadian Institutes of Health Research.

REFERENCES

1. M. Cooperberg, D. Lubeck, M. Meng, S. Mehta and P. Carroll. (2004) *"The changing face of low-risk prostate cancer: trends in clinical presentation and primary management."* J Clin Oncol, 22: 2141-2149.
2. A. Potosky, *et al.* (2004) *"Five-year outcomes after prostatectomy or radiotherapy for prostate cancer: the prostate cancer outcomes study."* J Natl Cancer Inst, 96: 1358-1367.
3. R. Chopra, N. Baker, V. Choy, A. Boyes, K. Tang, D. Bradwell, and M. Bronskill. (2008) *"MRI-compatible transurethral ultrasound system for the treatment of localized prostate cancer using rotational control."* Med Phys, 35 (4): 1346-1357.
4. A. Kinsey, C. Diederich, V. Rieke, W. Nau, K. Pauly, D. Bouley and G. Sommer. (2008) *"Transurethral ultrasound applicators with dynamic multi-sector control for prostate thermal therapy: in vivo evaluation under MR guidance."* Med Phys, 35(5): 2081-93.
5. R. Chopra, C. Luginbuhl, F. Foster and M. Bronskill (2003) *"Multifrequency ultrasound transducers for conformal interstitial thermal therapy."* IEEE Trans Ultrason Ferroelectr Freq Control, 50: 881-889.
6. A. Blana, B. Walter, S. Rogenhofer and W. Wieland. (2004) *"HIFU for the treatment of localized prostate cancer: 5-year experience."* Urology, 63: 297-300.
7. T. Uchida, H. Ohkusa, H. Yamashita, S. Shoji, Y. Nagata, Y. Hyodo and T. Satoh. (2006) *"Five years of transrectal HIFU using the Sonablate device in the treatment of prostate cancer."* Int J Urol, 13: 228-233.
8. D. Grignon and W. Sakr. (1994) *"Zonal origin of prostatic adenocarcinoma: are there biologic differences between transition zone and peripheral zone adenocarcinomas?"* J Cell Biochem Suppl 19: 267-269.
9. M. Dewhirst, B. Viglianti, M. Lora-Michiels, M. Hanson and P. Hoopes. (2003) *"Basic principles of thermal dosimetry and thermal thresholds for tissue damage from hyperthermia."* Int J Hyperthermia; 19: 267-294.

Numerical Simulation of Shock Wave Propagation in Fractured Cortical Bone

Frédéric Padilla[a,b] and Robin Cleveland[a]

[a]Dpt of Mech Eng, Boston Univ., 110 Cummington St., Boston, MA 02115.
[b]CNRS UMR 7623 & University Paris 6, 15 rue de l'Ecole de Médecine, 75006 Paris, France.

Abstract. Shock waves (SW) are considered a promising method to treat bone non unions, but the associated mechanisms of action are not well understood. In this study, numerical simulations are used to quantify the stresses induced by SWs in cortical bone tissue. We use a 3D FDTD code to solve the linear lossless equations that describe wave propagation in solids and fluids. A 3D model of a fractured rat femur was obtained from micro-CT data with a resolution of 32 μm. The bone was subject to a plane SW pulse with a peak positive pressure of 40 MPa and peak negative pressure of -8 MPa. During the simulations the principal tensile stress and maximum shear stress were tracked throughout the bone. It was found that the simulated stresses in a transverse plane relative to the bone axis may reach values higher than the tensile and shear strength of the bone tissue (around 50 MPa). These results suggest that the stresses induced by the SW may be large enough to initiate local micro-fractures, which may in turn trigger the start of bone healing for the case of a non union.

Keywords: Shock waves, Bone Healing, Numerical Simulation.
PACS: 87.50.Y, 43.80.Gx, 43.80.Sh

INTRODUCTION

In vitro and *in vivo* studies published over the last two decades have provided considerable evidence that shock wave therapy (SWT) can treat non-unions and pseudarthrosis. SWT is a noninvasive procedure with low complication rates. For non-unions and pseudarthrosis indications, SWT would spare patients from surgery, mainly fixation with autogenous bone grafting, and from the associated with donor site morbidity.

The mechanisms of action of the shock wave (SW) are poorly understood, which in turn makes it difficult to assess an appropriate treatment strategy for patients. An early rationale for the use of SWs to treat nonunion was the potential of SWs to create microdamage in the cortical bone tissues [1] paralleling their ability to fragment kidney stones in lithotripsy. The creation of micro-fissures and bony fragments was reported when SWs were incident on sites of delayed and nonunion fractures [1]. Microdamage in intact cortical bone have also been observed at the interface between bone and cement during attempts to reduce the interfacial strength of the bone and bone cement with SWs for arthroplasty applications [2, 3]. Another piece of indirect evidence of SW induced microdamage is a report that SWs can cause enough damage to cortical bone in vitro to result in complete fracture of the cortex [4]. It is likely that this gross damage observed was preceded by micro-fractures which could not be

CP1113, *8th International Symposium on Therapeutic Ultrasound*, edited by E. S. Ebbini
© 2009 American Institute of Physics 978-0-7354-0650-6/09/$25.00

observed by the radiographic examination technique used by the authors. The assumption that SW-induced microdamage might play a role in the SW treatment of healing bone is supported by experimental evidence that favors the hypothesis that microdamage evokes local remodeling [5].

The objective of the present study is to assess the potential of SWs to induce stresses in bone tissues large enough to induce micro-damage. We propose to simulate SWs propagation through fractured rat bones to estimate the induced stresses, and to compare these last ones with bone tissue strength.

MATERIAL AND METHODS

Computational scheme

For the numerical simulation of shock waves propagation, the bone tissue was assumed to be a homogeneous, isotropic, elastic medium characterized by the mass density ρ, the lame coefficients λ and μ. The underlying elasto-dynamics equations are:

$$\frac{\partial v_i}{\partial t} = \frac{1}{\rho} \frac{\partial \tau_{ij}}{\partial x_j} \tag{1}$$

$$\frac{\partial \tau_{ij}}{\partial t} = \lambda \delta_{ij} \frac{\partial v_k}{\partial x_k} + \mu \left(\frac{\partial v_i}{\partial x_j} + \frac{\partial v_j}{\partial x_i} \right) \tag{2}$$

which can be interpreted as Newton's second law and Hooke's law respectively. In Eqs. (1) and (2), v_i represents the particle velocity, τ_{ij} the stress tensor, and δ_{ij} the Kronecker delta function. The equations are written in tensor notation employing Einstein's convention for implicit summation with subscripts varying from 1 to 3. These equations can be solved by finite difference and here we use a numerical program (Simsonic) which employs Virieux scheme developed in geophysics community to accurately model propagation in inhomogeneous media with a mix of both fluids and solids [6]. Note that in this code, absorption both in fluids and solids is neglected.

For the simulations, the incident wave was plane, propagating perpendicular to the longitudinal axis of the bone. Given the typical dimensions of a rat femur (around 3/4 mm in diameter) and given the typical beamwidth of the emitted sock wave at the focus (typically 8 mm), this assumption is justified.

Input Data

Three input data are required for the computations.

The first one is the geometry of the specimens. We used micro computed-tomography 3D reconstructions of rat bones to model the 3D structure of the fracture gap. The 3D μCT dataset was thresholded and binarized to simulate homogeneous tissue with an isotropic voxel size of 32 μm.

The second required input data is the mechanical properties for bone tissue and fluid. The computations were performed assuming that the bone specimen was placed in water. The mechanical constants used were, for water: $\rho = 1$ g/cm^3, $V_c = 1500$ m/s; and for bone: $\rho = 1.85$ g/cm^3, $V_c = 4000$ m/s and $V_s = 1800$ m/s; where ρ is the density, V_c and V_s the compressionnal and shear waves velocities.

The third input data is the incident signal. We used a signal with characteristics identical to the ones measured with our experimental system : peak positive pressure of 40MPa, peak negative pressure of -8 MPa, rise time 190 ns.

Output Data

From a material failure point of view, the principal stresses and strains and maximum shear stress and strain are important indicators of fracture. In these 3D simulations, there are 3 principal stresses σ_1, σ_2, and σ_3 that can be obtained from stress analysis. The principal tensile stress is defined as $\sigma_T = \max(\sigma_1, \sigma_2, \sigma_3)$, the principal compressive stress $\sigma_C = -\min(\sigma_1, \sigma_2, \sigma_3)$, and the maximum shear stress $\tau_{max} = (\sigma_T - \sigma_C)/2$.

The mechanical bone tissue properties are anisotropic. Cortical bone is weak both in tension and shear. The shear strength is almost isotropic and around 50 MPa, while the tensile strength exhibit highly anisotropic behaviour with lower value in transverse plane of 50 MPa [7].

We therefore computed from the 3D simulations the principal shear stress and the principal tensile stress in the transverse plane.

We also computed the divergence and the curl modulus of the particle velocity, to be able to follow the propagation of compressionnal and shear waves in water and in the bone tissue.

RESULTS AND DISCUSSION

The figure 1 displays the propagation of a shock wave. These are 2D snapshots from a 3D simulations. At t= 1.98µs, the wave just reached the bone. It can be seen from t=2.31 µs, that part of the wave transmitted in the bone as a longitudinal wave is accelerated compared to the wave propagating in water. Part of the wave will be transmitted through the bone segment, part of it will be guided by the cortex. It is observed that propagation of the guided longitudinal waves is associated with the generation and propagation of shear waves (see the curl modulus frames).

divergence

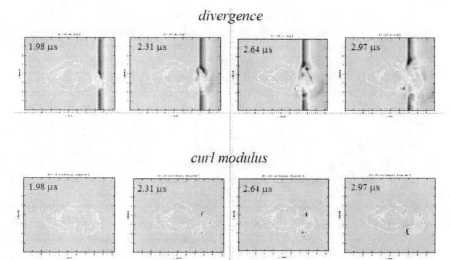

FIGURE 1. Divergence (top) and curl modulus (bottom) of the particle velocity. The amplitude are displayed using a pseudo-color scale in arbitrary units. The time indicated in the top-left corner of each frame indicate the time elapsed since the beginning of emission by the source. The contour of the bone section is depicted in white. The field of view is _8*10 mm^2.

Figure 2 depict propagation in the second part of the bone section. We present here divergence and curl modulus of the particle velocity, but also the principal tensile stress in a the transverse plane and the principal shear stress. It is observed at t = 4.95 and 5.28 µs, that maximum of the stresses will take place in the second part of the bone section (upper left part). It might be that the first part of the bone, as seen on figure 1, act as a screen to prevent the shock wave to properly couple with the bone located just behind the fracture gap. The apparition of the high stresses are associated with the propagation of both compressionnal and shear waves, which seem to be guided by the cortex.

In these simulations, typically 6% of the total bone volume experienced a tensile stress above the tensile strength of 50 MPa, and 1% a shear stress above 50 MPa.

To test the influence of the shear waves propagation in the generation of these high stresses, we preformed the same simulations, but changing the material constants in order to prevent propagation of shear waves in the solid, leaving compressionnal wave velocity unchanged. The result was that the threshold of 50 MPa was never reached for both tensile stress in the bone tissue. This suggests that the high values of stresses produced result from an interaction between compressionnal and shear waves in the bone.

The results presented in Fig 2 suggest that SW can create stresses which are above the strength of the material, both in tension and in shear, with more regions of the bone experiencing high tensile stress. These results therefore suggest that SW-induced stresses might be able to provoke locally micro-fractures.

This study has limitations, because the fatigue behaviour of bone tissue, cavitation effects associated with propagation of SWs and absorption by the bone tissue were not taken into account. Experiments are currently undergoing to compare precise location of SWs induced micro-damage with location of numerically predicted regions of high stresses.

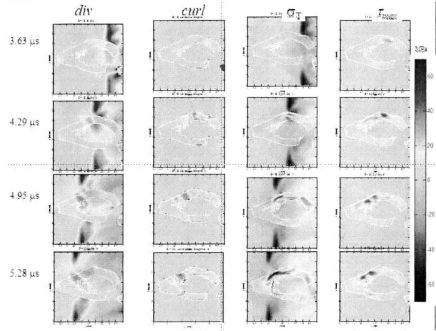

FIGURE 2. Divergence, curl modulus, principal tensile stress and principal shear stress as function of time. The amplitudes of stresses are displayed using a pseudo-color scale according to the scale bar on depicted on the right. The contour of the bone section is depicted in white. The field of view in each frame is 8*8 mm^2.

ACKNOWLEDGMENTS

This work was supported by the DGA/DAS/MRIS (French Army), the Fulbright Program and the National Institutes of Health NIH DK 43881.

REFERENCES

1. V.D. Valchanou and P. Michailov. Int Orthop 15 181-4 (1991).
2. J.N. Weinstein, D.M. Oster *et al.*. Clin Orthop Relat Res 235 261-7 (1988).
3. R.R. Karpman, F.P. Magee *et al.* Clin Orthop Relat Res 387 4-7 (2001).
4. D.M. Kaulesar Sukul, E.J. Johannes *et al.* J Surg Res 54 46-51 (1993).
5. D.B. Burr. Calcif Tissue Int 53 Suppl 1 S75-80; discussion S-1 (1993).
6. J. Virieux. Geophysics 51 889-901 (1986).
7. C.H. Turner, T. Wang, and D.B. Burr. Calcif Tissue Int 69 (6) 373-8 (2001).

A Simulation Model for Local Harmonic Motion Monitoring of Focused Ultrasound Surgery

Janne Heikkilä[a], Laura Curiel[b] and Kullervo Hynynen[b]

[a]Department of Physics, University of Kuopio, FIN-70211 Kuopio, Finland
[b]Imaging Research, Synnybrook Health Science Centre, M4N 3M5 Toronto, ON, Canada

Abstract. A computational model for local harmonic motion (LHM) imaging-based monitoring of high-intensity focused ultrasound surgery (FUS) is presented. LMH technique is based on a focused ultrasound radiation force excitation, which induces local mechanical vibrations at the focal region. These pulse-echo imaged vibrations are then used to estimate the mechanical properties of the sonication region. LHM has been proven to be feasible for FUS monitoring because changes in the material properties during the coagulation affect the measured displacements. The presented model includes separate models to simulate acoustic fields, sonication induced temperature elevation and mechanical vibrations, and pulse-echo imaging of the induced motions. These simulation models are based on Rayleigh integral, finite element, and spatial impulse response methods. Simulated temperature rise and vibration amplitudes have been compared with in vivo rabbit experiments with noninvasive MRI thermometry.

Keywords: Simulations, Radiation force, Localized Harmonic Motion Imaging, Ultrasound surgery monitoring.
PACS: 43.35.Yp; 46.40.-f

INTRODUCTION

Many applications in which focused ultrasound surgery (FUS) is used for non-invasive thermal therapy have been published [1-3]. The temperature rice must be monitored during FUS because temperature elevation may have local variations. Currently, the temperature distribution monitoring around the sonication point is based on magnetic resonance imaging (MRI), but because of the cost and technical limitations of MRI monitoring, alternative treatment monitoring techniques have been studied. Most of these alternative approaches to real-time temperature monitoring are based on diagnostic ultrasound and the detection of changes in temperature-dependent properties of tissue, such as backscattered power [4], speed of sound [5] and stiffness [6-8]. Estimation of stiffness changes has been proven to be feasible for FUS monitoring since the mechanical properties are different for thermally coagulated and surrounding tissues.

Localized harmonic motion imaging (LHM) [9] is one of the techniques recently developed to investigate mechanical properties of soft tissue. In LHM, mechanical properties of tissue are estimated by using pulse-echo imaging to detect tissue harmonic displacements induced by a time-varying ultrasound radiation force. Finally, the displacement analysis is made based on time-delay estimation between the echoes acquired during harmonic motion. The LHM technique is considered as an

CP1113, *8th International Symposium on Therapeutic Ultrasound*, edited by E. S. Ebbini
© 2009 American Institute of Physics 978-0-7354-0650-6/09/$25.00

elastographic tool because the characteristics of the induced harmonic motions at the sonication point are dependent on mechanical properties of tissue. Other techniques to estimate stiffness-related tissue parameters using radiation force have been published, such as ARFI [10] and USAE [11]. A common factor of all of these elastographic techniques is that they are based on the analysis of externally induced motion at the region of interest within a target tissue.

In this study, FUS monitoring that is based on LHM imaging was investigated. It has been shown that LHM is feasible for FUS monitoring [8, 12, 13]. This study combines our existing simulation models [13,14] with a bioheat model such that LHM-monitored FUS could be modelled. We are finally comparing the prediction of the simulations to in vivo experiments results.

THEORY

We have developed a simulation model for LHM-based FUS monitoring, which consists of the following separate models: acoustic model, thermal model, mechanical model and pulse-echo imaging model. These models have been solved in series such that for example temperature dependences of some tissue parameters can be taken into account into the mechanical model. The acoustic model yields the time-averaged intensity distribution. This intensity distribution is then used to compute the source terms for both the thermal and mechanical model. The solutions of the thermal model at different time moments have then been used to scale the material parameters for the mechanical model. Finally, the pulse-echo imaging model has been used to detect changes in the mechanical vibrations at the sonication region.

The intensity field produced by a sonication transducer was modelled using the Rayleigh-Sommerfield integral. This model included three flat medium layers that can have different attenuations and sound speeds. These three homogeneous layers are used to model different media between the transducer and the focal point, such as coupling medium, skin layer and target tissue.

In an absorbing medium, part of the energy of a propagating wave is absorbed into the medium which then increases its temperature. In soft tissue, the temperature evolution induced by a known heat source can be modelled using the Pennes' bioheat equation [15]. The temperature distribution T caused by a temporal-averaged absorbed power density Q_{av} $(=2\alpha I_{av})$ can be found as a solution of the following equation:

$$\rho C_t \frac{\partial T}{\partial t} = k\nabla^2 T - w_b C_b (T - T_a) + Q_{av},$$ (1)

where C_t is the heat capacity of tissue, k is the thermal conductivity, w_b is the arterial perfusion, T_a is the arterial blood temperature, C_b is the heat capacity of blood, α is the absorption coefficient of tissue and I_{av} is the time-averaged acoustic intensity.

The mechanical behaviour of tissue can be described using the equation of dynamic equilibrium. The equation of motion for a general volume element can be written in the following form:

$$\rho \frac{\partial^2 \mathbf{u}}{\partial t^2} - \nabla \cdot \sigma = \mathbf{F} \qquad (2)$$

where $\mathbf{u}$ is the displacement, σ is the visco-elastic stress tensor and $\mathbf{F}$ ($=2\alpha\mathbf{I}_{av}/c$) is the radiation force induced by a sonication beam with c being the speed of sound.

In the displacement detection model, we used the zero phase technique [16] to estimate the time differences between rf-signals received at different time points. The delay between two signals can be obtained from the point where the phase of the correlation function of signals is zero. The displacement that caused the detected time shift can be computed by using the sampling frequency, delay and speed of sound.

MATERIALS AND METHODS

Equations (1) and (2) were solved using the semi-discrete finite element method. The time-dependent solutions of the thermal and displacement models were computed using the implicit Euler integration and the Newmark's integration method, respectively. The diagnostic ultrasound bursts and the echoes were computed using Field II [17] codes in the same domain as the previous models. All parameters in the simulation models were chosen to be as close as possible to experiments.

In vivo experiments were made on rabbit muscle thigh after approval of the local ethics committee. A FUS transducer (1.485 MHz, 100-mm diameter, 80-mm focal length) was used. It was excited by a square-modulated signal (50% on/off duty cycle) at 23W time-averaged power. Movements were tracked with a diagnostic transducer (5 MHz, 47-mm focal length, Imasonic, France) placed at the center of the FUS transducer excited at 3 kHz PRF. The echoes were acquired at 125 MHz sampling frequency and signal tracking was performed using cross-correlation techniques. LHM measurements were performed before, after and during FUS exposure at different modulation frequencies. Lesions were made at 100 Hz modulation frequency with a continuous 42.8-s sonication while MR thermometry was performed with fast gradient echo sequence using phase change method (FGRE, 256x256, TE/TR=17.3/34.9, FOV=16cm, Slice=3mm, im. time=4.6 s, ETL=1, 1NEX, 30 images, temp. coeff. = 0.00909). Base temperature for the thermometry was obtained by a rectal probe.

RESULTS

Figure 1 shows results from our thermal model and *in vivo* experiments. Both the simulated and measured temperature rises have been show as a function of time during 43.8-second sonication. The simulated lesion (a contour of 240 equivalent minutes at 43°C) and the average of the measured dimensions have also been shown. The dimensions of the *in vivo* lesions were analyzed using MRI after lesion formation.

When comparing the simulated and measured temperature rises, the simulation model over-predicted the temperature rise. The simulated temperature elevation after the sonication was about 1.6 times higher than the measured temperature elevation. It can also be seen that the width of the simulated lesion is congruent with the average width of the experimental lesions. However, the length of the simulated lesion is smaller than the experimental lesions. The length of the simulated lesion was about

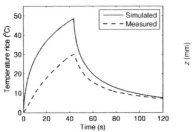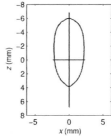

FIGURE 1. (left) The simulated and average of the measured temperature rises at the focal point as a function of time. (right) Simulated lesion (thermal dose = 240 equivalent minutes at 43 °C) and the mean dimensions (horizontal and vertical lines) of the experimental lesions. The centre axis of the transducer points to the positive z-direction.

77% of the average length of the experimental lesions.

Figure 2 shows the normalized differences between the maximum and minimum displacements during the vibration cycle. These normalized LHM amplitudes are shown before and after the 43.8 s sonication as a function of burst frequency. In addition, the measured displacements during the sonication are shown for all eight experiments. Fig. 2 also shows the normalized mean value of the measured and the simulated amplitudes during the sonication.

When the normalized simulated amplitudes were compared with the normalized measured values they were in good agreement showing that the simulated and measured results behaved very similarly. However, the simulated LHM amplitudes were lower (~40%) than the measured amplitudes. It can also be seen that both measured and simulated amplitudes start to decrease very similarly after about 6.5 s of sonication and behave quite similarly during the sonication.

In Fig. 3, simulated pulse-echo detection of the induced displacements is shown. The pulse-echo imaged displacements along the central axis of the transducer before and after sonication are shown. Three different echo frequencies have been used.

Figure 3 shows that simulated displacements and changes in displacements caused by the lesion can be easily detected using a pulse-echo technique. In addition, these results show that, in this case, 3 MHz seems to be the lowest useable frequency of the tracking beam and 3 MHz and 5 MHz yields very similar profiles.

CONCLUSIONS

We have compared our complete simulation model for LHM controlled FUS with in-vivo experiments in rabbit thigh muscle. Results show that simulated temperature rise and displacements are in order to the measured amplitudes and simulated trends are close to measured results. Based on these results, this simulation model can be used to test and optimize parameters for experiments.

ACKNOWLEDGMENTS

This study was funded by the Academy of Finland.

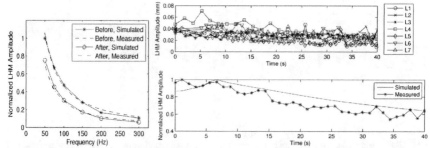

FIGURE 2. (left) Normalized LHM amplitude (difference between maximum and minimum displacement during the displacement cycle) as a function of burst frequency before and after sonication. (right) Measured LHM amplitudes during seven sonications and normalized mean value of the measured and the simulated amplitudes.

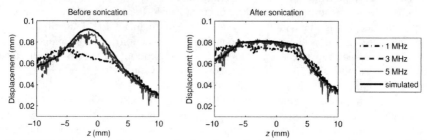

FIGURE 3. Simulated displacements and pulse-echo tracked displacements along the central axis of the transducer at the instant that the LHM reaches its maximum value before and after sonication.

REFERENCES

1. W. J. Fry, J. W. Barnard, F. J. Fry and J. F. Brennan, *Am. J. Phys. Med.* **34**, 413-423 (1955).
2. K. Hynynen, A. Darkazanli, E. Unger and J. F. Schenck, *Med. Phys.* **20**, 107-115 (1993).
3. G. ter Haar, *Ultrasound Med. Biol.* **21**, 1089-1100 (1995).
4. W. L. Straube and R. M.Arthur, *Ultrasound Med. Biol.* **20**, 915–922 (1994).
5. R. Maass-Moreno, C. A. Damianou and N. T. Sanghvi, *J. Acoust. Soc. Am.* **100**, 2522-2530 (1996).
6. R. Righetti, K. Kallel, R. J. Stafford, R. E. Price, T. A. Krouskop, J. D. Hazle and J. Ophir, *Ultrasound Med. Biol.* **27**, 1099-1113 (1999).
7. F. L. Lizzi, R. Muratore, C. X. Deng, J. A. Ketterling, S. K. Alam, S. Mikaelian and A. Kalisz *Ultrasound Med. Biol.* **29**, 1593-1605 (2003).
8. L. Curiel, R. Chopra and K. Hynynen, *Ultrasound Med. Biol.*, accepted for publication (2008).
9. E. E. Konofagou and K. Hynynen, *Ultrasound Med. Biol.* **29**, 1405–1413 (2003).
10. K. Nightingale, M. Soo, R. Nightingale and G. Trahey, *Ultrasound Med. Biol.* **28**, 227-235 (2002).
11. M. Fatemi and J. F. Greenleaf, *Science* **280**, 82-85 (1998).
12. E. Konofagou, J. Thierman, K. Hynynen, *Physics Med. Biol.* **46**, 2967-2984 (2001).
13. J. Heikkilä and K. Hynynen, *Ultrasonics*, in press (2008).
14. J. Heikkilä and K. Hynynen, *Ultrason. Imaging* **28**, 97-113 (2006).
15. H. H. Pennes, *J appl. Physiol.* **1**, 93-132 (1948).
16. A. Pasavento, C. Perrey, M. Krueger and H. Ermert, *IEEE Trans. Ultrason. Ferroelactr. Freq. Control* **46**, 1057-1067 (1999).
17. J. Jensen and N. Svendsen, *IEEE Trans. Ultrason. Ferroelec. Freq. Contr.* **39**, 262-267 (1992).

A New Design Approach for Dual-Mode Ultrasound Arrays

Yayun Wan and Emad Ebbini

Department of Electrical and Computer Engineering
University of Minnesota Twin Cities

Abstract. Advances in piezocomposite transducer technology have made it possible to design and fabricate therapeutic phased arrays with sufficiently high bandwidth and low element cross coupling to produce high-quality HIFU beams. These improvements have also allowed for the use of such arrays in dual-mode operation as imaging and therapy arrays. We have reported on a 1-MHz, 64-element concave dual-mode ultrasound array (DMUA) prototype with 100-mm radius of curvature. However, the imaging capabilities of this prototype remain limited by the coarse sampling of the large, concave aperture, i.e. the therapeutic performance of the DMUA was maintained at the expense of degradation in the imaging performance. We have conducted a simulation study of a new design approach for DMUAs that significantly improves their imaging performance without compromising their therapeutic capabilities. The approach is based on the use a finely sampled aperture in imaging mode (to optimize the spatial and contrast resolutions) and a coarsely sampled aperture in therapeutic mode (to optimize the therapeutic gain and driver efficiency). We will describe a 128 × 8 DMUA structure that can be configured as a 64 × 1 array in therapeutic mode and 128 ×1 in imaging mode. Pulse-mode simulations of wire targets and cyst phantoms using the Field II program show that the new DMUA design offers significant improvement in both spatial and contrast resolutions compared to the existing prototype design. These results provide initial validation of our approach toward the design and fabrication of piezocomposite DMUAs which are simultaneously optimized for therapeutic and imaging operations.

Keywords: Dual-Mode Ultrasound Arrays, Transducer Design
PACS: 87.50.yt

INTRODUCTION

Several image-guided high intensity focused ultrasound (HIFU) systems have been introduced for minimally invasive treatment of cancer and other tissue abnormalities [1]. We have reported on a 1-MHz, 64-element concave DMUA prototype which is able to operate in dual-mode operation as imaging and therapy arrays. Improving the imaging capabilities of DMUAs to levels comparable with diagnostic guidance systems will allow a unique paradigm in image-guided surgery. The inherent registration between the therapeutic and imaging coordinate systems will allow the physician to define the target point(s) where the power deposition is to be maximized directly on B-mode images produced by the DMUA.

DMUAs have some characteristic geometric features that are dictated by the need for high intensity focusing gain in the *ThxOF* and electrical-to-acoustic power conversion efficiency. These characteristics are: 1) non-planar concave apertures, 2) large directive elements (width $> \lambda$), and 3) low f-number (≈ 1 or lower). In addition to the geometrical characteristics, therapeutic arrays typically operate at relatively low frequencies

CP1113, *8th International Symposium on Therapeutic Ultrasound*, edited by E. S. Ebbini
© 2009 American Institute of Physics 978-0-7354-0650-6/09/$25.00

compared with diagnostic imaging array, e.g. 1 - 1.5 MHz is commonly used in abdominal applications [2]. Even with fractional bandwidths in the 30 - 40 % range, the resulting axial resolution is poor, in the range of 2 - 3 mm.

Advances in piezocomposite transducer technology allow for a choice of materials to meet a variety of power/bandwidth constraints. In addition, fine array lattice definition is now possible with improved manufacturing techniques. These advances open the door for a paradigm shift in the design of DMUAs for optimization of their performance in both imaging and therapy modes. Field II simulation program [3] is widely used in the ultrasound imaging community with a number of diagnostic array geometries supported. We have used a modified version of the program to allow for the simulation of concave large-aperture DMUAs. In this paper, a modified DMUA design with different aperture sampling in imaging and therapy modes is presented. Simulation results from the modified DMUA design are also provided to illustrate the improvements in imaging performance.

CURRENT DMUA PROTOTYPE

Current prototype DMUA has 64 elements, and each element is 1.5 mm wide and 50 mm long. The center-to-center spacing between adjacent elements is 2 mm. The shape of this transducer is a section of a spherical surface. Both lateral and elevation focal lengths are 100mm. The aperture size is 119mm. The geometry of the array is primarily determined by therapeutic HIFU applications. It has a fairly low $f_\#$ of 0.8 and the elements are not finely sampled as a pure imaging transducer. Furthermore, the transducer operates on 1.1MHz with about 37% bandwidth using a matching circuit [4].

NEW DMUA DESIGN

Transducer Bandwidth

In this section, we investigate the effect of bandwidth on the PSF and contrast ratio in imaging a variety of cyst phantoms. The bandwidth was varied from 40% to 90% with 10% increments. Figure 1 shows 50-dB images of the PSF in a 140×140 mm^2 region centered at the geometric center for bandwidth values of 40% (a), 60% (b) and 80% (c). Both axial and lateral dimensions of the PSF are reduced with increased bandwidth indicating improved resolution. In addition, sidelobe levels are also reduced with increased bandwidth indicating improved dynamic range as shown in Figure 1 (d). These results are further quantified in Figure 2 (left). As expected, improvement in axial resolution is directly proportional to $1/FBW$ while the improvement in lateral resolution is much less dramatic. To further illustrate the effect of increased bandwidth on image quality, we formed images as shown in Figure 2 (right) from simulated data from a phantom (40 mm in axial direction and 140 mm in lateral direction) with statistically random-distributed scatterers and a 12mm-diameter cyst. One can clearly see the improvement in geometric representation of the cyst with increased resolution as well as the reduction in clutter inside the cyst. The cyst diameter was measured at

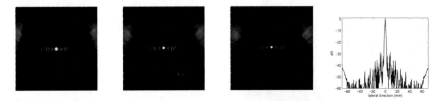

FIGURE 1. Grayscale images (50 dB) of the PSF with 40%, 60% and 80% bandwidths, (a) - (c). A lateral profile of the 40% PSF is shown in (d) to demonstrate the sidelobe structure.

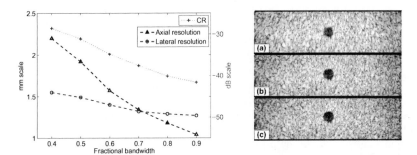

FIGURE 2. Left: axial & lateral resolutions and lateral sidelobe level vs. bandwidth for the 1 MHz DMUA. Right: hrayscale images (50 dB) of a simulated phantom with a cyst at [0 0 100] mm with radius = 6 mm; (a) 40% bandwidth; (b) 60% bandwidth; (c) 80% bandwidth.

-33 dB to be 8.0, 9.3, and 9.8 mm, and the contrast ratio was also evaluated to 21.2, 23.0, and 23.7 dB for 40%, 60%, and 80% bandwidth values, respectively. We have also performed cyst phantom images for a variety of cyst locations [5].

Transducer Geometry – Lateral Sampling

The quality of the beam patterns of the DMUA can be improved by increasing the lateral sampling of the aperture. For the same aperture size, doubling the number of array elements results in element-to-element spacing of $0.6\bar{6}$-λ (instead of $1.3\bar{3}$-λ in the current prototype). This is expected to significantly reduce the grating lobes of the array. To quantify this improvement, we simulated the PSF of a 128-element array having the same geometry as the current DMUA, but with double the lateral sampling of the aperture and assuming a 40% bandwidth. The PSF of the 128-element array is shown in Figure 3 (left) (50 dB). Comparing this result with Figure 1 (a) shows a significant reduction in the near-end grating lobes and a dramatic reduction in the far-end grating lobes. This results in an overall improvement in the imaging dynamic range. Comparing the near-end grating lobes in Figure 1 (d) and Figure 3 (right), one can see a reduction in peak value from -28.6 to -35.4 dB. The far-end grating lobes are reduced by more than

20 dB.

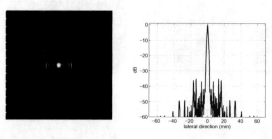

FIGURE 3. Left: grayscale image (50 dB) of the PSF of a 128-element, 40% bandwidth DMUA using the same aperture as the current DMUA. Right: a lateral profile of the PSF to demonstrate the sidelobe structure.

Transducer Geometry – Elevation f-number

The elevation focus has an obvious effect on the image quality obtained by the DMUA prototype. Specifically, the slice thickness is nearly 2 mm near the geometric center, but it is significantly larger in the prefocal and postfocal regions. We have simulated the current DMUA prototype with element height $h = 50$ mm. In addition, we simulated an array with the same geometry but with $h = 25, 10$, and 5 mm. The results of this simulation are summarized in Table 1, which shows that increasing the elevation f-number from 2 to 4 improves the lateral resolution and reduces the near-end grating lobes. It should be noted that the slice thickness near the geometric center with $h = 25$ mm will be double that of the current DMUA (about 4 mm), but it will be more uniform throughout the *IxFOV*.

TABLE 1. PSF Characteristics for 64-Element DMUA with Different Elevation Heights.

	50 mm	25 mm	10 mm	5 mm
Axial resolution	2.2 mm	2.27 mm	2.28 mm	2.28 mm
Lateral resolution	1.55 mm	1.22 mm	1.2 mm	1.2 mm
Lateral sidelobe level	-28.6 dB	-32 dB	-32.2 dB	-32.2 dB

Modified DMUA Design for Improved Image Quality

The simulation results indicate that a more finely sampled aperture with f-number = 4 in the elevation direction (at the geometric focus) with $\approx 70\%$ bandwidth offers improved imaging performance compared with the current prototype geometry as shown in Figure 4 (Left). In therapy mode, a group of 4×2 subelements can be connected to form 1 low-impedance element, resulting in a 64×1 array similar to the current prototype. In imaging mode, 2×1 subelements (from the two center rows of elements in the elevation directions) can be connected to form one imaging element, resulting in a 128×1 imaging array. Figure 4 (middle) and (right) show images of the PSF and the wire target array of the modified DMUA design, respectively. The 50-dB dynamic range images of the PSF and wire-target array show clearly the reduction in grating lobes, increased target visibility away from the geometric center, and improved axial and lateral resolution compared with the exsiting prototype.

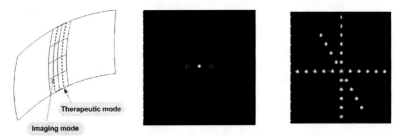

FIGURE 4. Left: geometry of a modified DMUA: a 128×4-element array that can be configured as 64×1 array in therapy mode and 128×1 array in imaging mode. Middle: grayscale image (50 dB) of the point spread function for the modified DMUA design. Right: grayscale image (50 dB) of the wire target array using the modified DMUA design.

CONCLUSION

We have proposed a modified DMUA design that results in significant enhancement in the imaging performance in terms of spatial and contrast resolution as well as expanded IxFOV. Using simple element interconnection schemes in imaging and therapy modes, the modified DMUA can achieve this enhancement while simultaneously maintaining the therapeutic aperture sampling of the existing DMUA design that has been optimized for therapy.

ACKNOWLEDGMENTS

This work is funded by Grant EB8191 from the National Institutes of Health. This work was carried out in part using computing resources at the University of Minnesota Supercomputing Institute.

REFERENCES

1. N. Sanghvi, K. Hynynen, and F. Lizzi, *IEEE Eng. Med. Biol. Mag.* pp. 83 – 92 (1996).
2. C. M. Tempany, E. A. Stewart, N. McDannold, B. J. Quade, F. A. Jolesz, and K. Hynynen, *Radiology* **226**, 897 – 905 (2003).
3. J. Jensen, and N. Svendsen, *IEEE Trans. Ultrason., Ferroelect., Freq. Contr.* **39**, 262–267 (1992).
4. C. Simon, P. VanBaren, and E. S. Ebbini, "Combined imaging and therapy with piezocomposite phased arrays," in *IEEE Ultrason. Symp.*, 1998, vol. 2, pp. 1555–1558.
5. Y. Wan, and E. S. Ebbini, *IEEE Trans. Ultrason., Ferroelect., Freq. Contr.* **55**, 1705–1718 (2008).

Transrectal Array Configurations Optimized For Prostate HIFU Ablation

Ajay Anand[a], Balasundar I. Raju[a], Shriram Sethuraman[a], and Shunmugavelu Sokka[b]

[a]*Philips Research North America, 345 Scarborough Road, Briarcliff Manor, NY 10510, USA.*
[b]*Philips Healthcare, 3000 Minuteman Road, Andover, MA 01810, USA.*

Abstract. The objectives of this study were to evaluate and compare steering and ablation rates from several types of transrectal arrays operated at different frequencies for whole prostate ablation. Three-dimensional acoustic and thermal modeling (Rayleigh-Sommerfield and Penne's BHTE) were performed. Treatment volumes up to 70cc and anterior-posterior distances up to 6 cm were considered. The maximum transducer dimensions were constrained to 5 cm (along rectum) and 2.5 cm (elevation), and the channel count was limited to 256. Planar array configurations for truncated-annular, 1/1.5D, and 2D random arrays were evaluated at 1, 2, and 4 MHz for capability to treat the entire prostate. The acoustic intensity at the surface was fixed at 10 W/cm^2. The maximum temperature was restricted to 80°C. The volumetric ablation rate was computed to compare the treatment times amongst different configurations. The 1.5D Planar array at 1 MHz ablated the whole prostate in the shortest amount of time while maintaining adequate steering. The higher frequency arrays required smaller elevation apertures for a fixed channel count to maintain a single focal spot at the desired location. Consequently, these arrays resulted in slower heating rates with increased near-field heating. The 1 MHz 1.5D array would also be advantageous compared to single-element transducers since only one mechanical degree of motion is required. This study demonstrates the selection of an optimal array geometry and frequency for transrectal HIFU, resulting in faster ablation rates and reduced treatment times.

Keywords: HIFU, ultrasound therapy, transrectal, prostate.

INTRODUCTION

Prostate cancer is the most common non-skin cancer among males in the US with an incidence of 186,320 cases and 28660 deaths in 2008. Transrectal HIFU is currently used in many countries and is in Phase III trials in the US. These HIFU systems use a single element transducer that is mechanically moved and positioned. Phased arrays have the advantage over mechanically steered transducers due to reduced planning and treatment time, improved reliability, and the avoidance of motion related artifacts when used under MR guidance and monitoring. Previous works on transrectal arrays include Sokka and Hynynen [1], Curiel et al [2], Seip et al [3] and Saleh and Smith [4]. The previous studies have primarily focused on feasibility of steered arrays, but have not dealt with optimization of the array geometry and frequency to account for a number of requirements such as reduced treatment time and reduced mechanical motion, in addition to having sufficient steerability to cover large prostates. Accordingly, in this work, we performed a systematic analysis of

CP1113, *8th International Symposium on Therapeutic Ultrasound*, edited by E. S. Ebbini
© 2009 American Institute of Physics 978-0-7354-0650-6/09/$25.00

various array configurations and sonication frequencies in order to develop an array that has sufficient steering capability with reduced sonication duration.

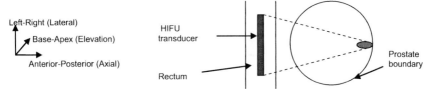

FIGURE 1. Coordinate axes convention used in this work.

METHODS

Three-dimensional acoustic fields and temperature distributions were simulated using the Rayleigh-Sommerfield and Pennes bioheat equations respectively (geometry shown in Figure 1). The propagation medium was assumed to be homogeneous except for the rectum which was assumed to be filled with water. The following properties were used for the prostate: Density = 1050 kg/m^3, speed of sound = 1530 m/s, ultrasound attenuation = 5.3 Np/m/MHz, specific heat = 3639 J/Kg/K, thermal conductivity = 0.56 W/m/K, blood perfusion rate = 5 Kg/m^3/s, specific heat capacity of blood = 3650 J/Kg/K. The therapy was turned off when the maximum temperature at the focus reached 80°C as a safety measure to avoid undesired tissue boiling.

TABLE 1. Different array configurations evaluated in this work.

Array type	Degrees of freedom for electronic steering of HIFU beam	Degrees of freedom for mechanical movement of HIFU beam
Annular arrays	1 (anterior-posterior)	2 (left-right; along rectal axis)
1D/1.5D arrays	2 (anterior-posterior, along rectal axis)	1 (left-right)
2D arrays	3 (anterior-posterior, along rectal axis; left-right)	0

Three planar transducer configurations were evaluated in this study: 1D/1.5D linear array, 2D Random array, and truncated annular array (Table 1). The size of the array was kept at 5 cm along the rectum and a maximum of 2.5 cm across the rectum. The output acoustic intensity was set to 10 W/cm^2 over the face of the transducer for all the work described here. The 1D/1.5D arrays had lateral inter-element spacing of λ/2, where λ is the acoustic wavelength. Due to the fixed channel count (maximum of 256), higher frequencies required more elements per row to maintain the same aperture width, which in turn decreased the number of rows (Table 2). At 1 MHz, a 1.5D array with 4 independent rows (8 rows total) is possible (Figure 2). At a frequency of 4 MHz, only a 1-D array with 256 elements is possible.

Designing a 2D array with λ/2 spacing in both dimensions is not feasible as this would require an extremely large channel count. Instead, a random array with two types of square elements (200 elements with 1.05 mm and 56 elements with 1.95 mm size) was used.

TABLE 2. Transducer configuration (1/1.5D) at different frequencies with 256 channels.

Freq (MHz)	Element Spacing mm	Elements per row	Number of independent rows
1	0.75	64	4
2	0.375	128	2
4	0.1875	256	1

The annular phased array transducers were designed such that the rings were of equal area, truncated to a 5 cm x 2.5 cm size. The criteria used to assess the performance of each transrectal array were the lack of secondary hot spots, ability to sonicate the extremities of the prostate, and the treatment duration.

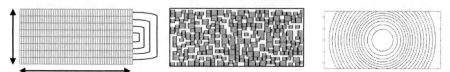

FIGURE 2. 1/1.5D (1 MHz), 2D-random, and annular arrays studied in this work.

RESULTS

Results from simulation studies with 1D/1.5D arrays are first described. The key design goal at each of these frequencies was to determine the largest elevation aperture that results in a homogenous single focal spot with no secondary heating. At each frequency the performance at 60 mm axially (deepest focal spot) was analyzed. For the 1 MHz case with 25 mm elevation aperture and all rows turned on, the peak focal temperature of 80 degrees C was reached within 4 s (Figure 3).

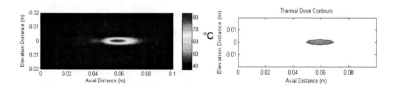

FIGURE 3. Spatial temperature profiles and thermal dose contours for the 1 MHz 1.5D Linear array at time t=4 s after HIFU therapy was turned ON.

Figure 4 illustrates the acoustic beam plots for 2 MHz array operation for elevation apertures of 25 mm, 18 mm and 12.5 mm at a focal depth of 60 mm. For elevation apertures of 18 and 25 mm, there are secondary lobes having intensities similar in magnitude to that at the focus. To avoid these effects, an elevation aperture of 12.5 mm is proposed for operation at 2 MHz. Similar analyses indicated that at 4 MHz the elevation aperture size should be about 6 mm in order to avoid the secondary lobes. A quantitative study was performed to determine the volumetric ablation rate at 25 mm and 60 mm axially which represent the extreme locations of the treatment zone. The total ablated volume based on the thermal dose was computed continuously during heating up to a maximum temperature of 80° C and an additional cooling period (Figure 5). The heating rate is superior at 1 MHz in that for the same sonication time, the treated volume is larger.

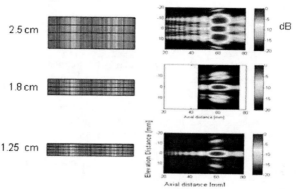

FIGURE 4. Acoustic beam plot in the axial plane for the 2 MHz 1.5D phased array. Note the secondary focal spots for the 2.5 cm and 1.8 cm height configurations.

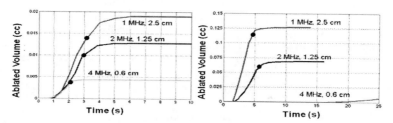

FIGURE 5. Comparison of volumetric ablation rates at frequencies of 1, 2 and 4 MHz with elevation apertures of 2.5, 1.25 and 0.6 cm respectively at focal depths of (a) 25 mm and (b) 60 mm. The dots indicate time points at which heating was stopped (maximum temperature reached 80° C).

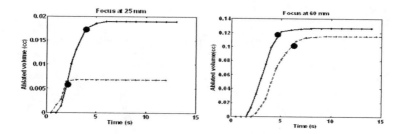

FIGURE 6. Comparison of volumetric heating rates for 1 MHz 256 element random array (dashed red) and 1.5D linear array (solid blue) at the same spatial location.

A comparison of the performance of the 2D random array relative to the 1.5D linear array is presented in Figure 6 for focal depths of 25 mm and 60 mm. The results demonstrate superior volume ablation rates for the 1.5D array compared to the random array. For the case of annular arrays, it was found that 16, 32, and 48 rings were needed at 1, 2, and 4 MHz to ensure beam steering without secondary axial lobes.

DISCUSSION AND CONCLUSIONS

A variety of configurations were considered for the design of a transrectal applicator for whole prostate ablation. The designs were a trade-off between the need for multi-dimensional mechanical movement and electronic steering. The simulation results for the 1.5D linear phased array illustrated that with increasing frequency from 1 to 4 MHz, a smaller elevation aperture for each row was required to produce a homogenous heating spot with no secondary lobes. Comparing the ablation rates at different frequencies, the 1 MHz 1.5D array configuration produced the best performance.

The 2D random array required no mechanical movement and allowed beam steering in all three dimensions. Within the constraint of 256 channels, it was determined that the 2 MHz random array produced grating lobes when steered in the lateral and elevation directions. The operation at 1 MHz was found to be suitable, but the heating rate was inferior to the 1.5D 1 MHz linear array.

The annular array provided the simplest configuration in terms of channel count and electronic steering capabilities, but required 2 degrees of mechanical movement. The best candidate in terms of optimal heating rate was the 1 MHz 16 ring configuration. The heating rate with this array was comparable to the 1 MHz 1.5D linear array case.

In a MR imaging environment for therapy monitoring and control, a linear 1.5D array with electronic steering in 2 dimensions would be most suitable. The annular array would preferable due to its simplicity when alternate imaging modalities are used for monitoring. In summary, this study showed that a suitable transrectal array can be designed to meet various requirements such as sufficient steering capability, treatment duration and the imaging modality for guidance and monitoring.

REFERENCES

1. S. D. Sokka and K. H. Hynynen, "The Feasibility of MRI-guided Whole Prostate Ablation With a Linear Aperiodic Intracavitary Ultrasound Phased Array", *Phys. Med. Biol*, 45, 3373-3383 (2000).
2. L. Curiel, F. Chavier, R. Souchon, A. Birer, J. Y. Chapelon, "1.5-D, High Intensity Focused Ultrasound Array for Non-Invasive Prostate Cancer Surgery", *IEEE. Trans. Ultrason. Ferroelect. Freq. Contr*, 49, 231-242 (2002).
3. R. Seip, W Chen, R Carlson, L Frizzell, G Warren, N. Smith, K. Saleh, G. Gerber, K .Shung, H. Guo, and N. T. Sanghvi, "Annular and Cylindrical Phased Array Geometries for Transrectal High-Intensity Focused Ultrasound (HIFU) using PZT and Piezocomposite Materials", *Proceedings of the 4th International Symposium on Therapeutic Ultrasound*, 229-232 (2004).
4. K. Saleh and N. B. Smith, "A 63 element 1.75 dimensional ultrasound phased array for the treatment of benign prostatic hyperplasia", *BioMedical Engineering Online*, 4 (2005).

On the Applicability of the Thermal Dose Cumulative Equivalent Minutes Metric to the Denaturation of Bovine Serum Albumin in a Polyacrylamide Tissue Phantom

Sacha D. Nandlall, Manish Arora, Heiko A. Schiffter and Constantin-C. Coussios

Institute of Biomedical Engineering, Department of Engineering Science, University of Oxford, Oxford, Oxfordshire, United Kingdom OX3 7DQ

Abstract. Thermal dose has been proposed for various hyperthermic cancer treatment modalities as a measure of heat-induced tissue damage. However, the applicability of current thermal dose metrics to tissue is not well understood, particularly at the temperatures and rates of heating relevant to ablative cancer therapy using High-Intensity Focussed Ultrasound (HIFU). In this work, we assess whether the most widely employed thermal dose metric, Cumulative Equivalent Minutes (CEM), can adequately quantify heat-induced denaturation in a tissue-mimicking material (phantom) consisting of Bovine Serum Albumin (BSA) proteins embedded in a polyacrylamide matrix. The phantom is exposed to various temperature profiles and imaged under controlled lighting conditions against a black background as it denatures and becomes progressively more opaque. Under the assumption that the mean backscattered luminous intensity provides a good measure of the extent of BSA denaturation, we establish a relationship between the amount of thermal damage caused to the phantom, exposure time, and temperature. We demonstrate that, for monotonically increasing and bounded temperature profiles, the maximal degree to which the phantom can denature is dependent on the peak temperature it reaches, irrespective of exposure duration. We also show that when the CEM is computed using the commonly employed piecewise-constant approximation of the parameter R, the CEM values corresponding to the same degree of damage delivered using different temperature profiles do not agree well with each other in general.

Keywords: Thermal dose; biological effects; hyperthermia.
PACS: 43.35.Wa, 43.80.Gx, 43.80.Sh, 87.19.Pp, 87.50.yk

INTRODUCTION

Thermal dosimetry aims to quantify heat-induced tissue damage based on knowledge of the tissue's temperature profile. This quantitative framework is particularly useful for assessing the biological effects of hyperthermia cancer treatments in clinically-relevant terms. The goal of these treatments is to denature malignant tissue, which involves imparting enough damage to the tissue's morphology or structure so that it can no longer function normally. One such treatment is thermal ablation using High-Intensity Focussed Ultrasound (HIFU), which is rapidly emerging as a promising technique for treating deep-seated solid tumours non-invasively [1].

The damage that a biological medium undergoes due to heat is quantified by measuring the medium's thermal dose, which may be defined as the amount of time for which the tissue has been maintained at a given, constant reference temperature [2].

CP1113, *8th International Symposium on Therapeutic Ultrasound*, edited by E. S. Ebbini
© 2009 American Institute of Physics 978-0-7354-0650-6/09/$25.00

Unfortunately, this definition does not specify how to compare thermal doses at different reference temperatures, nor does it readily apply to the time-varying temperature profiles that occur in practical scenarios. Thus far, the most popular method for dealing with these limitations has been to compute the Cumulative Equivalent Minutes (CEM), which was proposed by Sapareto and Dewey in 1984 [3] and converts an arbitrary temperature profile into an ostensibly equivalent thermal dose at any desired reference temperature. The CEM at reference temperature T_{ref} (denoted $CEM_{T_{ref}}$) is given by the formula

$$CEM_{T_{ref}} = \int_0^{t_{tot}} R(T(t))^{T_{ref}-T(t)} \, dt, \tag{1}$$

where the placeholder function R is defined as

$$R(T) = \exp\left[-\frac{E_a}{R_{gas}T(T+1\,K)}\right] \tag{2}$$

and where:

- $T(t)$ denotes the temperature in the tissue as a function of time;
- t_{tot} is the length of the treatment session, which is assumed to start at time $t = 0$;
- E_a is the activation energy of the single chemical reaction that best describes the biological medium's mechanism of thermal damage; and
- R_{gas} denotes the ideal gas constant of $8.314\,J \cdot K^{-1} \cdot mol^{-1}$.

The most common reference temperature used in the literature is $43\,°C$. Also, the exponential function defining R in Equation (2) is typically approximated using the piecewise-constant function

$$R(T) = \begin{cases} 0.5\,°C^{-1} & \text{if } T \geq 43\,°C \\ 0.25\,°C^{-1} & \text{if } 37\,°C \leq T < 43\,°C \\ 0 & \text{otherwise} \end{cases} \tag{3}$$

Although the CEM metric has been used essentially without modification for establishing dose parameters in HIFU therapy, its applicability to this therapeutic modality is not entirely clear. Issues surrounding the application of the CEM metric to HIFU therapy include the following:

- The CEM metric was developed to characterise cell culture hyperthermia up to $46\,°C$ [3], which is far below the temperatures achieved during HIFU ablation. In particular, the piecewise-constant approximation to R in Equation 3 may be inaccurate beyond $46\,°C$ and thus potentially inapplicable to HIFU therapy.
- The CEM metric was originally tested for warm-up times on the order of minutes [3], which correspond to heating rates much lower than those encountered in HIFU therapy. Since the CEM model does not account for the rate of heating [3], it is possible that the CEM metric does not apply as-is at HIFU-relevant heating rates.
- The CEM model's assumption of a single activation energy may be an oversimplification for complex biological media such as tissue [4].

As a first step towards addressing these issues, this paper presents an assessment of the applicability of the CEM metric at lower rates of heating to a simplified, single-protein model of tissue for which an objective metric of denaturation exists. The aim of this work is to motivate further investigations into the applicability of this metric to the more complex context of HIFU thermal ablation in tissue.

MATERIALS AND METHODS

Although biological tissue would be the best choice of test medium from the point of view of clinical relevance, it is difficult to obtain an objective, quantitative assessment of tissue denaturation in real time during heating. Therefore, a tissue surrogate made of Bovine Serum Albumin (BSA) proteins dissolved in a polyacrylamide matrix was used as the testing medium instead. This tissue-mimicking phantom possesses an objective indicator of denaturation, whereby the material changes from optically transparent to opaque white in places where the BSA has denatured, as shown in Figure 2. The procedure for manufacturing this phantom has been described by Lafon *et al.* [5]; in this study, the phantom contained 7% BSA (weight by volume) and was moulded into square slices with 5 cm edges and 5 mm thickness.

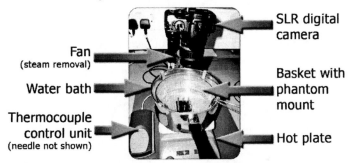

FIGURE 1. Experimental setup for characterising the thermal dosimetry of BSA phantom.

The experimental setup that was used is shown in Figure 1, and consisted of a constant-temperature water bath that was heated using a hot plate and was rigidly mounted to an optical test bench. The water bath contained a removable basket that housed a mount for the phantom slice. The mount held the phantom slice in place by impaling it onto spaced rods, which allowed circulation of water all around the slice. A camera placed above the bath imaged the plane of the phantom slices against a matte black background every 5 seconds, as shown in Figure 2. An objective measurement of the degree of damage sustained by each phantom slice over time was then computed based on the grayscale pixel intensities in the slice's central area, with 256 levels of resolution for the chosen image format. The pixel intensity histograms in all cases were found to be Gaussian in shape, with well-defined means and standard deviations of less than 10 levels; hence, the mean pixel intensity was chosen as a quantitative, overall measure of denaturation throughout the slice. These mean intensity values were normalised to a "percentage of denatured protein" using an affine transformation, with

0% corresponding to an undenatured slice (measured at the start of each run of the experiment) and 100% corresponding to a slice that had been denatured at the highest possible temperature and under identical lighting conditions until its mean pixel intensity had stabilised. A needle thermocouple was also inserted into the phantom slices to measure temperature, which was found to be uniform throughout the slice's central area. This allowed calculation of the slice's CEM over time using Equations (1) and (3).

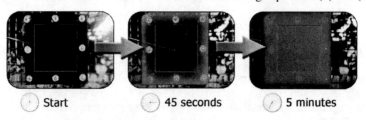

FIGURE 2. Time-lapse sequence of BSA denaturation in a 78 °C water bath. The square indicates the central area of the phantom slice in which the pixel intensity histograms were computed. The inclusion of the thermocouple needle in this area does not noticeably influence the histograms.

RESULTS

Analysis of data acquired for 7 runs of the experiment at various water bath temperatures from 70 to 90 °C yields two observations of interest. The first is that the percentage of denatured protein reaches a temperature-dependent steady-state value. Figure 3 illustrates this phenomenon by graphing the percentage of denatured protein over time for one run of the experiment at 70 °C and another at 85 °C. The curves are roughly S-shaped, with the portion past their inflection points following an exponentially-decaying pattern (fitted by minimising the least-squared error). It is clear from the graphs that both curves reach and plateau at significantly different steady-state values: in fact, the steady-state percentage of denatured protein consistently increases with temperature, as shown in Table 1. Yet this should not be the case according to the CEM model: indeed, CEM predicts that the 70 °C curve should eventually be able to attain the same percentage of denatured protein achieved at 85 °C, just in a longer time. It should be noted that this discrepancy was still present when the phantoms cooled to room temperature, suggesting that this observation is not merely a temperature-related effect. Furthermore, this phenomenon is also present in similar results obtained by Lafon *et al.* [5] using a phantom of identical composition at temperatures in the 58–66 °C range.

The second observation of interest pertains to the numerical CEM values. If the CEM metric is a valid descriptor of thermal damage for BSA phantom, then its value at a given percentage of denatured protein should be the same in any run of the experiment, regardless of the temperature profile and the amount of time that were required to attain this degree of damage. However, this is found not to be the case in general: for example, the distribution of the $CEM_{43 °C}$ values for 40% denatured protein spans $10^{7.47}$–$10^{9.76}$ s with a mean of $10^{8.96}$ s and a standard deviation of $10^{9.33}$ s, indicating that the values do not agree well.

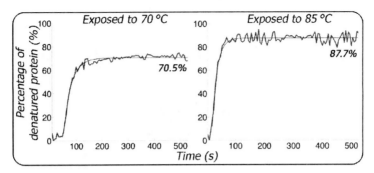

FIGURE 3. The percentage of denatured protein versus time during heating at 70 °C and 85 °C. An exponentially-decaying curve of best fit is overlaid on both curves starting at their inflection points, and the steady-state value of this curve is indicated on the graphs. Both plots are displayed at the same scale.

TABLE 1. Steady-state percentage of denatured protein versus temperature.

Temperature of the water bath	70 °C	78 °C	85 °C	90 °C
Steady-state percentage of denatured protein	69.6%	78.3%	87.7%	96.9%

CONCLUSION

In this work, the thermal dose Cumulative Equivalent Minutes (CEM) metric was shown to yield potentially misleading results when applied to the quantification of denaturation in a single-protein model of tissue at HIFU-relevant temperatures. Specifically, the existence of a temperature-dependent maximum achievable degree of damage was demonstrated, and it was also shown that the CEM values for the same degree of damage do not agree well for the commonly used piecewise-constant approximation to R. These observations indicate the need for additional research into the applicability of the CEM metric at the higher temperatures and rates of heating encountered in HIFU therapy. Future work in this direction could include generalising the results presented herein to cells or to biological tissue, enhancing the experimental setup to accommodate HIFU-relevant rates of heating, and examining the effect of using the formal definition of R instead of its piecewise-constant approximation to compute thermal dose.

REFERENCES

1. J. E. Kennedy, *Nature Reviews—Cancer* **5**, 321–327 (2005).
2. M. W. Dewhirst, B. L. Viglianti, M. Lora-Michiels, M. Hanson, and P. J. Hoopes, *International Journal of Hyperthermia* **19**, 267–294 (2003).
3. S. A. Sapareto, and W. C. Dewey, *International Journal of Radiation Oncology, Biology, Physics* **10**, 787–800 (1984).
4. C. C. Church, "Thermal Dose and the Probability of Adverse Effects from HIFU," in *Proceedings of the 6th International Symposium on Therapeutic Ultrasound*, 2006.
5. C. Lafon, V. Zderic, M. L. Noble, J. C. Yuen, P. J. Kaczkowski, O. A. Sapozhnikov, F. Chavrier, L. A. Crum, and S. Vaezy, *Ultrasound in Medicine and Biology* **10**, 1383–1389 (2005).

Transient Fields Generated by Spherical Shells in Viscous Media

James F. Kelly and Robert J. McGough

Department of Electrical and Computer Engineering, Michigan State University, East Lansing, MI 48824

Abstract. The lossless impulse response method models transient wave propagation generated by finite apertures, including focused radiators, while neglecting frequency-dependent attenuation. Therefore, an analytical time-domain expression that incorporates loss, diffraction, and focusing is needed for calculations of transient pressures produced by spherical shells in attenuating media. To derive an impulse response expression in lossy media, the Green's function to the Stokes wave equation, which models viscous loss, is decomposed into into diffraction and loss factors. By utilizing a previously derived fast nearfield expression for a baffled, spherical shell, a single integral expression, involving the error function, is derived for the lossy impulse response. This expression generalizes a previous expression that was derived for on-axis pressures (Djelouah et. al., 2003). The resulting impulse response simultaneously accounts for frequency-squared dependent attenuation and diffraction and is straightforward to evaluate numerically. Transient fields, both on and off-axis, are produced by convolving the lossy impulse response with a known incident pulse. The effect of frequency-squared attenuation on focusing is evaluated, thereby facilitating transducer modeling in lossy media.

Keywords: viscous, spherical shell, transient
PACS: 43.20.Px, 43.20.Hq, 43.35.Bf

INTRODUCTION

Simulation of pulsed ultrasound requires a numerical model that accounts for the simultaneous effects of time-domain diffraction, focusing, and frequency-dependent loss. The lossless impulse response method [1] accounts for time-domain diffraction by finite apertures and focusing by geometrically curved apertures such as the spherical shell [2], but attenuation is neglected. Time-domain modeling in attenuating media was considered in [3] using the dispersive tissue model developed in [4] within the Field II program. However, the Field II model 1) is not a closed-form solution and 2) approximates frequency-dependent attenuation as constant for all points on the surface of the radiator.

The impulse response generated by a spherical shell in viscous media, developed in [5], partially mitigated these limitations by developing closed-form, analytical expressions. However, only observation points on-axis were considered in [5], thus only providing a partial description of the transient field generated by a pulsed spherical shell. To address this deficiency, the lossy impulse response method, which has been developed for circular [6] apertures, is applied. This methodology facilitates the analytical modeling of pulsed fields in lossy media. The purpose of this paper is to extend the lossy impulse response to spherically curved shells, which are commonly used in thermal therapy calculations.

CP1113, *8th International Symposium on Therapeutic Ultrasound*, edited by E. S. Ebbini
© 2009 American Institute of Physics 978-0-7354-0650-6/09/$25.00

THEORY

An isotropic, homogeneous, Newtonian fluid, bounded by an infinite, rigid baffle in the $z = 0$ plane, is considered. Under the linear adiabatic hypothesis, small disturbances are governed by the viscous wave equation, or Stokes equation [7], characterized by the thermodynamic speed of sound c_0 and the viscous relaxation time γ. The relaxation time γ is proportional to the attenuation per frequency squared in the low-frequency limit. As shown in [6], the lossy impulse response function may be expressed as a convolution of the lossless impulse response $h(\mathbf{r},t)$ and a loss function $g_L(t,t')$, where the convolution is evaluated over t'. For viscous media, loss function is a Gaussian with zero mean and variance $t\gamma$ [6]

$$g_L(t,t') = \frac{u(t)}{\sqrt{2\pi t\gamma}} \exp\left(-\frac{t'^2}{2t\gamma}\right). \tag{1}$$

The lossy impulse response function $h_L(\mathbf{r},t)$ in the homogeneous half space is obtained by integrating the Green's function over the surface of the radiating aperture S and multiplying by two to account for the infinite, planar baffle in the $z = 0$ plane. The lossy impulse response function is then expressed as a convolution of the lossless impulse response with a loss function given by Eq. (1):

$$h_L(\mathbf{r},t) = g_L(t,t') \otimes h(\mathbf{r},t') \tag{2}$$

SPHERICAL SHELL

A spherical shell with radius a and radius of curvature R, centered at $(0,0,-R)$ and surrounded by an infinite rigid baffle, is displayed in Fig. 1. The radial coordinate is denoted by $r = \sqrt{x^2+y^2}$, and the axial coordinate is indicated by z.

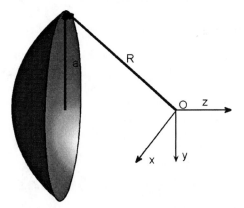

FIGURE 1. A spherical shell with radius a and radius of curvature R, surrounded by an infinite rigid baffle. The origin is located at the geometric focus of the shell, the radial coordinate denoted by $r = \sqrt{x^2+y^2}$, and the axial coordinate is indicated by z.

Lossless Media

The lossy impulse produced by a rigid spherical piston embedded in a viscous medium was evaluated in [5]. An exact expression was given in the on-axis case; however, observation points off-axis ($r > 0$) were not considered. In this section, an exact nearfield solution is provided for all field points. The solution is derived for a spherical shell centered at $(0,0,-R)$ and surrounded by an infinite, rigid baffle. As shown in [8], the transient solution for a spherical shell with radius a and radius of curvature R is given by

$$h(r,z,t) = \frac{2aRc_0}{\pi} \int_0^{\pi} N_{a,R}(r,\psi)\left[u(t - \tau_1) - u(t - \tau_2)\right] d\psi \qquad (3)$$

where the kernel function $N_{a,R}(r,z,\psi)$ is given by

$$N_{a,R}(r,z,\psi) = \frac{r\cos\psi\sqrt{R^2 - a^2} + za}{R^2 r^2 + 2arz\cos\psi\sqrt{R^2 - a^2} - a^2 r^2 \cos^2\psi + z^2 a^2} \qquad (4)$$

and the delays τ_i are given by

$$\tau_1 = \sqrt{R^2 + r^2 + z^2 - 2ar\cos\psi + 2z\sqrt{R^2 - a^2}}/c_0 \qquad (5a)$$

$$\tau_2 = (R + \text{sign}(z)\sqrt{r^2 + z^2})/c_0, \qquad (5b)$$

Eq. (3) is valid at all observer locations except the geometric focus $(0,0,0)$, where the impulse response is given by

$$h(0,0,t) = 2\left(R - \sqrt{R^2 - a^2}\right)\delta(t - R/c_0) \qquad (6)$$

Viscous Media

Convolving Eq. (3) with Eq. (1) via Eq. (2) yields

$$h_L(r,z,t) = u(t)\frac{aRc_0}{\pi} \int_0^{\pi} N_{a,R}(r,z,\psi)\left[\text{erf}\left(\frac{t - \tau_1}{\sqrt{2t\gamma}}\right) - \text{erf}\left(\frac{t - \tau_2}{\sqrt{2t\gamma}}\right)\right] d\psi \qquad (7)$$

where $\text{erf}(z)$ is the error function [9]. Eq. (7) is valid for all points in the acoustic half-space excluding $(0,0,0)$. The impulse response at the focus is computed by inserting Eq. (6) into Eq. (2). The ensuing integration yields the closed-form expression

$$h_L(0,0,t) = u(t)\sqrt{\frac{2}{\pi t\gamma}}\left(R - \sqrt{R^2 - a^2}\right)\exp\left(\frac{(t - R/c_0)^2}{2t\gamma}\right) \qquad (8)$$

Unlike the lossless case, the lossy impulse response is not infinite at the geometric focus. Evaluating Eq. (7) for $r = 0$ and $z \neq 0$ yields the closed-form expression

$$h_L(0,z,t) = u(t)\frac{Rc_0}{z}\left[\text{erf}\left(\frac{t - \sqrt{R^2 + z^2 + 2z\sqrt{R^2 - a^2}}/c_0}{\sqrt{2t\gamma}}\right) - \text{erf}\left(\frac{t - (R+z)/c_0}{\sqrt{2t\gamma}}\right)\right]$$

$$(9)$$

which corresponds to Eq. (6) in [5] multiplied by a factor of two (the baffled boundary condition was not utilized in [5]). The delay in the first term of Eq. (9) corresponds to the greatest distance from the observation point and the shell, whereas the second delay term corresponds to the shortest distance from the observer to the shell.

NUMERICAL RESULTS

To display the effect of loss on pulse propagation, the velocity potentials in a water-like medium and a liver-like medium are evaluated by convolving the lossy impulse response $h_L(\mathbf{r}, t)$ with an input pulse $v(t)$. In the following simulations, $v(t)$ is given by a five-cycle Hanning-weighted toneburst with center frequency $f_0 = 5$ MHz. For water, $c_0 = 1.54$ mm/μs and $\gamma = 10^{-6}$ μs. For liver, the attenuation coefficient α given in [10] is converted via the relation $\gamma = c_0\alpha/(2\pi^2 f^2)$, yielding $c_0 = 1.58$ μs / mm and $\gamma = 7 \times 10^{-5}$ μs. Thus, the viscous relaxation time in liver is almost two orders of magnitude larger than that in water. The velocity potential is evaluated on-axis at a) $z = -20$ mm and b) $z = 0$ mm by performing FFT based convolutions, yielding the waveforms displayed in Figure 2. As shown, the effect of loss has little effect in water, allowing a the pulse to form a geometric focus near $z = 0$ mm. In the liver-like medium, however, loss noticeably impacts the focusing of the pulsed waveform. In the pre-focal regions, shown in a), the pulse has been attenuated and slightly stretched due to the absorption of sonic energy by the medium. In the focal region shown in b), the amplitude of the waveform relative to water is diminished by about a factor of 5.

Examples of off-axis propagation are displayed in Figure 3. The velocity potential is shown in the focal plane $z = 0$ mm at lateral positions a) $x = a/2 = 4$ mm and b) $x = a = 8$ mm in both water-like and liver-like media. Relative to the on-axis velocity potential shown in Fig. 2, the duration of the off-axis velocity potential is longer due to differences in phase from the finite extent of the radiating shell. As expected, this destructive interference increases as the observation point moves for $x = 4$ mm to $x = 8$ mm. In the liver-like media, there is additional broadening of the waveform due to viscous absorption, as well as a down-shift in center frequency.

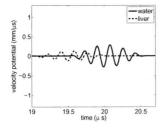 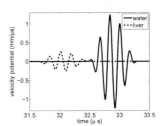

FIGURE 2. Velocity potential generated by a spherical shell with radius $a = 8$ mm and radius of curvature $R = 50$ mm in a lossless, water-like medium, and a lossy, liver-like medium. Velocity potentials are displayed on axis at a) $z = -20$ mm and b) $z = 0$ mm.

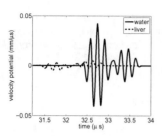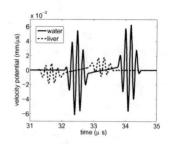

FIGURE 3. Velocity potential generated by a spherical shell with radius $a = 8$ mm and radius of curvature $R = 50$ mm in a lossless, water-like medium, and a lossy, liver-like medium. Velocity potentials are displayed off-axis at $z = 0$ mm and a) $x = 4$ mm and b) $x = 8$ mm.

DISCUSSION AND CONCLUSION

Simulations of transient pressure fields for ultrasonic thermal therapy applications typically neglect the effect of attenuation, thereby producing an 1) estimates of the axial and lateral resolution that do not account for viscous spreading and 2) an overestimate of energy delivered to the focal region. Eqns. (7) and (8) may be used as first-order models for the transient pressure produced by thermal therapy devices in biological media.

By utilizing a previously derived fast nearfield expression for a baffled, spherical shell [8], a single integral expression, involving the error function, is derived for the lossy impulse response, thereby generalizing a previously derived on-axis expression [5]. The effect of frequency-squared attenuation on focusing is evaluated, thereby facilitating transducer modeling in tissue-like media.

ACKNOWLEDGMENTS

This work was funded in part by NIH Grant No. 1R21 CA121235.

REFERENCES

1. J. C. Lockwood, and J. G. Willette, *J. Acoust. Soc. Am.* **53**, 735–741 (1973).
2. M. Arditi, F. S. Foster, and J. W. Hunt, *Ultrason. Imaging* **3**, 37–61 (1981).
3. J. A. Jensen, D. Gandhi, and W. D. O'Brien, *Proceedings of the IEEE Ultrasonics Symposium, Baltimore, MD* pp. 943–946 (1993).
4. K. V. Gurumurthy, and R. M. Arthur, *Ultrason. Imaging* **4**, 355–377 (1982).
5. J. Djelouah, N. Bouaoua, A. Alia, H. Khelladi, and D. Belgrounde, *2003 World Congress on Ultrasonics, Paris* pp. 1347–1350 (2003).
6. J. F. Kelly, and R. J. McGough, *J. Acoust. Soc. Am.* **123**, 2107–2116 (2008).
7. L. E. Kinsler, A. R. Frey, A. B. Coppens, and J. V. Sanders, *Fundementals of Acoustics*, John Wiley and Sons, Inc., New York, 2000, pp. 210–213, fourth edn.
8. R. J. McGough, *J. Acoust. Soc. Am.* **114**, 2346 (2003).
9. M. Abramowitz, and I. A. Stegun, *Handbook of Mathematical Functions, with Formulas, Graphs, and Mathematical Tables*, Dover Publications, Inc., New York, 1972, pp. 295–309.
10. F. A. Duck, *Physical Properties of Tissue*, Academic Press, London, 1990, pp. 99–124, first edn.

Model Predictive Control of HIFU Treatments in 3D for Treatment Time Reduction

A. Blankespoor[a], A. Payne[a,b], N. Todd[b], M. Skliar[c], S. Roell[d], J. Roland[d], D. Parker[b] and R. Roemer[a,b]

[a]University of Utah, Dept of Mechanical Engineering, 50 S. Central Campus Dr.,
Salt Lake City, UT 84112
[b]Utah Center for Advanced Imaging Research, 729 Arapeen Dr., Salt Lake City, UT 84108
[c]University of Utah, Dept. of Chemical Engineering, 50 S. Central Campus Dr.,
Salt Lake City, UT 84112
[d]Siemens Medical Solutions, Erlangen, Germany

Abstract. A real time model predictive feedback controller has been integrated with a combined Magnetic Resonance (MR) scanner and 256-element ultrasound phased array system to improve High Intensity Focused Ultrasound (HIFU) treatments. The objective of this research is to use a model based feedback controller to improve the quality of HIFU treatments by adjusting the power, heating time and cooling time of each applied pulse based on the measured MR temperatures. A prototype controller has been evaluated in simulations and agar phantom experiments. The results demonstrate the feasibility of the proposed real time MR control, including a 65% reduction in treatment time, and increase dose uniformity in the treatment volume with all normal tissue safety constraints satisfied.

Keywords: Model based control, MR temperature, ultrasound phased array
PACS: 87.61.Tg

INTRODUCTION

Current clinical applications of MR guided HIFU treatment protocols specify a sequential movement of the heating pulse throughout the tumor to cover the prescribed volume. The pulses generally consist of 10-30 seconds of heating followed by a cooling time of 60-120 seconds. The interpulse cooling intervals are required to maintain safe temperatures in the ultrasound near field and are also used in the clinic to achieve uniform temperatures in the tissue so each subsequent heating pulse has a predictable outcome. However, there are still large variations in the maximum temperatures among the heating pulses [1], which makes it difficult to prescribe the necessary cooling times to balance safety and overall treatment time.

As a step towards reducing treatment times, we have built on our previous hyperthermia and HIFU control experience [2-5] to develop a controller that uses the flexibility of a 256-element phased array inside a 3T MR scanner to automatically control the thermal dose delivered to the tumor. The controller uses a model, identified during a pretreatment test, and the current temperature measurements to make on-line predictions in order to reduce the heating and cooling times while keeping the normal tissue temperatures below a specified threshold. By using this

CP1113, *8th International Symposium on Therapeutic Ultrasound,* edited by E. S. Ebbini
© 2009 American Institute of Physics 978-0-7354-0650-6/09/$25.00

model base feedback controller, both the heating and cooling times can be reduced to near optimal values.

METHODS

Experiments with a real time model predictive controller (MPC), seen in Figure 1, have been performed with an integrated with a 3T MRI scanner and 256-element ultrasound phased array system seen in Figure 2. The power level applied and duration of the heating pulse are optimized in real time using a full order model. The model is a finite difference approximation of the Pennes' BHTE, with the power deposition and perfusion parameter empirically derived with MR temperature measurements. An example power deposition is shown in Figure 3.

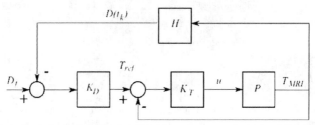

FIGURE 1: Block diagram of the 3-D MPC. KD = dose controller, KT = MPC temperature controller, P = patient, H = dose prediction and calculation. Tref is the reference temperature, D(tk) is the current dose, Df is the desired dose, u is the optimal power value and TMRI is the temperature map from the MR measurements.

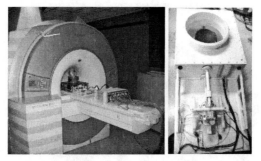

FIGURE 2: MRI guided HIFU system with 256 element phased array transducer (IGT, Inc.) and 3T Siemens TIM Trio MR scanner.

The input power and heating period length are determined from the empirically derived 3D Pennes' model. The length of the cooling time between pulses is optimized in real time using an exponential decay model, as detailed in Figure 4. The MPC uses the full order tissue model to calculate the thermal dose that would accumulate during the cooling period if the power was terminated at the current time. The cooling dose is added to the previously delivered dose to produce the total cumulative dose each time a new temperature measurement is available. This feature of pre-accounting for this cooling dose represents a significant time savings in the total treatment time because the dose accumulated during the cooling portion can account for over half the desired dose. While the controller predicts the future cooling dose at the current location and keeps track of the dose previously delivered while treating past locations, it does not predict the dose accumulated during the treatment of future locations.

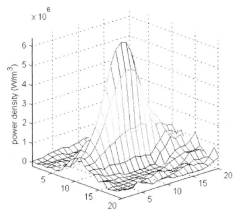

FIGURE 3. Experimentally measured applied power distribution for a 256-element phased array transducer (100W electrical input). Shown is a transverse central plane at the geometric focus.

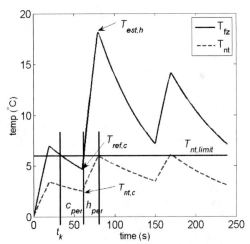

FIGURE 4: Representation of the optimal values used to optimize the interpulse cooling period. Five unknown variables are solved for simultaneously: c_{per} = cooling period, h_{per} = heating period, $T_{ref,c}$ = current pulse cooling reference temperature, $T_{nt,c}$ = current pulse normal tissue cooling temperature, $T_{est,h}$ = estimated next pulse reference temperature. $T_{nt,limit}$ is the user defined normal tissue safety limit and t_k is the current time.

A nine position (3x3) sonication pattern was tested in agar phantom experiments. Two paths were tested: a raster pattern and an alternating pattern. The experiments were performed using a normal tissue temperature constraint 1 cm from the tumor volume in the ultrasound near field.

RESULTS

1) Open Loop test: The results from an open loop, nine position HIFU treatment (both heating and cooling times were fixed at typical clinical values) are shown in Figure 5(a). For these values, significant overdosing and occasional normal tissue constraint violations occurred.

2) MPC test: The results from the nine position MPC test, using the alternating path are shown in Figure 5(b) and Table 1. A 65% reduction in treatment time is seen when comparing the open loop raster to the MPC alternating treatment time. While overdosing still occurred, it is not as large of an overdose, and the tumor dose is much more uniform throughout the volume. In addition to the results presented here, the MPC has been successfully implemented in an ex vivo perfused kidney model, with similar reductions in treatment time. These experimental results verified the time reduction seen in 3D treatment simulations.

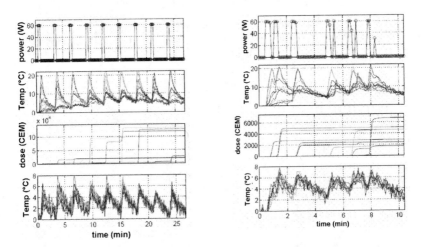

FIGURE 5: (a) Open loop agar phantom results for nine position raster scan. (b) Agar phantom experimental MPC results using the alternating scan path. Shown, from top to bottom, is the phased array electrical input power over time, the temperature elevations in the nine focal zone locations, the minimum dose delivered in the nine focal zone locations, the normal tissue temperatures, located 1 cm from the focal zone area in the ultrasound near-field.

218

TABLE 1. Agar phantom experimental results

	Open Loop raster	MPC raster	MPC alternating
Treatment time (min)	23.7	10.1	7.9
Heating time (min)	3.7	2.4	2.3
Cooling time (min)	20.0	7.7	5.6
Min dose (CEM)	3.7e3	1.6e3	1.7e3
Max dose (CEM)	1.3e5	7e3	6.8e3
Max NT temp. (°C)	8.0	7.5	7.8

CONCLUSIONS

The use of optimized, 3D model predictive control provides significant reductions in treatment time and more uniform distributions of thermal dose while ensuring normal tissue safety. The presented, advanced 3-D MPC includes 3-D MR temperature measurements, models and treatment volumes. The controller has been implemented experimentally with a 3T MR scanner and a 256-element ultrasound phased array system, showing significant reductions in treatment time and more uniform distributions of thermal dose while ensuring normal tissue safety. Such gains in treatment time reduction are not possible with pure feedback control.

ACKNOWLEDGMENTS

We gratefully acknowledge the support of NIH-1-R01-CA87785, Siemens Medical Solutions, the Focused Ultrasound Foundation, the University of Utah, and the Ben B. and Iris M. Margolis Foundation.

REFERENCES

1. K. Hynynen et al., *Radiology*: **219** 176-185 (2001).
2. D. Arora et al., *Int. J. Hyperthermia*: **22** 29-42 (2006).
3. D.Arora et al., *IEEE Trans. Biomedical Engineering*: **49** 629-639 (2002).
4. A. Payne et al., *Phys. Med. Biology*: submitted.,
5. C. Johnson et al., *Phys Med Biol*: **35** 781-786 (1990).

TREATMENT MONITORING AND GUIDANCE

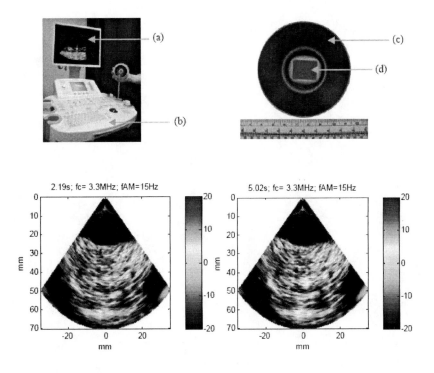

Fast Referenceless PRF Thermometry Using Spatially Saturated, Spatial-spectrally Excited Flyback EPI.

Andrew B. Holbrook[1,2], Elena Kaye[2,3], Juan M. Santos[3], Viola Rieke[2], Kim Butts Pauly[2]

[1]Department of Bioengineering, Stanford University, Stanford, CA
[2]Department of Radiology, Stanford University, Stanford, CA
[3]Department of Electrical Engineering, Stanford University, Stanford, CA

Abstract. High intensity focused ultrasound (HIFU) is a promising technique for noninvasive treatment of liver tumors. To safely monitor HIFU, accurate temperature measurements must be acquired. However, respiratory motion impairs the performance of conventional MR-guided PRF-thermometry sequences, leading to inaccurate temperature measurements and locations. We developed an MR imaging system to minimize these with the following key elements: imaging at 3.62 frames/sec and utilizing real-time referenceless thermometry processing. A spatially saturated, spectral-spatially excited flyback echo planar readout pulse sequence that allows rapid temperature acquisition was developed. The spatial-spectral pulse ignores lipids, and other off-resonance effects are mitigated with linear delays of the EPI readout. The saturation pulse restricts the field of view in the phase encode direction, allowing for increased resolution without aliasing. The pulse sequence was constructed in RTHawk, a real time MR environment, and tested by creating lesions in a phantom using the ExAblate 2000 (Insightec, Haifa, Israel). The experiment was performed when the transducer and phantom were stationary and when both were manually moved back and forth to simulate respiratory motion. Both lesions mainly followed the same shape, and the lesion appeared as a round growing spot during motion. The real-time sequence in conjunction with referenceless thermometry is promising for HIFU in the presence of motion.

Keywords: high intensity ultrasound, fast MRI imaging, referenceless thermometry.

INTRODUCTION

Hepatocellular carcinoma (HCC) is a cancer of increasing occurrence in the United States, and in the world more than one million people are diagnosed annually [1]. In the United States, the 21,370 new cases of liver and intrahepatic bile duct cancers are estimated for 2008, with 18,410 deaths estimated [2].

High intensity focused ultrasound (HIFU) is a potential noninvasive therapy for treating HCC. HIFU is capable of depositing high amounts of energy deep inside tissue while minimally depositing energy elsewhere along its path. This noninvasive method has been used successfully for treatments of the prostate and uterine fibroids and is being investigated for treatment protocols elsewhere in the body, including the abdomen. These HIFU treatments can be monitored with MRI, utilizing the temperature dependent proton resonant frequency (PRF) shift that occurs in water

CP1113, *8th International Symposium on Therapeutic Ultrasound*, edited by E. S. Ebbini
© 2009 American Institute of Physics 978-0-7354-0650-6/09/$25.00

molecules. Temperatures can be monitored by analyzing the phase difference between two time points of a heated area:

$$\Delta T = -\frac{\Delta \phi}{2\pi \cdot \gamma \cdot \alpha \cdot B_o \cdot TE}, (1)$$

where $\Delta\phi$ is the change of phase, γ is the gyromagnetic ratio, α is the PRF shift (-.01 ppm/°C), Bo is the magnetic field, and TE is the echo time. Temperature images can be created by subtracting pre-heated images (baselines) from heating images. Similarly, referenceless temperature images can be obtained by estimating the background phase from the non-heated regions of the image and subtracting that phase from the heated area. These methods can show how much a tissue has been heated over time, and thermal doses for each voxel can be calculated to determine if enough energy has been deposited for necrosis.

HIFU ablations typically take many seconds to a minute of sonication time to create enough heat inside tissue to cause coagulation necrosis. During this time, respiratory motion can cause the liver to move 10-26 millimeters in the cranio-caudal direction during quiet inspiration, while even more during deep inspiration [3]. If imaging temperature with a baseline subtraction technique, the baseline image is no longer registered to the current image, leading to an unreliable temperature image. Such motion can also lead to distortions from how k-space data is acquired and blurring in the motion direction, leading to inaccuracies in thermal dose prediction both from temperature mis-registration and from partial volume effects.

Utilizing a referenceless based thermometry technique solves the problems resulting from baseline subtraction [4]. With respect to blurring and distortion effects, one could decrease the resolution to decrease scan time and mitigate the motion and fast heating problem, however now the high resolution temperature information is lost not from motion errors but from averaging over larger voxels. Low frequency boundaries might be preserved, but high temperature centers of the lesion could be lost.

In our approach to overcoming motion in HIFU treatments, we designed a method that provided a high frame rate to minimize motion blurring, had a high resolution to minimize voxel blurring, and would not require baselines for temperature calculations. We have developed a high speed referenceless imaging technique utilizing high time bandwidth polynomial phase spatial saturation bands to limit our field of view, a spatial-spectral excitation pulse to excite only water in our slice, and a flyback EPI pulse sequence to read multiple k-space lines at once. This method was tested with HIFU treatments in motion and at rest in a gel phantom.

MATERIALS AND METHODS

A spatially saturated, spatial-spectrally excited, flyback EPI sequence, shown in Figure 2, was designed for use in the real time RTHawk scanner control environment

[5]. The spatial saturation pulse was a cosine modulated SLR designed polynomial phase saturation pulse with two saturation bands of 15 cm surrounding a 6 cm region of unsaturation in the phase encode direction [6]. The high order phase design allows for greater TBW while still operating under peak B1 constraints.

The excitation RF was a three subpulse spatial-spectral pulse. The 1-2-1 binomial pulse designed allowed for only water excitation with a slice thickness of 4.7 mm. Saturating fat was desirable since it does not exhibit a PRF shift, and its short T1 could result in fat from the outer volume

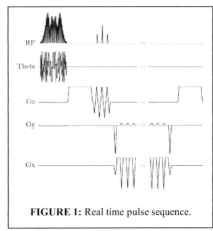

FIGURE 1: Real time pulse sequence.

relaxing in the milliseconds between saturation and excitation to alias back into the final images.

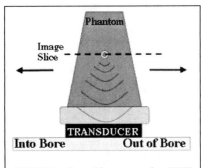

FIGURE 2: Diagram of HIFU experiment. Both the transducer and the phantom are moved inside the magnet.

In the following experiment, a seven interleave flyback EPI sequence was used, giving imaging parameters in Table 1. The real time sequence was tested with a HIFU experiment on a polyacrylamide gel phantom with and without motion as shown in Figure 2. Imaging was performed on a 3T GE Signa Excite MR Scanner (GE Healthcare, Waukesha, WI). An InSightec ExAblate 2000 (InSightec Ltd., Tirat Carmel, Israel) HIFU system with a 1000 element extracorporeal planar transducer was used to heat the phantom. Sonications were performed for 50 seconds, at a

frequency of 550 kHz with 40 W electrical power applied. For the first sonication, the hot spot was created in the phantom at rest. For the second sonication, the ultrasound was started with the phantom at rest, then manually moved back and forth along the bore direction, stopping during the post-heating imaging. The motion distance ranged from 0 mm to 32 mm, with speeds ranging from 0 mm/s to greater than 15 mm/s. The hot spot motion was parallel to the saturation band direction.

TABLE 1: Real Time Imaging Parameters.

# Shots	7
FOV	6.3 cm x 12.6 cm
Resolution	1 mm x 1 mm x 4.7 mm
TE	14.1 ms
TR	40 ms
Frame Rate	3.62 fps

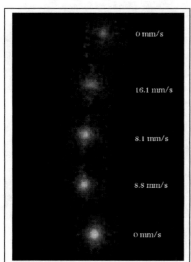

0 mm/s

16.1 mm/s

8.1 mm/s

8.8 mm/s

0 mm/s

FIGURE 3: Frames of sonication over time at various speeds. The images are scaled from 0 to 18 degrees, with time increasing from top to bottom.

The phase images were converted to temperature images offline using referenceless thermometry. Motion was measured by determining the center of the sonication lesion and tracking its location relative to the previous frame. All calculations were performed in MATLAB (The Mathworks, Natick, MA).

RESULTS

Images of the spot during heating at various speeds are shown in Figure 3. During these times the shape was depicted as a round, growing region. In our previous experiments, when the frame rate was slower the temperature rises would no longer appear as growing circular regions; instead they might elongate and have a more distorted shape.

Figure 4 shows a plot of the maximum calculated temperature through the moving and stationary hot spot over time. The corresponding motion of the moving sonication is shown below, indicating speeds as great as 20 mm/s. The measured temperatures matched each other when the set-up was stationary and also during the period of motion.

The images of Figure 3 and plots of Figure 4 show that it is possible to closely determine temperatures of moving sonications with our real-time sequence. For the most part, the referenceless thermometry algorithm could determine the temperature, regardless of location within the field of view. The one exception to this was around 30 seconds in Figure 4, at which point the spot was very close to the edge of the field of view. In this case the referenceless region of

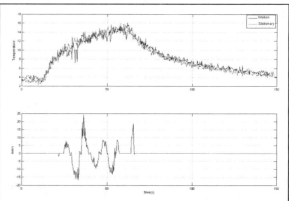

FIGURE 4: Maximum temperature in sonication region over time for both stationary (green) and moving (green) experiments (top), and the speed of motion for the moving phantom over time (bottom).

interest used to determine the background phase polynomial did not completely surround the lesion, potentially leading to this cause of error. Another reason could still be the speed, yet these speeds (greater than 15 mm/s) are greater than those we measured from normal volunteers free breathing and are less critical.

CONCLUSIONS

We have utilized referenceless thermometry with a high resolution and high frame rate pulse sequence to provide temperature imaging of HIFU ablations even in the presence of respiratory motion. Discrepancies between stationary and moving temperatures still need to be understood to determine if they are a function of the motion, position, or something else. The combination of this sequence with our RTHAWK real time system can make our treatment very dynamic with its ability to quickly change slice orientation, acquisition parameters, and the pulse sequence, thus making this a promising technique for monitoring abdominal HIFU ablations.

ACKNOWLEDGMENTS

The authors acknowledge funding from NIH grants R01 CA092061 and P41 RR009784, as well as funding and support from Lucas Foundation and GE Healthcare.

REFERENCES

1. "Adult Primary Liver Cancer Treatment." 03 Mar 2008. National Cancer Institute. 26 Sep 2008 <http://www.cancer.gov/cancertopics/pdq/treatment/adult-primary-liver/HealthProfessional/page2>.
2. American Cancer Society. Cancer Facts & Figures 2008. Atlanta: American Cancer Society; 2008.
3. Clifford, MA, Banovac F, Levy E, and K Cleary. Assessment of hepatic motion secondary to respiration for computer assisted interventions. Computer Aided Surgery 2002; 7(5): 291-299.
4. Rieke V, Vigen KK, Sommer G, Daniel BL, JM Pauly, and K Butts. Referenceless PRF Shift Thermometry. Magn Reson Med 2004; 51: 1223-1231.
5. Santos JM, Wright GA, and JM Pauly. Flexible Real-Time Magnetic Resonance Imaging Framework. 26th Annual Int. Conference IEEE EMBS, 1048, 2004.
6. Schulte RF, Henning A, Tsao J, Poesiger P, and KP Pruessman. Design of broadband RF pulses with polynomial-phase response. J. Magnetic Resonance 2007; 186(2): 167-175.

Volumetric HIFU Ablation guided by Multiplane MRI Thermometry

Max O. Köhler[a], Charles Mougenot[b,c], Bruno Quesson[c], Julia Enholm[a], Brigitte Le Bail[d], Christophe Laurent[e], Chrit T.W. Moonen[c], and Gösta J. Ehnholm[a,f]

[a]*Philips Healthcare, Äyritie 4, 01510 Vantaa, Finland*
[b]*Philips Healthcare, 33 rue de Verdun, 92156 Suresnes, France*
[c]*Laboratory for Molecular and Functional Imaging, 146 rue Léo Saignat, 33076 Bordeaux, France*
[d]*Pathology Department, Pellegrin Hospital, 1 place Amélie Raba-Léon, 33000 Bordeaux, France*
[e]*Department of digestive surgery, Saint André Hospital, 1 rue Jean Burguet, 33000 Bordeaux, France*
[f]*Philips Research North America, 345 Scarborough Road, New York 10510*

Abstract. High Intensity Focused Ultrasound (HIFU) is commonly performed using an iterative point-by-point approach with the sonications interleaved by delays to allow for cool-down of tissue. Although a safe sonication strategy, it remains rather slow due to the suboptimal utilization of deposited heat energy. As an alternative, we propose a volumetric ablation method where volumes larger than a focal spot are ablated per sonication by electronically steering the focal-spot along multiple outwards-moving concentric circles. A common problem of large volume ablations has been their safety with regards to nearfield heating. To this end, rapid multiplane thermometry is also introduced with coverage both parallel and perpendicular to the beam-path. Our approach monitors the temperature rise during sonication at a temporal resolution comparable to that of heat-development. Experiments were performed in an *in vivo* porcine model to assess the usefulness of the proposed volumetric sonication strategy and multiplane thermometry.

Keywords: hyperthermia, HIFU, MR thermometry, volume ablation
PACS: 87.50.Y-, 87.61.-c, 43.80.Sh

INTRODUCTION

The relatively recent introduction of magnetic resonance imaging (MRI) for guidance and monitoring of HIFU therapy[1] has aided HIFU in emerging as a feasible procedure of tumor treatment. In addition to providing planning of the therapy, MRI may be used for monitoring the temperature evolution as several MR parameters are known to be temperature sensitive. Monitoring of the proton resonance frequency (PRF) shift is the most commonly used approach for so-called MR thermometry, as this parameter is more or less tissue independent and linearly dependent on temperature[2].

Recent developments in phased-array transducers have allowed for the possibility to ablate larger volumes per sonication than a single focal-spot, for example by using

CP1113, *8th International Symposium on Therapeutic Ultrasound*, edited by E. S. Ebbini
© 2009 American Institute of Physics 978-0-7354-0650-6/09/$25.00

multiple simultaneous foci that can also be switched temporally[3]. We here introduce a new volumetric sonication approach that uses a single focus that is electronically moved along predetermined trajectories.

As larger volume ablations require larger amounts of energy to be deposited per sonication, a multiplane thermometry approach is introduced that is specifically designed for monitoring volume ablation and thus reduce the risks associated with the longer exposures.

This animal study addresses the efficacy and usefulness of the multiplane thermometry and volumetric ablation strategy. The relevancy of the thermal dose, both parallel and perpendicular to the beam-axis, as a predictor for thermally ablated tissue volume is also evaluated.

MATERIALS & METHODS

Nine (n=9, 50 kg) pigs were used for this study. The animals were kept ventilated and under general anesthesia throughout the HIFU session. At the end of the MRgHIFU session, the animal was quickly euthanized and targeted parts of the thigh muscles extracted for histological analysis. This protocol was approved by the local Ethical committee (Agreement AP1/01/2007).

The animals were placed on a Philips clinical HIFU platform, which was inserted into a 1.5T Achieva MR scanner. The platform consisted of three main parts: a table-top (with a phased-array HIFU transducer), an RF-generator cabinet, and a therapy control workstation.

Volumetric ablations were achieved by electronically steering the focal-spot along outwards-moving concentric circles positioned in a plane perpendicular to the beam-axis. Differently sized ablations were achieved by either adding or removing outside circles to the trajectories. The larger sonication trajectories required more energy to be deposited in order to induce necrosis within the entire trajectory. This energy increase was achieved by increasing the sonication duration.

Multiplane thermometry was performed with six slices simultaneously to sonication. Three coronal slices were positioned perpendicularly to the beam-axis, with the middle slice centered on the target region. One sagital slice, which was also centered on the target region, was placed along the beam-axis. Two additional coronal slices were placed in the nearfield for monitoring off-focus temperature rise, whose risk is increased with the increased energy deposit of the volumetric sonications. The sequence used was a segmented water selective FFE-EPI (TE = 20 ms, EPI-factor = 11), with a spatial and temporal resolution of 2.5 x 2.5 x 7 mm^3 and 2.9 sec, respectively. The resulting phase images were used to reconstruct online temperature images using the PRF-shift method. Thermal dose maps were also calculated online using the generally accepted Sapareto-Dewey equation[4], with units given in equivalent minutes at 43°C (abbreviated EM below).

229

RESULTS

No technical failure was seen during the 31 ablations of different diameter. The volume of the resulting thermal lesions increased with the diameter of the trajectory, as did the deposited energy. However, the ablated volume increased faster. Hence, the ratio of ablated volume per applied unit of energy increased with trajectory size, resulting in an approximately 13-fold increase in efficiency for the 16 mm diameter trajectory as compared to the 4 mm diameter trajectory. This indicates improved treatment efficiency for the larger trajectories when employing the proposed volume ablation strategy. The induced apparent thermal lesions were verified via histology.

The validity of the thermal dose provided by the multiplane thermometry method was evaluated by correlating the thermal lesion diameter and length as seen in the thermal dose images to that seen in the post-sonication images. A regression analysis of the thermal lesion dimensions seen as the non-enhancing volume in the post-sonication images was performed with the corresponding 240 EM thermal dose volume dimension as the only variable. Similarly, a regression analysis was also performed on the thermal lesion volume dimensions identified as the enhancing oedematous volume in the T_2-weighted images with the corresponding 30 EM thermal dose volume dimension as the only variable. The resulting fits for both thermal lesion diameter and length were very good (r^2 above 0.9), with near unit slopes and zero offsets.

CONCLUSIONS

The animal study demonstrated that the proposed volumetric ablation strategy does allow for efficient utilization of heat-deposition. Different thermal dose thresholds of the multiplane thermometry were shown to be relevant predictors of different levels of thermal tissue damage. Volumetric ablation coupled with rapid multiplane thermometry thereby allows for a precise, reproducible, and safe therapeutic procedure.

ACKNOWLEDGMENTS

This work was supported by: Ligue Nationale Contre le Cancer (France), Conseil Régional d'Aquitaine (France), and Philips Healthcare.

REFERENCES

1. K. Hynynen, W. R. Freund, H. E. Cline, A. H. Chung, R. D. Watkins, J. P. Vetro, and F. A. Jolesz, *Radiographics* **16**, 185-195, (1996).
2. Y. Ishihara, A. Calderon, H. Watanabe, K. Okamoto, Y. Suzuki, K. Kuroda, and Y. Suzuki, *Magn. Reson. Med.* **34**, 814-823, (1995).
3. X. Fan and K. Hynynen, *Ultrasound Med. Biol.* **22**, 471-482, (1996).
4. S. A. Sapareto and W. C. Dewey, *Int. J. Radiat. Oncol. Biol. Phys.* **10**, 787-800, (1984).

MRgHIFU: Feedback temperature control with automatic deduction of BHT tissue parameters

Charles Mougenot[a,b], Luis Kabongo[a,c,d], Bruno Quesson[a], Chrit T.W. Moonen[a]

[a]*Laboratory for Molecular and Functional Imaging: From Physiology to Therapy, ERT CNRS/Université Bordeaux 2 – 146, rue Léo Saignat, 33076 Bordeaux, France.*
[b]*Philips Systèmes Médicaux, 33 rue de Verdun, 92156 Suresnes, France*
[c]*LaBRI, UMR 5800 CNRS/Université Bordeaux 1 – 351, cours de la Libération, 33405 Talence, France*
[d]*Image Guided Therapy – 2, allée du Doyen Georges Brus 33600 Pessac, France*

Abstract. The Bio Heat Transfer Equation (BHTE) has been shown to be an efficient tissue representation during HIFU heating. This model requires knowledge of the following tissue parameters: ultrasound absorption, thermal diffusion and perfusion. The proposed technique, comparing BHTE simulation with MR thermal map, provides in real time an accurate and stable measurement of the ultrasound absorption and thermal diffusion and can be used to measure also perfusion. Therefore, temperature feedback control is significantly improved with more stable and faster convergence of the temperature.

Keywords: HIFU, MRI, temperature control, ultrasound absorption, thermal diffusion
PACS: 43.80.Sh

OBJECTIVES

MRgHIFU combined with real time temperature feedback algorithms (proportional integral and derivative) provides efficient local energy deposition. However, underestimation of the ratio between ultrasound absorption and thermal diffusion produces overshooting followed by unstable oscillations of tissue temperature. This study presents a method to perform robust measurement of tissue parameters based on the Bio Heat Transfer Equation (BHTE) in real time, in order to improve temperature control accuracy and stability.

MATERIAL&METHOD

HIFU heating was produced by a single channel transducer sonicating at 1.5MHz into an ex-vivo pig leg muscle. The transducer, manufactured by Imasonic with a focal length 80mm and a radius aperture 51mm, was integrated into a 1.5T Intera Philips magnet.

MRI temperature images based on PRF technique[1] were acquired using a receive coil with 10cm diameter and echo time T_E of 18ms. Every 2.7s, 6 adjacent slices of

CP1113, *8th International Symposium on Therapeutic Ultrasound*, edited by E. S. Ebbini
© 2009 American Institute of Physics 978-0-7354-0650-6/09/$25.00

128×128 voxels (voxel volume of 1.2×1.2×5mm³) were transferred on-line to a personal computer in charge of temperature control processing.

From this relative temperature cartography, the temperature increase is regulated at the center of the focal point by adjusting the ultrasound power intensity. This intensity is computed with a proportional integral derivative control algorithm based on the equation (1).

$$\frac{\partial \xi}{\partial t} + q\xi + \frac{q^2}{4}\int_0^t \xi = 0 \quad \text{with} \quad \xi = \theta - T \tag{1}$$

The parameter ξ in equation (1) corresponds to the difference between the target temperature θ and the measured temperature T. This differential equation (1) is named proportional integral and derivative control because it's composed of three terms. The first term, the derivation of ξ defines the temperature variation in order to reach the future target temperature. The second term proportional to ξ takes into account the instantaneous error between the measured and the targeted temperature. The third term including an integration of ξ corresponds to the sum of the past temperature errors. The parameter q offers the possibility to balance the relative importance of those three terms, it also defines the response time of this system being equal to 2/q.

The PID control was also combined [2] with the Bio-Heat Transfer Equation (2) [3] in order to anticipate the tissue reaction.

$$\frac{\partial T}{\partial t} = D \cdot \nabla^2 T + \alpha \cdot P + w \cdot T \tag{2}$$

Parameters D, α and w correspond respectively to the diffusion, absorption and perfusion coefficients. In order to simplify this expression, the temperature T is referenced to initial temperature measurement. In case of ex vivo experimentation, the perfusion is assumed to be equal to zero into this study.

Since the PID system feedback loop efficiency depends on tissue parameters, ultrasound absorption and thermal diffusion, a real time automatic method was used to deduce them. To obtain an accurate measurement of those tissue parameters the proposed approach consists to compare an HIFU simulation done with different tissue parameters with the current MR thermal map acquired.

In a first preprocessing step, the acoustic pressure and the intensity distribution is computed based on a Rayleigh Integral according to the transducer design.

In a second step, the temperature increase is deduced in real time with the BHTE (2) using variables tissue parameters. This equation was processed using the Fourier transform of thermal maps and the acoustic intensity distribution. The absorption and diffusion values of the tissue are deduced by looking for the simulation which minimizes the difference with the current MR thermal map. Theoretically, this method could be extended to the quantification of the perfusion value. This iterative search of tissue parameters is optimized using multi-dimensional local minimum search with parabolic interpolation[4].

RESULTS

Several feedback experimentations have been done in order to reach the target temperature of 15°C during 140s with a sinusoidal power increase starting at time 50s as described figure 3. An example of absorption and diffusion computed for each thermal map acquisition during such experiment is reported in figure 1. Tissue parameters could not be estimated before 65s when the temperature increase is larger than the noise of the measurement in several voxels in order to deduce several tissue parameters. Optimal tissue parameters estimation is obtained during the maximal temperature increase from 120s to 260s. During this time interval absorption is quantified at 0.339K/J with a standard deviation of 1.5% and diffusion is quantified at 0.175mm²/s with a standard deviation of 2.5%.

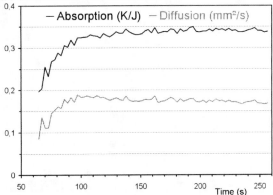

FIGURE 1. Ultrasound absorption and thermal diffusion deduced during a temperature increased controlled at 15°C

Figure 2 presents simulations comparatively to MR thermal maps for 3 orthogonal slices centered on the focal point when the maximal temperature of 15°C is reached. On the last row, the difference between theory and practice is mainly composed of measurement noise and never exceed 2°C. However a slightly negative difference on the right and positive negative difference on the left indicates a small shift of the focal point of one half voxel. In addition the temperature difference is mainly positive into the transversal probably due to the lack of ultrasound attenuation model.

To compare the improvement of tissue parameter, the figure 4 reports 18 experimentations performed at the same location successively with automatic tissue parameters adjustment (black line) and with constant tissue parameters (grey line). Initial or constant absorption and diffusion coefficients used have been modified by a factor 0.5 or 2. In case of constant tissue parameters used, similarly to the observation done into previous publication[2], the PID feedback control adjusts the temperature correctly if the ratio absorption to diffusion is correctly estimated. However if this ratio absorption to diffusion is underestimated, the temperature increase is lower than the target temperature. If this ratio is overestimated, the opposite effect occurs and the system could even become unstable. By including this automatic quantification of absorption and diffusion values into the temperature controller, the feedback control remains stable independently of tissue parameters estimation. If absorption and diffusion values are underestimated or overestimated, those parameters are progressively adjusted to correct values. With this method, errors between temperature increase and target temperature and risk of instability are removed.

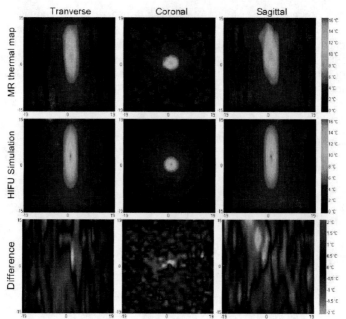

FIGURE 2. Ultrasound absorption and thermal diffusion deduced during a temperature increased controlled at 15°C

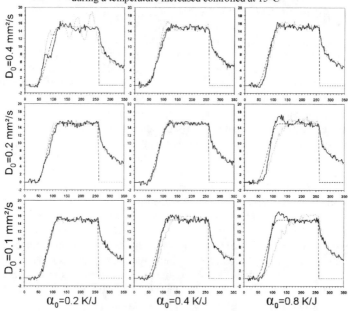

FIGURE 3. PID-control temperature obtained with predefined tissue parameters (solid grey lines) and automatic tissue parameters deduction (solid black lines) according to the target temperature (in dash lines) using absorption equal to 0.2 / 0.4 / 0.8 K/J and diffusion equal to 0.1 / 0.2 / 0.4 mm²/s

Discussion

In order to evaluate the stability of tissue parameters measurements relatively to the noise level, the same set of data was reanalyzed with additional white noise. As a consequence the same values of absorption and diffusion are obtained even with high noise level of 2°C.

However if we introduce a small baseline drift of +- 0.2°C/min, automatically deduced absorption and diffusion values deduced are strongly (up to factor 2) modified. Since MRI stability provides typical drifts of around 1°C/min, a baseline drift correction must be systematically used for tissue parameters quantification.

To summarize, this method offers the advantage to quantify precisely tissue parameters in real time with a low dependency on noise. This fast determination of tissue parameters improves significantly the stability of the temperature control process. However this method is valid for homogeneous tissue only, and requires significant processing resources. In addition the quantification of tissue parameters is strongly dependent of baseline drift.

The HIFU simulation could also include the perfusion effect without significant extra calculation duration. So this method may also be extended to real time deduction of perfusion coefficient in order to treat high perfused tissue like kidney or liver.

ACKNOWLEDGMENTS

European Union, NoE "Diagnostic Molecular Imaging" ; Ligue National Contre le Cancer, Conseil Régional d'Aquitaine, CDTU canceropôle network.

REFERENCES

1. J. Hindman, „J. Chem. Phys, **44**, 4582-4592 (1966).
2. R. Salomir, F. Vimeux, J. de Zwart, N. Grenier, C.T.W. Moonen, *Magnetic Resonance in Medicine,* **43**, pp. 342-347 (2000).
3. H.H. Pennes, J. *Appl. Physiol,* **1**, 93–122. (1948).
4. W.H. Pres, S.A. Teukolsky, W.T. Vetterling, B.P. Flannery, , "Chapter 10 Minimization or Maximization of Functions" in *Numerical Recipes in C*, Cambridge University Press, pp. 394-455 (1992).

Real-time Focused Ultrasound Surgery (FUS) Monitoring Using Harmonic Motion Imaging (HMI)

Caroline Maleke[a] and Elisa E. Konofagou[a,b]

[a]Department of Biomedical Engineering, Columbia University, New York, NY
[b]Department of Radiology, Columbia University, New York, NY

Abstract. Monitoring changes in tissue mechanical properties to optimally control thermal exposure is important in thermal therapies. The amplitude-modulated (AM) harmonic motion imaging (HMI) for focused ultrasound (HMIFU) technique is a radiation force technique, which has the capability of tracking tissue stiffness during application of an oscillatory force. The feasibility of HMIFU for assessing mechanical tissue properties has been previously demonstrated. In this paper, a confocal transducer, combining a 4.5 MHz FUS transducer and a 3.3 MHz phased array imaging transducer, was used. The FUS transducer was driven by AM wave at 15 Hz with an acoustic intensity (I_{spta}) was equal to 1050 W/cm^2. A lowpass digital filter was used to remove the spectrum of the higher power beam prior to displacement estimation. The resulting axial tissue displacement was estimated using 1D cross-correlation with a correlation window of 2 mm and a 92.5% overlap. A thermocouple was also used to measure the temperature near the ablated region. 2D HMI-images from six-bovine-liver specimens indicated the onset of coagulation necrosis through changes in amplitude displacement after coagulation due to its simultaneous probing and heating capability. The HMI technique can thus be used to monitor temperature-related stiffness changes of tissues during thermal therapies in real-time, i.e., without interrupting or modifying the treatment protocol.

Keywords: Displacement, FUS, HMI, monitoring, radiation force, sonication.
PACS: 43.80.Gx

INTRODUCTION

Researchers have investigated the potential of focused ultrasound surgery (FUS) for non-invasive or minimally invasive modalities for cancer treatment. FUS produces an acoustic wave that propagates through the tissue and deposits high acoustic energy only at the localized focus of the transducer. High acoustic energy at the localized focus can cause temperature elevation that is sufficient to initiate coagulation necrosis (thermal lesions), while the surrounding tissues remain unheated. The ability of FUS to cause irreversible cell damage in tissues has received attention from researchers as a potential technique for non-invasive cancer treatment.

The limitations of FUS applications constitute the difficulty in efficiently monitoring changes in temperature or tissue mechanical properties, and the lack of capability of optimally interrupting the treatment upon lesion formation. Currently, Magnetic Resonance Imaging (MRI) is being used for noninvasive guidance and monitoring of thermal therapies, because it can provide quantitative spatial maps of

CP1113, *8th International Symposium on Therapeutic Ultrasound*, edited by E. S. Ebbini
© 2009 American Institute of Physics 978-0-7354-0650-6/09/$25.00

the induced temperature rise at high spatial resolution. This technique is more widely known as MR-guided (MRg) FUS, or MRgFUS, [1-5]. However, while FUS is a relatively low-cost technique, an MRI system is a high-cost monitoring device. Our motivation is thus to implement a low-cost, real-time monitoring system of the tissue mechanical changes during treatment. We have therefore recently introduced an *all-ultrasound* based system for both ablation and monitoring, Harmonic Motion Imaging for Focused Ultrasound (HMIFU) [6].

Harmonic Motion Imaging (HMI) is a radiation-force-based technique that induces vibration at the focal zone of a FUS transducer for the detection of localized stiffness changes [7]. An amplitude-modulated (AM) signal was used to drive the FUS transducer that produced a constant harmonic radiation force at the focal zone [8, 9]. The resulting motion at the focus is also periodic with a frequency equal to twice the modulation frequency. This motion is tracked and estimated using a speckle tracking method on the RF ultrasonic signals acquired by a confocal phased array (Fig.1 (d)).

The purpose of this study was to investigate the tissue mechanical properties changes during FUS sonication in *in vitro* bovine livers using the HMIFU system (Fig. 1). The results were completed in six specimens with two different locations in each. The phased array imaging transducer and speckle tracking technique were used to track the motion, in replacement of previously used a single element (pulse-echo) transducer [6], and provide 2D imaging for better treatment and visualization. The HMIFU system (Fig. 1) could optimize the treatment time and lesion size, to avoid overheating, or boiling. This technique is suitable for thermal cancer treatment in the breast, liver, or prostate.

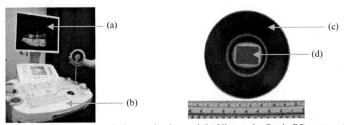

FIGURE 1. (a) 2D B-mode image during sonication and (b) Ultrasonix, Sonix RP system. (c) HMIFU transducer consists of a single-element FUS transducer and (d) a phased array imaging transducer.

Methods

All *in vitro* bovine liver specimens were degassed in Phosphate Buffered Saline (PBS) solution for 30 minutes prior to the experiment. The specimens were then placed into a glass container and submerged in a PBS solution. A hot plate was positioned underneath the glass beaker and a magnetic stirrer was placed to maintain a temperature of 37°C throughout the entire tissue specimen to simulate human body temperature. A silicone absorber (McMaster-Car, Dayton, NJ, USA) was placed beneath the specimen to further reduce the specular reflection from the glass container.

A 4.5 MHz FUS transducer (Imasonic, Voray sur l'Ognon, France) was used to generate an oscillatory radiation force using a low-frequency amplitude-modulated (AM) signal. The acoustic intensity (I_{spta}) at the focus was equal to 1050 W/cm^2. In all experiments, the FUS sonication time was approximately equal to 8 s, with a temperature rise up to 14°C. A function generator (Agilent (HP) 33120A, Palo Alto, CA, USA) was used to produce a carrier signal at the frequency of 4.5 MHz. The amplitude of the carrier signal was then modulated using a second function generator (Agilent 33220A) that generated a low frequency at 15 Hz.

The capability of monitoring tissue displacements during heating indicated the time occurrence of thermal lesion formation. By analyzing the displacement variations the relative tissue stiffness change during FUS sonication could be unveiled in real time. The speed of sound change due to heating was simply indicated by the DC offset in the displacement. The speed of sound effect on the estimated displacement could thus be removed [9].

A phased array imaging transducer on the Ultrasonix-Sonix RP system (Ultrasonix Medical Corporation, Richmond, Canada) with a center frequency of 3.3 MHz and bandwidth of 60% was mounted through a central opening in the FUS transducer; hence the beams of the two transducers were confocal (Fig. 1). The consecutive RF frames (Fig. 2) were acquired at a sampling frequency of 40 MHz and a frame rate of 288 frames/s. A digital lowpass filter with a cutoff frequency of 4.2 MHz was applied on the acquired RF ultrasonic signals in order to filter out the high force beam interference, prior to displacement estimation (Fig. 2(c)). A cross-correlation method was used to estimate the resulting axial displacements between consecutive filtered RF frames with a correlation window equal to 2 mm and a 92.5% overlap.

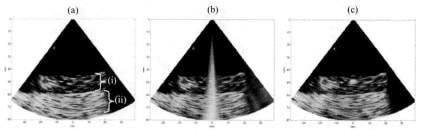

FIGURE 2. Acquired B-mode image (a) before sonication, (b) unfiltered B-mode image (during sonication), and (c) filtered B-mode image. Note: the force beam was successfully removed in (c). (i) liver specimen with a thickness approximately equal to 12 mm and (ii) was the gel phantom used to place the liver echoes at the focus.

Results

Fig. 2(a) shows B-mode image before sonication. The liver specimen was placed on to a gel so that the focus was positioned in the middle of the liver specimen, at a depth of 50 mm. Fig. 2(b) depicts the unfiltered B-mode during heating, where the bright region at the center of the B-mode image is the beam interference between imaging and FUS beams. After filtering, the hyperechoic region located inside the specimen at a depth of 50 mm was clearly seen. No hyperechoic region is present in Fig. 2(a), as expected. In order to follow and image the relative tissue stiffness change during heating, the axial displacements were estimated for consecutive filtered RF frames and the resulting displacements were overlaid onto the filtered B-mode images (Fig. 3). The axial displacements from each frame were used to quantitatively compare tissue stiffness before (Fig. 3(a)) and after (Fig. 3(b)) FUS sonication. The average displacement at the focal region (50 mm) was approximately 20 microns before treatment and 5 microns at the end of the sonication, i.e., underwent a 75% decrease.

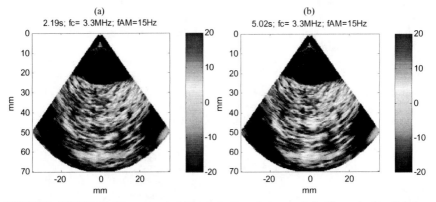

FIGURE 3. 2D HMI displacements overlaid onto the B-mode images during 8 s sonication. Colorbars represented displacements in microns. (a) Beginning of sonication, (b) end of sonication (displacement was smaller due to lesion formation).

If we take a closer look at the displacement at the beginning of heating, between 1.75 and 2.25 s, the amplitude displacement is approximately 40 microns (Fig. 4(a)). The amplitude displacement drops to 5 microns (Fig. 4(b)) after 4 s heating (between 4.75 and 5.25 s), as the tissue coagulates, i.e., becomes stiffer. The lesion size varies from 3 to 6 microns axially and 2 to 4 microns laterally over the 12 locations. The relationship between lesion location and size, and between the HMI image (Fig. 3(b)) and the gross pathology images (Fig. 5) are in good agreement.

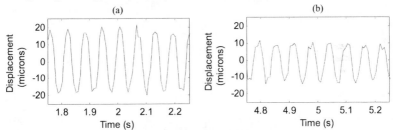

FIGURE 4. (a) Displacement at the beginning of heating and (b) displacement towards the end of the heating process. The displacements decrease by 75% due to lesion formation.

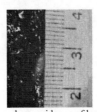

FIGURE 5. Gross pathology image show evidence of lesion formation deep inside the liver.

Conclusions

In this study, we presented tissue harmonic displacement variations resulting from temperature elevation during FUS sonication. The advantage of the HMIFU system using two distinct frequencies, i.e., force beam (high power beam) at 4.5 MHz and imaging beam at 3.3 MHz, lies in the fact that the high power beam can be filtered out prior to HMI processing.

Figure 3 confirmed that the protein-denatured lesion can be properly mapped due to its lower HMI response. Lesion location and size were highly correlated between the 2D HMI displacement and gross pathology images. Tissue displacement rapidly decreases by approximately 75% of the pre-treatment value, after 4 s sonication, indicating that a lesion was formed. Future study will include additional targeting and HMI visualization of tumor prior to thermal treatment *in vivo*.

ACKNOWLEDGMENTS

The study was supported by NIH under grant 1R21EB008521-01. The authors would like to thank Yao-Sheng Tung, MS and Wei-Ning Lee, MS, Ultrasound Elasticity Imaging Laboratory at Columbia University.

REFERENCES

1. H. E. Cline, K. Hynynen, R. D. Watkins, W. J. Adams, J. F. Schenck, R. H. Ettinger, W. R. Freund, J. P. Vetro, and F. A. Jolesz, *Radiology,* vol. 194, pp. 731-737, Mar 1995.
2. P. E. Huber, J. W. Jenne, R. Rastert, I. Simiantonakis, H. P. Sinn, H. J. Strittmatter, D. von Fournier, M. F. Wannenmacher, and J. Debus, *Cancer Research,* vol. 61, pp. 8441-8447, Dec 2001.
3. K. Hynynen, O. Pomeroy, D. N. Smith, P. E. Huber, N. J. McDannold, J. Kettenbach, J. Baum, S. Singer, and F. A. Jolesz, *Radiology,* vol. 219, pp. 176-185, Apr 2001.
4. D. Gianfelice, A. Khiat, M. Amara, A. Belblidia, and Y. Boulanger, *Breast Cancer Research and Treatment,* vol. 82, pp. 93-101, Nov 2003.
5. H. Furusawa, K. Namba, S. Thomsen, F. Akiyama, A. Bendet, C. Tanaka, Y. Yasuda, and H. Nakahara, *Journal of the American College of Surgeons,* vol. 203, pp. 54-63, Jul 2006.
6. C. Maleke and E. E. Konofagou, *Physics in Medicine and Biology,* vol. 53, pp. 1773-1793, 2008.
7. E. E. Konofagou and K. Hynynen, *Ultrasound in Medicine & Biology,* vol. 29, pp. 1405-1413, 2003.
8. C. Maleke, M. Pernot, and E. E. Konofagou, "A Single-element focused transducer method for harmonic motion imaging," in *IEEE Symposium Ultrasonics*, Rotterdam, Netherlands, 2005, pp. 17-20.
9. C. Maleke, M. Pernot, and E. E. Konofagou, *Ultrasonic Imaging,* vol. 28, pp. 144-158, Jul 2006.

Simultaneous Real-time Monitoring of Thermal and Mechanical Tissue Responses to Pulsed HIFU Using Pulse-Echo Ultrasound

Dalong Liu[*] and Emad S. Ebbini[†]

[*]Dept. of Biomedical Engineering, University of Minnesota, Minneapolis, MN 55455
[†]Dept. of Electrical and Computer Engineering, University of Minnesota, Minneapolis, MN 55455

Abstract. Pulsed HIFU beams are being increasingly used in a number of therapeutic applications, including thermal therapy, drug and gene delivery, and hemostasis. This wide range of applications is based on a range of HIFU-tissue interactions from purely thermal to purely mechanical to produce the desired therapeutic effects. We have developed a real-time system for monitoring tissue displacements in response to pulsed HIFU beams at high PRFs. The imaging component of the system comprises an FPGA-based signal processing unit for real-time filtering of M-mode pulse-echo data followed by real-time speckle tracking for tissue displacements before, during, and after exposure to pulsed HIFU. The latter can be used in evaluating temperature and/or viscoelastic response to the applied HIFU beam. The high acquisition rate of the M-mode system, together with the real-time displacement tracking are necessary for simultaneous estimation and separation of the thermal and viscoelastic tissue responses. In addition, the system provides a real-time link to MATLAB-based nonlinear spectral estimation routines for cavitation detection. The system has been tested in vitro bovine heart tissue and the results show that the displacement tracking captures the full dynamics of tissue displacements for the full range of HIFU exposures of interest.

Keywords: HIFU, Real-time Speckle Tracking, Thermal Imaging
PACS: 87.63.Hg

INTRODUCTION

Therapeutic and sub-therapeutic pulsed HIFU beams produce thermal and mechanical responses in target tissues that help determine the nature and extent of tissue damage. The intensity and pulse-repetition frequency (PRF) can be designed to produce largely thermal, largely mechanical, or mixtures the two leading to variability in lesion sizes, shapes, and damage profiles. Real-time monitoring of the thermal and mechanical responses during the application of pulsed HIFU may provide the essential component in feedback control of lesion formation leading to reduced variability and increased predictability of the lesion parameters.

Temperature Imaging. When a region of tissue is heated with high intensity focused ultrasound (HIFU) beam, the backscattered ultrasound RF-echo from the region experiences time-shifts. These are caused by thermally induced local speed of sound change [1] and thermal expansion [2, 3] in the heated region. To estimate the temperature change, the ultrasound echo from the region is continuously acquired, the time shifts are estimated using cross-correlation based speckle tracking technique [4], estimated time shifts are then differentiated along axial depth and spatially filtered to compute estimates of

CP1113, *8th International Symposium on Therapeutic Ultrasound*, edited by E. S. Ebbini
© 2009 American Institute of Physics 978-0-7354-0650-6/09/$25.00

temperature change [5, 6].

$$\Delta T(z) = c(z,T)k_m\frac{\partial}{\partial z}(\delta t(z)) \tag{1}$$

Current Limitations. A practical implementation for Equation 1 is to apply a low-pass differentiator to the estimated time shifts. Since HIFU beam generates both thermal and mechanical effects, in experiments that track the time shifts with a relatively low PRF, the above implementation could have these limitations:

1. The time-shifts induced by mechanical effects could be aliased into lower frequency, which distorted the temperature estimation
2. Increased time-shifts estimation artifacts due to abrupt change of speckle pattern. In extreme cases, this may result in complete loss of tracking

We have designed and implemented a system capable of high frame data collection with a RF sampling frequency of 200MHz. We have also designed the real-time processing hardware that can perform speckle tracking at the same rate as pulse-echo RF data.

MATERIAL AND METHODS

Experiment Setup. The system shown in Figure 1 was used for applying pulsed HIFU, monitoring of the tissue response and real-time processing of captured data. A Virtex2Pro board is dedicated for HIFU source generation and M-mode imaging control. These two units are also synchronized so that high quality, uninterrupted motion tracking can be done before, during and after the application of HIFU beams with a frame rate up to 10KHz. This is sufficient to capture tissue dynamics due to both mechanical and thermal effects. The raw RF data is then transfered to another Virtex5SXT board loaded with cross correlation based 1D speckle tracking algorithm [4]. This hardware engine has a sustained processing speed of 200 MSample/s which is more than adequate to handle the massive raw data produced by the previous stage. The estimated shift profile is transfered to host PC system via PCI Express DMA engine and further light-weight post processing (e.g. temperature estimation) are performed on the PC.

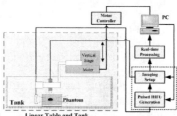

FIGURE 1. System Architecture

Fresh *ex vivo* bovine heart and elastography phantoms [7] were used in the heating experiment. For all experiments, HIFU beams are applied with a sub-therapeutic level (10W electrical power). Tracking starts 200ms before the application of HIFU beams,

242

then the HIFU beams ramp up to the set intensity in 200ms and stay for another 1.8 seconds. After this sequence, the HIFU source is shut down and another 2 seconds of relaxation response is monitored. A thermocouple placed near the focus is used as a reference with a sampling frequency of 250Hz.

Post Processing Method. Estimated shift results are first differentiated along axial direction and filtered in both spatial and time directions to get spatio-temporal temperature map. To suppress the mechanical artifacts in temperature estimation, we use a spatio-temporal matched filter derived from BHTE to "regularize" the axial derivative of the echo shifts:

$$h(\vec{r},t) = \frac{1}{(4\kappa(t-t_o))^{n/2}} e^{-\frac{|\vec{r}|^2}{2\kappa(t-t_o)}} \qquad (2)$$

where $\kappa = K/\rho C$, t_0 is the switch-on time and n=1,2,3 is the order of the filter.

To apply the filter, we use Projections Onto Convex Sets (POCS) method with non-negativity constraint.

$$T_{i+1}(z,t) = G(t)PT_i(z,t) \qquad (3)$$

P is the non-negativity constraint and G is the convolution with $h(z,t)$.

RESULTS AND DISCUSSIONS

Spatio-temporal echo-shift profiles resulting from heating the *ex vivo* bovine heart and the elastography phantom are shown in Figure 2. Note that the heating location is at an axial distance of 14 mm. In both cases, we can clearly see the shift pattern due to heat conduction proximal to the transducer. This the expected behavior based on the heat conduction equation. However, one can see spots where significant shifts occur instantaneously upon the application of the HIFU beam. This, of course, is not due to heat conduction. Rather, it is due to mechanical stresses in the tissue/phantom due to radiation force effects.

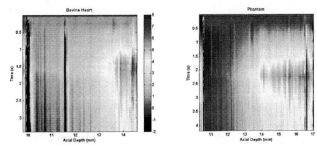

FIGURE 2. Spatio-temporal shift map of bovine heart (LEFT) and elastography phantom (RIGHT)

By differentiating the shift data in the axial direction and applying the POCS method, we obtain the spatio-temporal temperature map shown in Figure 3. One can see that the iterative algorithm achieves a well-behaved estimate of the temperature profile after only two iterations. It should be noted, however, that the algorith only partially removes the mechanical shifts.

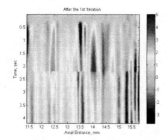 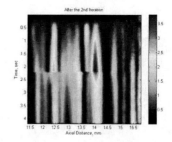

FIGURE 3. Spatio-temporal temperature map produced after 1st iteration (LEFT) and 2nd iteration (RIGHT)

The effect of the POCS iterative procedure with the physics-based regularization filter can be better appreciated by plotting the estimated temperature along the time axis. Figure 4 shows the estimated temperature at the heating spot (14.1 mm) and a proximal spot (12.5 mm) after the first and second POCS iterations. It is interesting to note that the artifact at the heating spot is smaller than the proximal spot. It is also interesting to note that, after the second iteration, the artifacts are reduced without excessive smoothing of the data. One can also observe that, after the initial sharp drop in temperature at the proximal point, the temperature continue to rise albeit slowly. This is due to temperature conduction away from the focal spot.

In a separate study [8], we used modulated ARF to excite the tissue to produce a largely mechanical response with insignificant heating. Extended Kalman Filter (EKF) was used to extract tissue viscoelastic property with a proper constitutive model. This on-line tracking method could produce tissue modulus measurement from our experimental data with reasonable accuracy and reliability. We plan to extend the current model to take both tissue mechanical and thermal properties into account. By utilizing the new model, the EKF could possibly separate the responses from these two different effects and produce more accurate mechanical and temperature estimation from a single measurement.

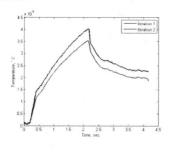 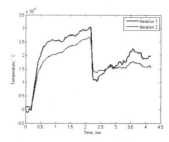

FIGURE 4. Iteration results at two locations. LEFT: at focus. RIGHT: with large mechanical artifacts

CONCLUSION

We have designed and implemented a high frame rate M-mode imaging system that can simultaneously capture thermal and mechanical tissue responses to pulsed HIFU beams. A cross-correlation based shift estimation algorithm was implemented fully in hardware to allow real-time data processing with high spatial and temporal resolution. The experiment setup make it possible to collect data at sufficiently high frame rate to capture the full dynamics of tissue response to both thermal and mechanical effects of the HIFU beam, this was validated with both *ex vivo* bovine heart and elastography phantom as heating target.

We also demonstrated the use of POCS method to reduce the temperature estimation artifacts due to mechanical effects. The result is quite satisfactory at locations that thermal effect is dominant. However, temperature estimation artifacts may still be significant even after several iterations at locations where the response is largely due to mechanical effects. We, therefore, propose to use the EKF with a properly designed tissue model to separate the two responses for more accurate temperature estimation.

ACKNOWLEDGMENTS

This work was funded by Grant EB006893 from the National Institutes of Health.

REFERENCES

1. R. Nasoni, and T. Bowen, *Non-invasive Temperature Measurement* **1**, 95–107 (1989).
2. R. Seip, and E. Ebbini, *IEEE Trans. Biomed. Eng.* **42**, 828–839 (1995).
3. R. Seip, *Ph.D. dissertation, EECS, Univ. of Michigan* (1996).
4. C. Simon, P. VanBaren, and E. Ebbini, *IEEE Trans. Ultrason., Ferroelect., Freq. Contr.* **45**, 989–1000 (1998).
5. R. Seip, P. VanBaren, C. Simon, and E. Ebbini, "Non-invasive spatio-temporal temperature change estimation using diagnostic ultrasound," 1995, pp. 1613–1616.
6. R. Seip, P. VanBaren, C. Cain, and E. Ebbini, *IEEE Trans. Ultrason., Ferroelect., Freq. Contr.* **43**, 1063–1073 (1996).
7. K. R. Nightingale, M. L. Palmeri, R. W. Nightingale, and G. E. Trahey, *J. Acoust. Soc. Am.* **110**, 625–634 (2001).
8. D. Liu, and E. S. Ebbini, *IEEE Trans. Ultrason., Ferroelect., Freq. Contr.* **55**, 368–383 (2008).

Experimental System Setup for HIFU under MRI for mouse experiments

Tao Long[a], Viren Amin[a], and Michael Boska[b]

[a]Dept. of Electrical and Computer Engineering, Center for Non-destructive Evaluation, Iowa State University.
[b]Dept. of Radiology, Univ. of Nebraska Medical Center.

Abstract. We describe an integrated system setup for HIFU and MRI thermometry for mouse experiments. The applications of such a system include MRI imaging and thermometry for evaluation and feedback during HIFU applications on mouse models of various diseases; and validation of temperature estimated by other methods, such as RF data. A 5 MHz geometrically focused (diameter of 16.1mm, focal length 35mm), MRI-compatible HIFU transducer is used, driven by a programmable signal generator and a power amplifier. The small animal MRI scanner has been programmed to acquire sequential phase information, which is used to determine frequency shift. Relative temperature rise is then calculated by proton resonance frequency (RPF) method. The current software development is done in C++ and Matlab. An integrated software is being developed to streamline the acquisition, analysis and visualization during HIFU delivery. Preliminary experiments have been performed using different phantoms. Performing HIFU (less than 100 watts) under MRI has had minimal interference for MRI data acquisition. The development is continuing for further characterizing and understanding the interference at the higher power level and accelerate data acquisition rate to achieve thermometry for a few frames per second. Further tissue experiments are under way with target of live mouse experiments. We present the overall design and discuss challenges encountered in the development of such system for experiments on mouse.

Keywords: HIFU, MRI-guided, Temperature mapping
PACS: 43.35.+d, 41.90.+e, 43.80.Sh

INTRODUCTION

Temperature mapping based on MRI is one of the most reliable, non-invasive methods for HIFU monitoring[1]. Several research groups have used MRI thermometry for HIFU studies but the discussion on challenges faced in developing such a system for mouse is limited. As compared to other temperature measuring methods such as thermocouple and RF backscattering data analysis, MRI based temperature mapping has several distinctive advantages. These include non-invasive effects of MRI for both *in-vitro* and *in-vivo* studies and temperature for a large area can be mapped in a single data acquisition [1]. We demonstrate an integrated system for HIFU and MRI thermometry for mouse experiments, whose applications include

CP1113, 8th International Symposium on Therapeutic Ultrasound, edited by E. S. Ebbini
© 2009 American Institute of Physics 978-0-7354-0650-6/09/$25.00

MRI thermometry for HIFU experiments and validation of temperature estimated by other methods, such as RF data.

Preliminary experiments have been performed using different animal tissues and phantoms. The development is continuing for further characterizing and understanding the interference at the higher power level and accelerate data acquisition rate to achieve thermometry for a few frames per second. Further tissue experiments are under way with target of live mouse experiments in the coming months. We present the overall design and challenges encountered in the development of such system for experiments on mouse.

Experiment Setup

Hardware Setup

In this study, A 5 MHz geometrically focused (diameter of 16.1mm, focal length 35mm), MRI-compatible HIFU transducer (Sonic Concepts, Inc.) is used. The transducer is driven by a programmable signal generator (Spetrasonics, Inc) and a power amplifier (AN762 HF amplifier from Communication Concepts, Inc.). The small animal MRI scanner (Bruker BioSpin system) has been programmed to acquire sequential phase information for temperature mapping. Figure 1 shows the overall system setup block diagram

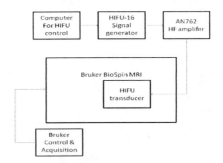

FIGURE 1. Hardware system setup block diagram

Software and Algorithms

Relative temperature rise is then calculated by proton resonance frequency (RPF) method [1]. The current software development is done in C++ and Matlab. MRI sequence has been programmed to acquire signals for later temperature mapping algorithm. Typical MRI parameters are listed in Table 1.

TABLE 1. Typical MRI parameters used

Parameter	Value	Unit
Slice number	3	
Slice thickness	1	mm
Slice separation	1.5	mm
Flip angle	35	degree
Echo time	4	ms
Repetition time	25	ms
Recover time	24.1	ms
Field of view	5 10	cm

Data from MRI scanner were stored as base maps (B_0 maps), which frequency response in the form of a matrix of complex number (pairs of 32bit real numbers). Such complex matrix was transformed from frequency domain to spatial domain by inverse FFT method. The phase of each pixel in spatial domain is calculated and unwrapped by algorithms describe in [2]. Unwrapped phase is then used to calculate the frequency shift and temperature change as compared to initial data set collected before HIFU exposure. Unwrapped phase is then used to calculate temperature change from initial data set collected before HIFU exposure [3]. Figure 2 shows the flow chart for algorithm implementation.

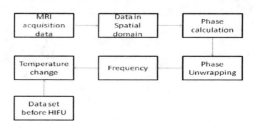

FIGURE 2. Data acquisition and algorithm flow chart

Temperature rise were calculated by water proton resonance frequency method according to [3][4]. The local magnetic field. Local magnetic field B_{nuc} as observed by the spins is a function of the main magnetic field B0 and the chemical shift $B_{nuc} = (1 + \sigma)B_0$, where the chemical shift σ is the sum of temperature independent contribution (B_0 field inhomogeneities) and temperature dependent contribution σ_T. $\sigma = \sigma_0 + \sigma_T$. The chemical shift can be calculated from the phase information Φ in RF-spoiled gradient-echo images $\Phi = \gamma\sigma T_E B_0$. The constant γ is the gyromagnetic ration of the observed nucleus ($42.58 * 10^6$ Hz T^{-1} for protons) and T_E is the echo time. The temperature rise is calculated as $\Delta T = T - T_{ref} = (\Phi - \Phi_0) / \gamma\alpha T_E B_0$, where α is the temperature-dependent water chemical shift.

Preliminary Results

A set of experiments were performed to evaluate the design of the system. Various types of animal tissues were used. Figure 3 shows the configuration of the upward facing HIFU transducer and the bore of the MRI machine. Tissue samples were placed on top of the transducer and then inserted in the MRI machine for imaging and HIFU exposure.

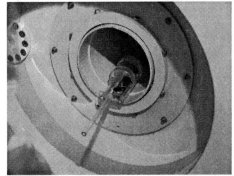

FIGURE 3. HIFU transducer and MRI machine configuration

Typical HIFU parameters were 5-20w power output in the form of continuous sinusoidal waves. MRI images were acquired before, during and after HIFU exposure. For tissue samples, we used chicken skeletal muscle for these experiments.

Figure 4 shows six sequential frequency shifts calculated from MRI images for an HIFU exposure of 10 seconds. The first two were acquired before HIFU exposure. The middle two were acquired during the HIFU exposure and the last two were acquired after HIFU exposure. All images were 64 by 64 in resolution in a FOV of 10 cm.

FIGURE 4. Frequency shift from MRI.

Discussion and Future Work

We have faced several issues challenges in operating HIFU under MRI. First of all, the HIFU transducer needs to be MRI compatible in construction. Since uniform magnetic field must be maintained in MRI machine during data acquisition, the transducer itself and connecting cable must contain no magnetic material.

During the MRI data acquisition, coupling of HIFU transducer can be an issue, in that not only the coupling need to fit into MRI machine and provide sufficient cooling and/or bubble filtering for HIFU exposure, it can also change the electrical impedance of the transducer. Driving the HIFU transducer with mismatched impedance not only reduces the power transfer efficiency but also pose a risk for the HIFU power amplifier. As a result, a tunable and MRI compatible matching circuit is desirable. Also, the matching circuit needs to be tested for any resonance closer to the MRI frequency as a close resonance can cause very poor signal-to-noise ratio.

Since most HIFU exposure usually lasts no more than a minute, the temperature rise in target tissue occurs within a few seconds in high power setting. In such cases, the data acquisition of MRI machine needs to be fast enough to capture the characteristics of temperature rise associated with certain HIFU parameter setting. The data acquisition process can be expedited with fewer slices and/or lower resolutions.

We have demonstrated a system setup for HIFU under MRI for thermometry. Such system has the potential to serve as a validation of other means of thermometry, such as backscattered RF based methods[5]. Future work also includes making the system viable for *in-vivo* studies for mouse and explores other effects of HIFU on tissues under MRI monitoring.

REFERENCES

1. Quesson, Zwart et al, *Journal of Magnetic Resonance Imaging*, Vol 12 Issue 4 Page 525-533, Wiley, 2008
2. Schofield, Zhu, *Optics Letters*, Vol. 28 No. 14, 2003
3. Miyasaka, Takshashi et al, *Magnetic Resonance in Medicine*, Page 198-202, 2006
4. Hindman, *Journal of Chemical Physics*, Vol 44, page 4582-4592, 1995
5. Anand, Kaczkowski, *Acoustics Research Letters*, Vol 5, Issue 3, Page 88-94, 2004

Bounds on Thermal Dose Estimates using Ultrasonic Backscatter Monitoring of Heating

Gavriel Speyer, Peter Kaczkowski, Andrew Brayman, Marilee Andrew and Lawrence Crum

Center for Industrial and Medical Ultrasound, Applied Physics Laboratory
University of Washington, Seattle WA 98105-6698

Abstract. Diagnostic ultrasound provides a means for estimating the spatial distribution of temperature in tissue in response to HIFU therapy. One approach to estimating the temperature is to distort backscattered ultrasound between two frames, one preceding and one following the treatment, in a manner consistent with the heat equation, the exposure protocol, the beam pattern, and the specific material properties of the tissue. Ascribing a probability distribution to the measurements taken after treatment, the Cramer Rao bound may be determined for coefficient estimates in a functional expansion for the applied heating during therapy. This formulation also identifies the function with coefficient estimates having least variance, providing the lower bound. We study the implications of this characterization for heat deposition from a linear scan, examining how estimation accuracy is influenced by the lesion length and the delay following treatment and preceding acquisition. It is shown that for these studies, temperature estimates with accuracy well below $1°C$ are possible. In addition, the thermal dose can be estimated to tens of equivalent minutes, referenced to $43°C$.

Keywords: HIFU, Temperature Estimation, Acoustic Backscattering, Therapy Monitoring
PACS: 43.10.Ce, 43.35.Yb

INTRODUCTION

Diagnostic ultrasound provides a means for temperature estimation [7]. The estimation paradigm holds that a change observed in the relative position of scatterers in frames acquired before and after HIFU treatment is due to temperature changes in the material. Accounting mechanistically for the source of heating and exposure protocol, the estimated temperature rise associated with the relative movement of scatterers can have its uncertainty tightly bounded. For therapy delivery, the thermal dose metric [6] is widely accepted, so a lower bound on performance for this metric is especially relevant.

MATERIALS AND METHODS

Consider the arrangement shown in Figure 1a. A tissue sample is treated continuously with high intensity focused ultrasound (HIFU) radiated from the transducer at the left, which moves in the plane perpendicular to its axis. A diagnostic ultrasound scanhead, mounted above the sample, captures two frames in the focal plane of the transducer, one frame preceding and one frame following HIFU treatment. The observed differences between the two frames are the result of time of flight changes experienced in regions of elevated temperature [7]. The temperature is in turn derived from the heating introduced

CP1113, *8th International Symposium on Therapeutic Ultrasound,* edited by E. S. Ebbini
© 2009 American Institute of Physics 978-0-7354-0650-6/09/$25.00

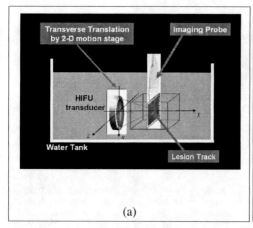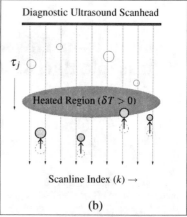

| (a) | (b) |

FIGURE 1. Temperature Estimation using Diagnostic Ultrasound. (a) A focused ultrasound transducer moves in the plane perpendicular to its axis, forming a lesion in its focal plane. A diagnostic ultrasound scanhead is mounted from above, and captures frames in the focal plane before and after therapy is administered. (b) Illustration of scatterers before and after treatment. Scatterers below the heated region appear to move towards the scanhead due to the effects of temperature on sound speed.

during therapy [1]. Figure 1b illustrates the displacements observed following treatment.

Let $i = a, b$ index the frame capture times t_i (slow time) before and after treatment. Let j index the delay τ_j into a given scanline (fast time), and let k index the position z_k of a scanline along the scanhead, oriented along the z axis. The ultrasound frames are indexed by (i, j, k), with t_i specifying a given backscattered data frame $\rho_{t_i}(\tau_j, z_k)$. For the kth scanline, a specular reflector at delay τ_j and time t_b corresponds to an initial delay τ^b_{ajk} at t_a, linearly adjusted for temperature along the propagation path by α_1, as [7]:

$$\tau_j = \tau^b_{ajk} - \alpha_1 \int_0^{c_0 \tau^b_{ajk}} T_{t_b}(\xi, y = R_0, z = z_k)d\xi \quad , \tag{1}$$

with c_0 the speed of sound at the equilibrium temperature. The temperature distribution $T_t(\mathbf{r})$ is linearly related to the heat source $Q_t(\mathbf{r})$ through the Green's function $\Gamma_{t|t_0}(\mathbf{r} \mid \mathbf{r}_0)$, providing the temperature rise at $(\mathbf{r}, t)$ in response to a heat source at $(\mathbf{r}_0, t_0)$ [3]:

$$T_t(\mathbf{r}) = \int_{t_a}^{t} \int_V Q_{t_0}(\mathbf{r}_0) \Gamma_{t|t_0}(\mathbf{r} \mid \mathbf{r}_0)dV_0 dt_0 \quad . \tag{2}$$

The heat source $Q_t(\mathbf{r})$ is highly focussed by the beam, allowing the decomposition $Q_t(\mathbf{r}) = q(t)Q(\mathbf{r} - \mathbf{r}_t)$. The spatial component $Q(\mathbf{r})$ follows the beam pattern of the transducer, and $\mathbf{r}_t$ is the path of the scan in the focal plane. The unknown heating rate is denoted by $q(t)$. Defining $g_{t|t_0}(\mathbf{r} \mid \mathbf{r}_0) \equiv \int Q(\mathbf{r}_0 - \mathbf{r}_{t_0})\Gamma_{t|t_0}(\mathbf{r} \mid \mathbf{r}_0)dV_0$, and with the diagnostic ultrasound capturing the focal plane $y = R_0$, Eq. (1) takes the form:

$$\tau_j = \tau^b_{ajk} - \alpha_1 \int_0^{c_0 \tau^b_{ajk}} \int_{t_a}^{t_{exp}} q(t_0) g_{t_b|t_0}(\xi, R_0, z = z_k \mid x_{t_0}, R_0, z_{t_0})dt_0 d\xi$$

$$= \tau_{ajk}^b - \alpha_1 \int_{t_a}^{t_{exp}} q(t_0) G_{t_b|t_0}(c_0 \tau_{ajk}^b, z_k \mid x_{t_0}, z_{t_0}) dt_0 \quad , \tag{3}$$

where $t_{exp} < t_b$ is the duration of the exposure. Observe that $G_{t|t_0}(x, z_k \mid x_{t_0}, z_{t_0})$ subsumes all known quantities, with the dependence on $y = R_0$ suppressed to simplify the discussion. The uncertainty in Eq. (3) is attributed to the time variation in $q(t)$, which is estimated using a functional expansion for $q(t)$ over the exposure interval (t_a, t_{exp}) of the form

$$q(t) = \sum_{n=1}^{N} q_n \phi_n(t) \quad . \tag{4}$$

The estimation problem is parameterized by $\mathbf{q} = \begin{bmatrix} q_1 & \cdots & q_N \end{bmatrix}^T$, with $\tau_{ajk}^b = \tau_{ajk}^b(\mathbf{q})$.

It is assumed that, adjusting for time of flight changes due to temperature, differences between the frame captured at time t_a before treatment and that captured at time t_b after treatment are due to measurement noise. The set of measurements $\rho_{t_b}(\tau_j, z_k)$ captured at time t_b are assumed normally distributed and conditionally independent given $\mathbf{q}$ and initial frame $\rho_{t_a}(\tau, z_k)$, with expected value $\rho_{t_a}\left(\tau_{ajk}^b(\mathbf{q}), z_k\right)$, and variance σ_ε^2:

$$\rho_{t_b}(\tau_j, z_k) \sim N\left(\rho_{t_a}\left(\tau_{ajk}^b(\mathbf{q}), z_k\right), \sigma_\varepsilon^2\right) \quad . \tag{5}$$

The Cramer Rao lower bound on parameter estimates $\hat{\mathbf{q}}$ is given by $\mathrm{var}(\hat{\mathbf{q}}) \geq \mathbf{I}^{-1}(\mathbf{q})$, with $\mathbf{I}(\mathbf{q})$ the Fisher Information matrix [4]. For the model in Eq. (5), $\mathbf{I}(\mathbf{q})$ is [4]:

$$I(\mathbf{q}) = \frac{1}{\sigma_\varepsilon^2} \sum_{j=1}^{J} \sum_{k=1}^{K} \left(\frac{\partial \rho_{t_a}(\tau, z_k)}{\partial \tau}\bigg|_{\tau = \tau_{ajk}^b(\mathbf{q})}\right)^2 \frac{\partial \tau_{ajk}^b(\mathbf{q})}{\partial \mathbf{q}} \frac{\partial \tau_{ajk}^b(\mathbf{q})}{\partial \mathbf{q}^T} \tag{6}$$

The derivative of ρ with respect to τ has finite second moment, because the measurements are bandlimited, and assuming a tissue block with uniform statistical properties, we may consider the expected value $\sigma_\rho^2 \equiv E_\rho\left\{(\partial \rho_t(\tau, z)/\partial \tau)^2\right\}$. Accordingly, an average Fisher information is computed over the ensemble of backscattered measurements $\rho_t(\tau, z)$. The bounds on parameter estimates for $\mathbf{q} = 0$ are used, for which $\tau_{ajk}^b = \tau_j$, $\forall(j, k)$. The expected information is

$$\bar{I}(\mathbf{q} = 0) = E_\rho\{I(\mathbf{q} = 0)\} = \frac{\sigma_\rho^2}{\sigma_\varepsilon^2} \sum_{j=1}^{J} \sum_{k=1}^{K} \frac{\partial \tau_{ajk}^b(\mathbf{q})}{\partial \mathbf{q}}\bigg|_{\mathbf{q}=0} \frac{\partial \tau_{ajk}^b(\mathbf{q})}{\partial \mathbf{q}^T}\bigg|_{\mathbf{q}=0} \quad . \tag{7}$$

Substituting Eqs. (3) and (4) into Eq. (7) provides the $(m, n)^{th}$ matrix component as:

$$\bar{I}_{m,n}(\mathbf{q} = 0) = \frac{\sigma_\rho^2}{\sigma_\varepsilon^2} \alpha_1^2 \int_{t_a}^{t_{exp}} \int_{t_a}^{t_{exp}} \phi_m(s) \phi_n(s') K_{t_b}(s, s') ds' ds \quad , \tag{8}$$

where $K_t(s, s') = \sum_{j,k} G_{t|s}(c_0 \tau_j, z_k \mid x_s, z_s) G_{t|s'}(c_0 \tau_j, z_k \mid x_{s'}, z_{s'})$. For cases of physical interest, $\int_{t_a}^{t_{exp}} \int_{t_a}^{t_{exp}} K_t(s, s') ds ds' < \infty$, and $K_t(s, s')$ is a self-adjoint Hilbert-Schmidt kernel

[2]. The kernel $K_t(s,s')$ thus has a spectral decomposition, and a greatest eigenvalue $\lambda_{max} \equiv \lambda_1$, so that the minimum possible variance for heating estimates is bounded as $\sigma_q^2 \geq \bar{I}_{11}^{-1} = \sigma_\varepsilon^2/(\sigma_\rho^2 \alpha_1^2 \lambda_1)$. As temperature is linearly related to the heating, this implies that the variance of a temperature estimate at given location $\mathbf{r}$ and time t is bounded as $\sigma_T^2(\mathbf{r},t) \geq c_T^2(\mathbf{r},t)\bar{I}_{11}^{-1}$, with $c_T(\mathbf{r},t) = \int_{t_a}^{\min(t,t_{exp})} \phi_1(t_0) g_{t|t_0}(\mathbf{r} \mid \mathbf{r}_{t_0}) dt_0$.

Thermal dose is defined over an interval (t_a, t_f) [6], and is related to the applied heating in an exponential manner, through temperature, as

$$TD(\mathbf{r}) = \int_{t_a}^{t_f} e^{\kappa(T_t(\mathbf{r}) - T_{ref})} dt \quad . \tag{9}$$

The theory of maximum likelihood estimation [4] states that the estimate $\hat{q}_1$ is asymptotically unbiased for the true parameter q_1, and normally distributed with variance $\bar{I}_{11}^{-1}$. With $c_{TD} = e^{-\kappa T_{ref}}$, the variance of thermal dose estimates has lower bound

$$\sigma_{TD}^2(\mathbf{r}) \geq \underbrace{\iint_{t_a}^{t_f} c_{TD}^2 e^{\kappa q_1(c_T(\mathbf{r},t) + c_T(\mathbf{r},t'))}}_{\text{minimize with small } q_1} e^{\frac{(c_T(\mathbf{r},t))^2 + (c_T(\mathbf{r},t'))^2}{2\bar{I}_{1,1}\kappa^{-2}}} \underbrace{\left(e^{\frac{2c_T(\mathbf{r},t)c_T(\mathbf{r},t')}{2\bar{I}_{1,1}\kappa^{-2}}} - 1 \right)}_{\text{minimize with large } \bar{I}_{1,1}} dt\,dt'. \tag{10}$$

RESULTS

The Green's function satisfying the bio-heat transfer equation in an infinite medium with thermometric conductivity χ and no perfusion is, with $U(t)$ the unit step function [3]:

$$\Gamma_{t|t_0}(\mathbf{r} \mid \mathbf{r}_0) = \frac{1}{8(\pi\chi(t - t_0))^{3/2}} e^{-\frac{|\mathbf{r} - \mathbf{r}_0|^2}{4\chi(t - t_0)}} U(t - t_0) \quad . \tag{11}$$

A Gaussian radiator [5] having beam pattern parameterized by aperture a, diffraction length $\ell_d = ka^2/2$ and focal length R_0, and drawing a linear track $\mathbf{r}_t = (h, 0, vt)$ is:

$$Q(\mathbf{r} - \mathbf{r}_t) = \left[\left(1 - \frac{y}{R_0}\right)^2 + \left(\frac{y}{\ell_d}\right)^2 \right]^{-1} e^{-\frac{2\left((x-h)^2 + (z-vt)^2\right)}{a^2} \frac{1}{\left(1 - \frac{y}{R_0}\right)^2 + \left(\frac{y}{\ell_d}\right)^2}} \quad . \tag{12}$$

A study is performed with focal length $R_0 = 3.5$ cm, HIFU frequency $f_0 = 3.5$ MHz, aperture $2a = 3.3$ cm, speed of sound $c_0 = 1,430$ m/s, diffraction length $\ell_d = \pi f_0 a^2/c_0 = 2.093$ m, $\alpha_1 = 0.0007$ /°C, $K = 128$ scanlines over a 2.2 cm scanhead, and $J = 1400$ samples per scanline. The thermometric conductivity is $\chi = 1.72 \times 10^{-7} \text{m}^2/\text{s}$.

Figure 2a shows lower bounds for the standard deviation of heating estimates as a function of wait time after treatment and for lesion lengths of 1, 2, 4, 8, or 16mm, drawn at $v = 2$mm/s. The lesion lies parallel to the scanhead, 20mm below, and is centered in the middle of the frame. Figure 2b depicts the bound for temperature estimates, obtained at points along the lesion at the moment of deposition, and Figure 2c shows the bounds for thermal dose estimates when the expected dose is 240 equivalent min at

$T_{ref} = 43°C$ and $T_0 = 37°C$. The lower variance associated with longer lesions reflects the contribution of more scanlines in forming the estimates. The figures also indicate that an acquisition delay of minutes after treatment still affords accurate inference, allowing frame capture at lower temperatures, for which Eq. (1) is more appropriate [1].

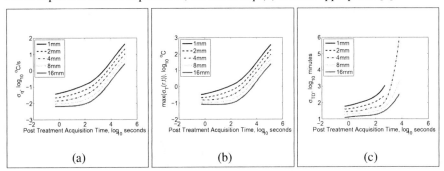

FIGURE 2. Lower bounds for linear scans of length 1, 2, 4, 8, or 16mm as a function of acquisition time, centered in frame at depth of 2cm. (a) Standard deviation of heating estimate. (b) Maximum standard deviation of temperature. (c) Standard deviation for thermal dose, for expected dose of 240 equivalent min.

ACKNOWLEDGEMENTS

This research was supported by NIH grant 5R01CA109557.

CONCLUSIONS

A method for characterizing the performance of treatment monitoring using diagnostic ultrasound is presented. From basic physical and statistical considerations, the accuracy of estimates is formulated from the parameters of the diagnostic ultrasound, the material properties, and the choice of protocol. Under the conditions studied, a thermal dose estimate near 240 equivalent minutes at 43°C can have accuracy to within tens of minutes. Similarly, temperature estimates with accuracy below 1°C are also possible.

REFERENCES

1. A. Anand *Noninvasive Temperature Estimation Technique for HIFU Therapy Monitoring Using Backscattered Ultrasound*, PhD Thesis, University of Washington, 2005.
2. J. P. Keener, *Principles of Applied Mathematics*, Addison Wessley, Reading, MA, 1988.
3. L. D. Landau, and E. M. Lifshitz, *Fluid Mechanics*, Elsavier, Burlington, MA, 2004.
4. E. L. Lehmann, and G. Cassella, *Theory of Point Estimation*, Springer, New York, NY, 1998.
5. B. K. Novikov, O. V. Rudenko, and V. I. Timoshenko, *Nonlinear Underwater Acoustics*, American Institute of Physics, New York, NY, 1987.
6. S. A. Sapareto, and W. C. Dewey, "Thermal Dose Determination in Cancer Therapy," *Int. J. Radiation Oncology Biol. Phys.*, Vol **10**, pp 787-800.
7. R. Seip, and E. S. Ebbini, "Non-invasive Estimation of Tissue Temperature Response to Heating Fields Using Diagnostic Ultrasound," *IEEE Trans Biomed Eng*, Vol. **42**, No. 8, August 1995, pp. 828-839.

Feasibility of Transient Image-guided Blood-Spinal Cord Barrier Disruption

Jeff Wachsmuth[a], Rajiv Chopra[a,b] and Kullervo Hynynen[a,b]

[a]Imaging Research, Sunnybrook Health Sciences Centre, 2075 Bayview Avenue,
Toronto, ON, Canada M4N3M5
[b]Medical Biophysics, University of Toronto, 610 University Avenue,
Toronto, ON, Canada, M5G2M9

Abstract. To evaluate the feasibility of disrupting the blood-spinal cord barrier (BSCB), 31 rats were exposed to focused 1.08 MHz ultrasound at electrical powers of 0.5W and 1.0W after injection of the ultrasound contrast agent Definity. T1-weighted images were acquired before and after ultrasound exposure using a 3T MRI and the MR contrast agent Gadovist. At 0.5 and 1.0W the average relative enhancements observed were $29.1 \pm 21\%$ and $57.5 \pm 34\%$ respectively. After recovery from ultrasound exposure, the rats did not show signs of motor impairment. The results demonstrate the feasibility of BSCB disruption using ultrasound together with ultrasound contrast agents. Further studies of this method are warranted.

Keywords: spinal cord, blood-spinal cord barrier disruption, preclinical, feasibility.
PACS: 87.14em, 87.15.rs, 87.19xr, 87.19um

INTRODUCTION

The blood-spinal cord barrier (BSCB) works in concert with the blood-brain barrier (BBB) to mediate the movement of substances between the blood and the central nervous system (CNS). Through a number of mechanisms such as endothelial cell tight junctions, the BSCB maintains the selective permeability of the spinal cord microvasculature, preventing a wide range of potentially harmful materials from accessing the spinal cord. While this makes the BSCB a valuable physiological asset, its presence renders the spinal cord relatively inaccessible to intravenous drug delivery methods [1] and therefore significantly increases the difficulty of chemically treating pathologies based in the spine

To our knowledge, no work on a physical means of controlled, targeted disruption of the BSCB has been reported to date, although significant attention has been paid to the BBB. Low-intensity pulsed ultrasound exposures applied in the presence of microbubbles have been shown to produce localized and transient disruption of the BBB [2-4]. Like the brain, the spine is readily accessible to microbubbles, suggesting that the same methodology used to for the BBB could be used to effect targeted disruption of the BSCB.

In the present study we investigated the use of MRI-guided focused ultrasound as a controlled and non-invasive means of disrupting the BSCB *in vivo* in a rat model. The capability of MRI to detect BSCB disruption was also evaluated.

CP1113, *8th International Symposium on Therapeutic Ultrasound*, edited by E. S. Ebbini
© 2009 American Institute of Physics 978-0-7354-0650-6/09/$25.00

METHODS

31 rats (Wistar, 300-500g) were exposed to focused ultrasound in a clinical 3T MRI in accordance with the guidelines of the local Animal Care Committee at Sunnybrook Health Sciences Centre. Animals were anesthetized using an IP injection of ketamine and xylazine. The animals were placed on a water tank in the path of an ultrasound beam such that the focus was coincident with the upper spine, as shown in Figure 1 below. After the exposures the rats were recovered and survived for 3 days to evaluate the impact of the ultrasound exposure on their motor function. Three rats were survived for three weeks, and were exposed weekly in approximately the same location in the spine.

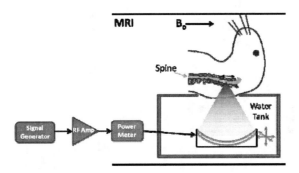

FIGURE 1. Experimental setup used for MRI-guided BSCB disruption experiments.

The ultrasound exposure consisted of 10ms bursts applied with a PRF of 1s. The ultrasound beam was produced with a frequency of 1.08MHz by a 7cm diameter transducer with a f-number of 0.8. Prior to the start of sonication, a bolus of ultrasound microbubbles (Definity, 0.043μl/kg) was administered, followed by a 0.5ml saline flush. The exposures were delivered in a linear raster scan comprised of 6 sonications each separated by 1mm, and the total exposure time was 300s. Electrical powers of 0.5 and 1.0W were applied in these experiments. MR imaging was performed in all animals to evaluate the location and extent of BSCB disruption. T1-weighted imaging was performed before and after the ultrasound exposure, and after injection of an MR contrast agent (Gadovist, 0.2mmol/kg). T2-weighted images were also acquired after each exposure to investigate the presence of tissue damage.

RESULTS

The typical appearance of BSCB disruption seen on T1-weighted MR images is shown below in Figure 2. A localized region of signal enhancement that extended over

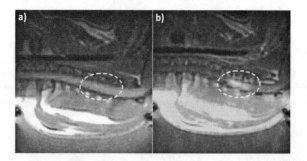

FIGURE 2. T1-weighted images acquired (a) before and (b) after ultrasound exposure of the upper spine. The region of BSCB disruption is shown in the region within the dotted circle. In these images the transducer was located below the animal and the ultrasound beam was approximately transverse to the spinal cord.

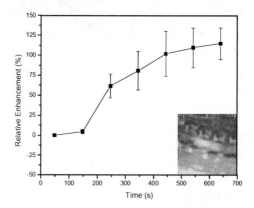

FIGURE 3. T1-weighted images acquired (a) before and (b) after ultrasound exposure of the upper spine. The region of BSCB disruption is shown in the region within the dotted circle

the 6mm region of exposure was observed for over 10 minutes in most animals. Figure 3 shows an example of the typical signal enhancement observed over time as the relative enhancement over the baseline value. There is a delay of approximately 2 minutes before an increase in signal enhancement is seen. The enhancement increases to what appears to be a plateau at about 10 minutes.

The average relative enhancement observed across the 31 animals exposed in this study was 29.1 ± 21% and 57.5 ± 34% at 0.5 and 1.0W respectively. The standard deviation represents the variation in enhancement observed between animals. The relative enhancement observed in this study is much larger than what has been observed in studies investigating BBB disruption, and the variability between animals is also higher.

Most rats showed normal motor function after recovering from the ultrasound exposures. Animals were able to move with all limbs without favouring any side, and were able to maintain balance when provided with mild challenges. This observation held even for the rats exposed weekly for three weeks. Approximately 5 rats did not recover properly from the exposures, but these animals were all from a single experimental day, and there were no signs (either MRI or histological) that indicated any significant spinal damage.

DISCUSSION

The preliminary results of this feasibility study were encouraging, with consistent enhancement observed in the spinal cord after focused ultrasound exposure in the presence of microbubbles. The magnitude of enhancement was significantly higher than that observed in similar exposures in the brain, however animals did not show signs of tissue damage on imaging, or impaired motor function after recovery. Variable enhancement was observed between rats and also among individual exposures, resulting in a large standard deviation in the relative signal enhancement. This was attributed to the effect of the bony vertebrae in the path of the ultrasound beam. The propagation of the acoustic wave is certainly affected by the presence of this bone, and so strategies to compensate for this effect are required.

CONCLUSIONS

Blood-spinal cord disruption is feasible using MRI-guided focused ultrasound in combination with ultrasound contrast agents, as observed previously in the brain. BSCB disruption was visualized using T1-weighted imaging on MRI, and rats did not show signs of impaired motor function after recovering from exposures. Further studies are warranted to better quantify the optimal exposures required to achieve BSCB disruption, and to verify the transient nature of this effect. Studies evaluating the capability of this method to delivery large molecular weight therapeutic agents to the spine are also necessary.

ACKNOWLEDGEMENTS

We would like to thank Shawna Rideout-Gros, Yuexi Huang, and Alex Garces for their technical assistance in performing these studies.

REFERENCES

1. H. S. Sharma, S. F. Ali, W. Dong, Z. R. Tian, R. Patnaik, S. Patnaik, A. Sharma, A. Boman, P. Lek, E. Seifert, and T. Lundsted, *Ann. N Y Acad. Sci.* **1122**, 197-218 (2007)
2. McDannold N, Vykhodtseva N, Hynynen K. *Ultrasound Med. Biol.* **33**, 584-590 (2007)
3. McDannold N, Vykhodtseva N, Hynynen K. *Ultrasound Med. Biol.* **34**, 930-937 (2008)
4. Vykhodtseva N, McDannold N, Hynynen K. *Ultrasonics* **48**, 279-296 (2008)

The Use of Susceptibility-Weighted Magnetic Resonance Imaging to Characterize the Safety Window of Focused Ultrasound Exposure for Localized Blood–Brain-Barrier Disruption

Hao-Li Liu[a,b], Po-Hong Hsu[a], Yau-Yau Wai[c], Jin-Chung Chen[d], Tzu-Chen Yen[b,e], and Jiun-Jie Wang[f]

[a]Department of Electrical Engineering, Chang-Gung University, Taiwan;
[b]Molecular Imaging Center, Chang-Gung Memorial Hospital, Linkou, Taiwan;
[c]Department of Diagnostic Radiology, Chang-Gung Memorial Hospital, Linkou, Taiwan;
[d]Department of Physiology and Pharmacology, Chang-Gung University, Taiwan;
[e]Departmemt of Nuclear Medicine, Chang-Gung Memorial Hospital, Linkou, Taiwan;
[f]Department of Medical Image and Radiological Sciences, Chang-Gung University, Taiwan.

Abstract. High-intensity focused ultrasound has been discovered to be able to locally and reversibly increase the permeability of the blood–brain barrier (BBB), which can be detected using magnetic resonance imaging (MRI). However, side effects such as microhemorrhage, erythrocyte extravasations, or even extensive hemorrhage can also occur. Although current contrast-enhanced T1-weighted MRI can be used to detect the changes in BBB permeability, its efficacy in detecting tissue hemorrhage after focused-ultrasound sonication remains limited. The purpose of this study was to determine the feasibility of using MR susceptibility-weighted imaging (SWI) to identify tissue hemorrhage associated with the process of BBB permeability increase and characterize the safety window of acoustic pressure level. Brains of 42 Sprague-Dawley rats were subjected to 107 sonications either unilaterally or bilaterally. Contrast-enhanced T1-weighted images, together with SWI were performed. Tissue damage and hemorrhage were analyzed histologically with light microscopy and staining by Evan's blue, HE staining as well as TUNEL staining. Our results showed that contrast-enhanced T1 weighted imaging is sensitive to the presence of the BBB disrupture, but was unable to differentiate from extensive tissue damage such as hemorrhage. Also, SWI proved to be a superior tool for the real-time monitoring of the presence of hemorrhage, which is essential to the clinical concerns. The safety operation window in vivo in our study indicated a pressure of 0.78 to 1.1 MPa. to increase the BBB permeability successfully without hemorrhage. Potential applications such as drug delivery in the brain might be benefited.

Keywords: Focused ultrasound, susceptibility-weighted imaging, blood–brain barrier, hemorrhage.
PACS: PACS 43.35.+d

CP1113, *8th International Symposium on Therapeutic Ultrasound*, edited by E. S. Ebbini
© 2009 American Institute of Physics 978-0-7354-0650-6/09/$25.00

INTRODUCTION

Focused ultrasound has been shown that the BBB may be transiently disrupted in the presence of microbubbles and the process may be monitored by means of contrast-enhanced magnetic resonance imaging [1], thereby opening a new era in central nervous system (CNS) drug delivery [2, 3]. However, that sonication used for focal BBB opening may result in erythrocyte extravasations and microhemorrhage, which is evidenced by observing from light microscopy [4] after conducting histological examination, but not directly monitored from in-vivo imaging. Contrast-enhanced T1-weighted MRI fails to detect possible hemorrhage caused by the focused ultrasound exposure, which makes the focused-ultrasound induced BBB disruption lacks of the in-vivo imaging tools for ultrasonic expose control and optimization. Therefore, there is a critical need to noninvasively monitor the occurrence of brain microhemorrhage in vivo during the focused-ultrasound induced BBB opening process. In this study, we intend to investigate the feasibility of using magnetic-resonance susceptibility-weighted imaging (MR-SWI) to in-vivo detect tissue hemorrhage associated with disruption of the BBB induced by focused ultrasound in a rat model, thereby utilizing for identify the safety window of ultrasonic exposure.

METHOD

A focused-ultrasound transducer (Imasonics, Besancon, France; diameter = 60 mm, radius of curvature = 80 mm, frequency = 1.5 MHz, electric-to-acoustic efficiency = 70%) was used to generate concentrated ultrasound energy. An arbitrary-function generator was used to generate the driving signal fed to a radio frequency power amplifier. For animal sonication, 42 adult male Sprague-Dawley rats were conducted with 107 sonication points either unilaterally or bilaterally of the brain. Craniotomy was performed prior to the ultrasound sonication to reduce distortion of the ultrasonic focal beam. A cranial window of approximately 1×1 cm^2 was fashioned using a high-speed drill. Skull defects were covered with saline-soaked gauze to prevent dehydration prior to the application of high-intensity focused ultrasound.

The animal brain sonications were conducted with the presence of an ultrasound microbubble (SonoVue, Bracco, Milan, Italy. SF6 coated with mean diameter = 2.0-5.0 μm), which was inject intravenously prior to sonications. Each bolus injection contains 0.025 mL/kg of microbubble mixed with 0.2 mL of saline then flushed by 0.2 mL heparin. In ultrasound energy delivery, burst-mode sonication was used (burst length = 10 ms, PRF = 1 Hz, sonication duration = 30 s). Negative peak pressure amplitudes ranging from 0.55 to 4.9 MPa was used.

All MRI images were acquired on a 3-T scanner. The contrast-enhanced T1-weighted imaging was acquired first (TR / TE = 534 /11 ms, slide thickness = 1.5 mm, 31 measurements with the contrast Magnevist® was inject bolus at the 16th measurement). The SWI imaging, which was modified from a heavy T2*-weighted gradient-recalled 3D-fast low-angle shot (FLASH) sequence with fully flow compensation in all three directions, was acquired following the T1-imaging (TR/TE/flip angle = 28 ms/20 ms/15 , slice thickness = 0.7 mm).

For histological examination, Evans blue was injected intravenously as a bolus immediately after sonication. BBB disruption was quantified according to the extravasations of the albumin-bound Evans blue dye injected immediately after MRI. Animals were sacrificed about 4 – 6 hours after sonication. Representative sections were stained by hematoxylin and eosin (H&E). Terminal deoxynucleotidyl transferase biotin-dUTP nick-end labeling (TUNEL) was used in selected slides to detect apoptotic neurons (ApopTag kit, Intergen, Purchase, NY).

RESULTS

Figure 1 shows typical MR images of rat brains after sonication with focused ultrasound applied in burst mode. The peak pressure of sonication was 1.9 MPa. Non-enhanced T1-weighted images is shown in Fig. 2(a). The presence of local hemorrhage in the same brain hemisphere was confirmed by frozen sections examination was shown in Fig. 2(b), and the corresponding SWI imaging is shown in Fi.g 2(c). It can be seen that the hemorrhage core occurred from brain section can be also identified from the SWI imaging.

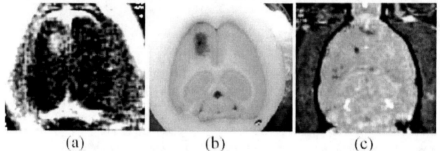

(a)   (b)   (c)

FIGURE 1. A typical example showing the comparison between contrast-enhanced T1-weithed imaging (a), coregistered brain section (b), and the coregistered SWI (c). Ultrasonic peak pressure of 1.9 MPa was employed in this case.

Figure 2 shows the SWI (upper row) and histology (lower row) patterns of local hemorrhage for different peak pressure levels (range: 0.78 – 2.45 MPa). The observed blue stains were due to local increase in BBB permeability, as evidenced by Evans blue leakage into the brain parenchyma. For peak pressure greater than or equal to 1.9 MPa, decreases in the SI are in keeping with the hemorrhage findings from Evans blue-stained slices (regions in red in Fig. 2(b) and 2(c)). The severity of hemorrhage increased proportionally with increasing electric power. However, the results at 0.78 – 1.1 MPa showed that an increased BBB permeability can be obtained without induction of cerebral hemorrhage. Further increases in pressure level lead to obvious hemorrhage detectable both by SWI and histology. In this regard, SWI images and histology findings showed a high degree of correlation.

We then plotted the occurrence and the severity of cerebral hemorrhage according to increasing peak acoustic pressure (Figure 3). The prevalence of intact brain (defined as "safe") decreased linearly with increasing peak pressure level. On the other hand, the percentage of mild (defined as "RBC extravasations") or severe (defined as "hemorrhage") increased proportionally to the peak pressure level. No increase in BBB permeability was detected with peak pressure below 0.78 MPa. However, RBC extravasations could be detected incidentally. Mild hemorrhage occurred in ~ 20% of cases with peak pressure of 0.78 – 1.1 MPa. Hemorrhage level became apparent with a peak pressure exceeding 1.9 MPa. Neuronal apoptosis as detected by TUNEL staining was evident with a peak pressure exceeding 2.45 MPa. The safety window of ultrasonic exposure for BBB disruption under this configuration was therefore considered to be 0.78 – 1.1 MPa from histological examination.

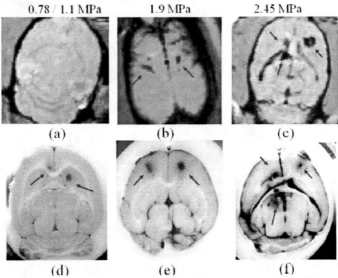

FIGURE 2. SWI images (upper row) and histology findings (lower row) according to different focused-ultrasound powers. Peak pressures used were as follows: 0.78 / 1.1 MPa (a, d), 1.9 MPa (b, e), and 2.45 MPa (c, f).

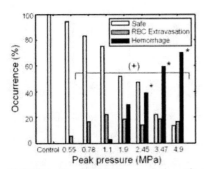

FIGURE 3. Statistical Analysis of the hemorrhage occurrence under different pressure levels (The level of RBC extravasations was considered to be mild and safe, and the level of hemorrhage were regarded as severe and unacceptable). Opening of BBB is labeled as (+).

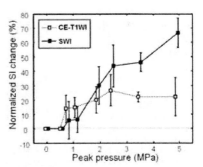

FIGURE 4. Normalized Signal Intensity curves (Mean ± S.D. are shown) for the contrast-enhanced T1-weighted images (dashed) and susceptibility weighted images (solid) under different applied peak pressures.

263

Detected cell apoptosis as assessed by the TUNEL assay is labeled as "*".

The normalized absolute SI changes for contrast-enhanced T1-weighted images (dashed) and susceptibility weighted images (solid) at sonication sites were plotted against the applied peak pressure (Fig. 4). In contrast-enhanced T1-weighted imaging analysis, the SI changes are statistically significant in difference with control when the peak pressure reached 0.78 MPa. The average SI change in the T1 weighted images was approximately 15% for 0.78 – 1.1 MPa. It subsequently reached a plateau of about 20% by application of higher pressures. In SWI analysis, the SI changes are statistically significant in difference with control when the peak pressure reached 1.9 MPa. Absolute SI changes in SWI were minimal between 0.78 – 1.1 MPa, with no apparent hemorrhage occurred. The safety window of ultrasonic exposure for BBB disruption found from in-vivo imaging also ranges from 0.78 to 1.1 MPa and matches the finding from histological examination shown above.

DISCUSSION AND CONCLUSION

Contrast-enhanced T1-weighted turbo-spin-echo imaging with bolus Gd-DTPA injection was used in this study to detect the focused ultrasound-induced BBB disruption. A monotonic increase in the averaged SI was evident with increasing peak pressure in the 0.78 – 2.45 MPa range. This finding is in keeping with previous found threshold pressure in rabbit experiments [1] and in rat experiments [4].

In conclusion, conventional contrast enhanced T1-weighted imaging serves as a reliable tool for detecting BBB disruption whereas MR-SWI. has the potential to be a complementary for brain tissue damage. In our case, a relatively safe window to induce BBB disruption with only few erythrocyte extravasations ranged between 0.78 – 1.1 MPa.

ACKNOWLEDGMENTS

This work was supported by grants from the National Science Council, Taiwan (94-2262-E-182-008-CC3) and the Chang-Gung Memorial Hospital (CMRPD34022 and CMRPD260041).

REFERENCES

1 K. Hynynen, N. McDannold, N. Vykhodtseva and F. A. Jolesz. Noninvasive MR imaging-guided focal opening of the blood-brain barrier in rabbits. *Radiology* **220**, 640-6 (2001).
2 N. D. Doolittle, M. E. Miner, W. A. Hall, T. Siegal, E. Jerome, E. Osztie, L. D. McAllister, J. S. Bubalo, D. F. Kraemer, D. Fortin, R. Nixon, L. L. Muldoon and E. A. Neuwelt. Safety and efficacy of a multicenter study using intraarterial chemotherapy in conjunction with osmotic opening of the blood-brain barrier for the treatment of patients with malignant brain tumors. *Cancer* **88**, 637-47 (2000).
3 W. M. Pardridge. Targeting neurotherapeutic agents through the blood-brain barrier. *Arch Neurol* **59**, 35-40 (2002).
4 L. H. Treat, N. McDannold, N. Vykhodtseva, Y. Zhang, K. Tam and K. Hynynen. Targeted delivery of doxorubicin to the rat brain at therapeutic levels using MRI-guided focused ultrasound. *Int J Cancer* **121**, 901-7 (2007).

The Feasibility of Integrating Elastography Measurements into MRI-Guided Transurethral Ultrasound Therapy

Arvin Arani[a], Yuexi Huang[b], Michael Bronskill[a,b], Rajiv Chopra[a,b]

[a]Department of Medical Biophysics, University of Toronto, Toronto, Ontario, Canada

[b]Rm C713, Imaging Research, Sunnybrook Health Sciences Centre, 2075 Bayview Avenue, Toronto, Ontario, M4N 3M5, Canada

Abstract. MRI-guided transurethral ultrasound therapy is being developed as a minimally invasive treatment for localized prostate cancer. The capability to identify target regions prior to therapy would provide an integrated diagnostic and therapeutic solution to the management of this disease. The objective of this project is to evaluate the feasibility of performing elastography using a transurethral actuator. Shear waves were generated in the prostate by vibrating the transurethral actuator longitudinally and resolving the tissue displacements with a 1.5 Tesla MRI. A piezoelectric actuator was used to vibrate the transurethral device with an amplitude of 32um at frequencies of 100 and 250Hz. GRE imaging sequences with displacement encoded along the direction of vibration were acquired transverse and parallel to the rod to visualize the dynamics of wave propagation. Experiments were performed in phantoms (8% gelatin) and in a canine model (n=5). Vibration was achieved in the MRI without significant loss of SNR in the images. The shear waves produced in the gel were cylindrical in nature, and extended along the length of the rod. Shear wave propagation in the canine prostate gland was observed at 100 and 250Hz, and shear modulus values agreed with previously published values.

Keywords: MR elastography, transurethral, prostate imaging, MRI, feasibility, Prostate Cancer

PACS: 87.19.rd, 81.40.Jj, 83.60.Uv

INTRODUCTION

MRI-guided transurethral ultrasound therapy is being developed as a minimally invasive treatment for localized prostate cancer. By combining the rotation of a multi-element ultrasound heating applicator with continuous MRI temperature feedback, a precise pattern of thermal damage can be generated in the prostate gland (Fig. 1). It would be desirable to have a rapid imaging technique capable of targeting cancer within the prostate immediately prior to therapy. The unique feature of this treatment with a transurethral device offers possibilities to explore elastographic imaging with MRI. MR elastography is an imaging technique that is capable of characterizing tissues with respect to their mechanical properties and could take advantage of the known changes in tissue stiffness associated with prostate cancer. Elastography may potentially be used to detect focal regions of stiffness in the prostate and evaluate and measure regions of coagulated tissue from thermal therapy.

CP1113, *8th International Symposium on Therapeutic Ultrasound*, edited by E. S. Ebbini
© 2009 American Institute of Physics 978-0-7354-0650-6/09/$25.00

Successful application of this technique could lead to a powerful integrated diagnostic and therapeutic tool.

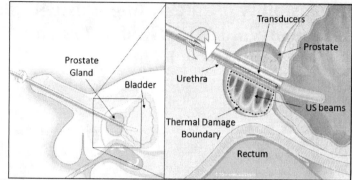

FIGURE 1. Conceptual illustration of MRI-guided transurethral ultrasound therapy device. (Image courtesy of Rajiv Chopra)

MRE is composed of two key components; namely, the creation of vibration in tissue, and the measurement of the tissue displacement with magnetic resonance (MR). The measured tissue displacement is related to tissue stiffness. Conventional approaches of prostate elastography rely on external actuators to create shear waves in the prostate gland. External approaches are only able to reach the prostate using low frequencies because of shear wave attenuation and obstructions in the path of the propagating waves. Unfortunately, low frequency shear waves result in long wavelengths, which correspond to lower resolution stiffness maps.

By utilizing the transurethral device as an actuator and generating shear waves directly in the prostate some limitations due to distance can be overcome. Previous work in which a needle was inserted into gels and used as an actuator for MRE was incorporated and the concept was applied to the transurethral probe [1] (fig. 2). Therefore, the objective of this study was to evaluate the technical feasibility of using a transurethral device to generate shear waves in the prostate gland for MRE.

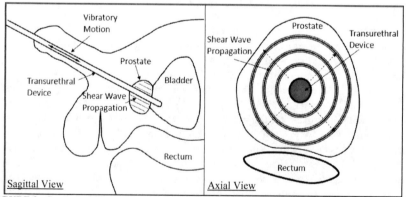

FIGURE 2. Conceptual illustration of transurethral MRE actuation.(Image courtesy of Rajiv Chopra)

METHODS

The technical feasibility of transurethral MRE was investigated in 8% gelatin from porcine skin (~300 bloom) and *in vivo* in a canine model (n=5).

Gelatin Experiments

The gelatin was poured into a 10cm x 10cm x 10cm box and a ¼ inch diameter brass rod was placed through the center of the box. A non-magnetic piezoceramic actuator (Physik Instruments, Germany) with maximum peak-to-peak displacement of 32 microns was used to cause the longitudinal vibration of the brass rod (fig.3).

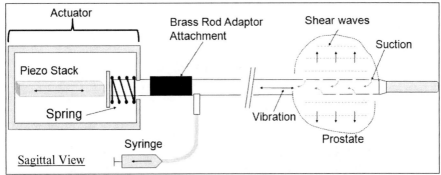

FIGURE 3. *In vivo* experimental setup including suctioning mechanism.

Imaging was performed on a 1.5T MRI (Signa, GE Healthcare), using a standard head coil. A fast GRE imaging sequence was used with a matrix size of 256x256, a field of view of 20 cm, TR = 100ms, TE = 30ms, a flip angle of 30 degrees, 1 to 3 bipolar gradients, and oscillation frequencies between 100 and 250 Hz. Images of the wave motion were acquired transverse and parallel to the rod to visualize the propagation of shear waves around the rod.

In Vivo Canine Experiments

An acute study was performed in five dogs to test the feasibility of transurethral MRE *in vivo*. Due to the anatomical differences between the urethra of canines and humans, a perineal urethrostomy procedure was needed to permit the insertion of the rigid transurethral applicator into the prostatic urethra. To accommodate for some expected differences *in vivo* and to maximize energy transfer between the actuator and the tissue, gentle suction was applied at the tip of the rod (fig.3). Imaging was performed using a 4 channel surface coil, a matrix size of 256x256, a field of view of 16 cm, TR = 100ms, TE = 30ms, a flip angle of 30 degrees, 1 to 3 bipolar gradients, 8 phase offsets, and oscillation frequencies of 100 and 250 Hz. Images were acquired transverse to and along the rod as in the gel experiments to visualize wave propagation.

Stiffness Maps (Elastograms)

Displacement images were converted to stiffness maps or elastograms using the publicly available 'MREwave' program developed by Ehman et al. at the Mayo Clinic in Rochester, Minnesota. The program utilizes a local frequency estimation algorithm to calculate shear modulus on a pixel-by-pixel basis [2].

RESULTS AND DISCUSSION

Wave images of the propagating shear waves perpendicular and parallel to the axis of the rod are shown in Fig.4a and Fig. 4b for the 8% gelatin experiments. The oscillation frequency was 150 Hz and displacements were on the order of 10 microns. Cylindrical radial propagating shear waves were measured throughout the gel, as anticipated. The corresponding stiffness maps for the perpendicular and parallel orientated wave images are shown in Fig. 4c and Fig. 4d, respectively.

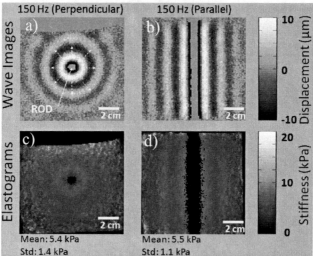

FIGURE 4. Wave images transverse (a) and perpendicular (b) to the rod in the gel experiments. The corresponding elastograms shown in (c) and (d) give consistent results.

The mean stiffness (± std.) of the transverse and parallel images was found to be 5.4±1.4 kPa and 5.5±1.1 kPa, respectively. The mean stiffness in both orientations agreed with one another, well within one standard deviation.

Oscillation frequencies of 100 Hz and 250 Hz were tested *in vivo*. Due to the low amplitudes of the piezocermic actuator, only 100 Hz waves could make it all the way out to the walls of the prostate. Fig. 5a shows the axial magnitude image of the *in vivo* experiments at 100 Hz. The corresponding elastogram is shown in Fig. 5b and each frame of the wave propagation is shown in Fig. 5c. At 100 Hz, even with a low amplitude actuator, cylindrical waves could be measured throughout the entire prostate. The mean shear prostate stiffness ± std. was 5.2±1.5 kPa and 5.7±1.9 kPa for

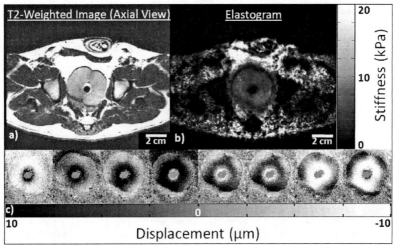

FIGURE 5. a) Axial T2-weighted image of canine pelvis. b) Corresponding MR elastogram. c) 8 frames of the 100 Hz *in vivo* wave propagation measured in the prostate.

the two dogs where 100 Hz data was obtained. These values are in the same range as previous data obtained in *ex vivo* human prostates [3] (4-6 kPa at 100 Hz) and *in vivo* human prostate data [4] (3.5-5 kPa at 65 Hz).

CONCLUSION

An integrated diagnostic and therapeutic applicator could prove to be a powerful tool in managing prostate cancer. Transurethral MRE has shown to be technically feasible for generating shear waves throughout the prostate and obtaining shear wave measurements that were consistent with literature. Further investigation is warranted for determining the diagnostic feasibility of transurethral MRE.

ACKNOWLEDGMENTS

This research was supported by the Prostate Cancer Research Foundation of Canada and the Ontario Graduate Scholarship for Science and Technology. The authors would like to thank Dr. Donald Plewes, Anthony Chau, Shawna Rideout-Gros, and Alex Garces for their technical support and valuable discussions.

REFERENCES

1. Chan, Q.C., Li. G., Ehman, R.L., Grimm, R.C., Li, R., Yang, E.S., *Magn.Reson.Med* **55**, 1175-1179 (2006).
2. A. Manduca, R. Muthupillai, P.J. Rossman, J.F. Greenleaf, R.L. Ehman, *SPIE* **2710**, 616-623 (1996)
3. R. Sinkus, T. Nisius, J.Lorenzen, J. Kemper, M. Dargatz, "In-Vivo Prostate Elastography", Proc. Intl. Soc. Mag. Reson. Med. 11 (2003).
4. M. A. Dresner, P.J. Rossman, S. A. Kruse, R.L. Ehman, "MR Elastography of Prostate", Proc. Intl. Soc. Mag. Reson. Med. 7 (1999).

Detection of HIFU lesions in Excised Tissue Using Acousto-Optic Imaging

Andrew Draudt, Puxiang Lai, Ronald A. Roy, Todd W. Murray, and Robin O. Cleveland

Dept. of Mechanical Engineering, Boston University, Boston, MA 02215

Abstract. Real-time imaging of the heating of tissue and lesion formation is a major barrier to the clinical application of HIFU. Tissue necrosis results in a change in the optical properties of the tissue. We have employed the acousto-optical (A-O) interaction to image HIFU lesions formed in excised chicken breast. The tissue was illuminated with infrared light (1064 nm wavelength) resulting in a diffuse optical field throughout the tissue. Simultaneously, the tissue was insonified with a diagnostic ultrasound imager running in B-mode. The photons that passed through the region of tissue where the pulsed 5 MHz ultrasound beam was present were phase modulated by the sound field. These modulated photons were detected by means of an interferometric detector employing a photorefractive crystal (PRC). To first order the amplitude of the output from the PRC is related to the optical absorption of the tissue where the sound was present. By firing multiple acoustic beams along different pathways, the spatially dependent optical absorption coefficient (uncalibrated) within a tissue region of interest is determined and presented in the form of a 2-D image. Images thus generated were recorded in chicken breast before and after HIFU exposure (1.1 MHz, 6 s duration, 6 MPa peak pressure). The acoustic and optical beams were scanned across the tissue, and the waveforms combined to form a 2-D AO image. The imaged lesion size of 9 x 2 mm^2 agreed well with the measured lesions size 10 x 3 mm^2.

Keywords: HIFU, lesion detection, Acousto-Optic Imaging
PACS: 43.35.Sx, 43.80.Sh, 78.20.Hp

INTRODUCTION

HIFU-induced tissue lesions show significant optical contrast with untreated tissue. The lesioned tissue has higher optical absorption and scattering [1]. Direct optical imaging of lesions generated at depth is impossible, however, due to the high level of scattering in the intervening tissue. Acousto-optic imaging provides a way to resolve optical contrast within structures with a spatial resolution equal to that of B-mode ultrasound [2]. Acoustic waves induce perturbations in density (and hence in optical index of refraction) as well as periodic translations of optical scattering sites Photons, whose diffuse random-walk passes through the ultrasound focal zone, will have their paths altered from what they would have been had the acoustic disturbance not been there, resulting in a periodic modulation in phase at the acoustic frequency. If these "tagged" photons can be monitored, then any changes in the tissue optical properties at the focal zone can be sensed and ultimately imaged.

The light emitted from a highly scattering media contains multiple speckle caused by interference of light propagating through different paths in the sample. The phase modulation induced by the interaction of ultrasound and light produces an intensity

CP1113, *8th International Symposium on Therapeutic Ultrasound*, edited by E. S. Ebbini modulation of the individual speckle, but this intensity modulation has a random phase across the speckle field. Early schemes for detecting tagged photons involved monitoring the intensity modulation in a single speckle [3]. The sensitivity of detection was later significantly improved by detecting multiple speckles using a CCD camera and summing the intensity modulation measured at each pixel [4] More recently, the detection of of the phase modulated signal using photorefractive crystal based interferometers has been demonstrated [5,6]. This approach allows for the use of a single photodetector and is thus not limited in light collection by the number of pixels on a CCD camera. In this work we apply the PRC-based detection scheme to the problem of detecting HIFU-induced lesions in tissue.

METHODS

Figure 1 depicts the experimental setup. The light source is a 700 mW Nd-YAG laser operating at 1064 nm (IRCL-700-1064-S, CrystaLaser, CA). The light passes through the sample and is collected by a lens and focused onto a GaAs photorefractive crystal (PRC) (MolTech GmbH). A beam-splitter is used to create a reference beam that does not pass through the sample and also illuminates the PRC creating an interference pattern in the PRC. Through the photorefractive effect, the local optical index of refraction changes as a function of the local optical intensity. The 3-D diffraction grating set up in the crystal diffracts the reference beam into a direction parallel to the signal beam, and with the same complex wavefront. These two beams coincide at the photodetector, and constructively interfere. When a perturbation (e.g, due to an ultrasound beam) changes the path of photons which pass through it, the wavefront of the signal beam will change. The signal and reference beams will no longer constructively interfere at the photodetector, and there will be a drop in the output.

Here the pulsed ultrasound field was created using a diagnostic ultrasound array transducer (Model 8802, BK Medical, Wilmington, MA). The scan-head was driven by an Analogic Ultrasound Engine (AN 2300, Analogic, Peabody, MA). The ultrasound system created 5 MHz pulsed ultrasound which had a nominal spatial extent of 1.5mm in the acoustic propagation axis (z-axis in Fig. 1) and 0.8mm in the lateral direction. As an ultrasonic pulse traverses the tissue that is illuminated, the flux of modulated photons increases resulting in an increasing negative voltage from the photodetector The profile of the A-O signal essentially tracks the local intensity of the illuminated region (typically Gaussian). If the pulse traverses a sub-region of higher optical absorption, such as a HIFU lesion, there will be less local photons available to "tag". This will diminish the AOI signal, and result in a blip in the overall decrease in photodetector output, giving it a characteristic "W" shape [5]. The ultrasound array is electronically steerable and by firing a sequence of acoustic pulses in different directions it is possible to create a 2D image of the AOI data. However for this study, restrictions in the set-up meant that the multiple lines were achieved by mechanical translating the sample.

In the experiments reported here the tissue sample consisted of store-bought chicken breast, cut into a 4 cm x 4 cm x 2 cm sample and then degassed for 40 min. in phosphate buffered saline (PBS). It was then transferred and mounted in the experimental tank, all under PBS. Before HIFU treatment the sample was imaged with AOI. To obtain sufficient signal-to-noise ratio it was necessary to average the AO signals for 10^4 acoustic pulses, however we believe that this figure can be significantly reduced by using long-pulsed lasers [7] and a more optimal wavelength. The sample was also imaged with the ultrasound scanner in standard B-mode.

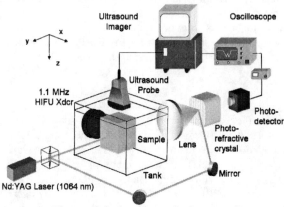

Figure 1. Experimental setup. The sample is placed in a tank of water to allow acoustic coupling of the HIFU transducer and ultrasound probe. The light passes through optically transparent walls into and out of the tank.

Single HIFU lesions were made in the center of the tissue sample, along the x-axis in Fig. 1. The lesions were made with a 1.1 MHz transducer (Model H-102, Sonic Concepts, 73 mm diam., 64 mm focal length,). The source was driven continuously for 6 s and pressure measurements in water yielded p+ = 6 MPa, p- = 4.32 MPa and I_{SPTA} = 880 W/cm^2. The depth of the HIFU focus into the tissue was 16 mm. After HIFU treatment the sample was re-imaged with AO and B-mode ultrasound.

RESULTS

Figure 2 shows time waveforms from the photodetector for a scan line through the center of a lesion. The width of the pre-lesion AOI dip, shown in Fig. 2(a), is 5 μs which, based on the speed of sound in the tissue, corresponds to a physical distance of 7.7 mm. This is the optically illuminated region and comprises the effective field of view of our current AO setup. Fig. 2(b) is the post-lesion waveform, showing a central region where the AOI effect is less. The width of the central blip is proportional to the width of the lesion region of increased optical absorptivity. By subtracting the two waveforms the resulting trace, Fig. 2(c), is essentially a 1-D line plot of the optical property contrast through the lesion. A 2-D image can be constructed by stacking the individual lines scanned across the sample (just as is done to create a B-mode ultrasound image). The result is an optical image of the interior of a diffuse medium, with a resolution determined by spatial extent of the acoustic pulse (typically of order 1 mm).

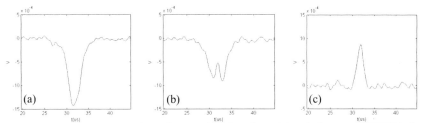

Figure 2. Photodetector waveforms for acoustic pulses directed though the center of HIFU lesion in chicken. (a) pre-lesion, (b) post-lesion, (c) difference.

Figure 3 shows the resulting image for one lesion. The white dotted line shows the location of the HIFU focal region, as determined by -6 dB pressure contours. The AO image indicates that the lesion "grew" toward the HIFU source—a phenomenon commonly reported in the literature. Shown at right is a B-mode image taken of the same sample, within five minutes post sonication. The dashed line indicates the region of the AOI image at left, and a similar oval marks the focal region. No evidence of the lesion can be seen, consistent with the known difficulty in detecting HIFU lesions with standard ultrasonic imaging. Any gas bubbles that may have been created during the HIFU insonation have dissolved by the time the B-mode image was taken.

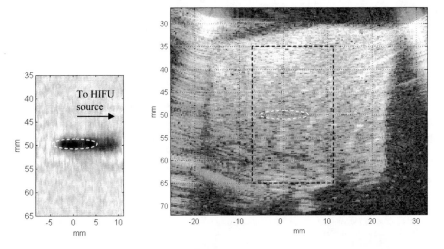

Figure 3. Left: AOI image of HIFU lesion in chicken breast. The HIFU focal zone is shown by the white dashed oval. The tissue was scanned in increments of 1/3 mm in the horizontal dimension. Right: A standard B-mode ultrasound image of the same tissue where the dashed rectangle represents the area of the AOI image shown at left. The lesion was not visible in the B-mode image.

The experiment was repeated on three separate chicken breasts. After AO imaging a "post-mortem" measurement was made by partially freezing the chicken samples, cutting them into 2 mm slices with a razor blade, and observing where the lesion occurred. For the three lesions the AOI measurements yielded lengths of 9, 14 and

273

8 mm and the "post-mortem" measurements 10, 17 and 9 mm. The location of the start of the lesion was within 1 mm for the two methods. The agreement between the AO and the measured properties of the lesion, both the position and length, are within the uncertainty of the measurements.

CONCLUSION

We have shown that HIFU lesions in ex-vivo chicken breast can be detected using AO imaging. The imaging technique exploited the changes in the optical properties of the lesions and the resolution was governed by the ultrasonic B-mode imaging (~1 mm). These lesions were invisible in standard B-mode images, due to the absence of the persistent gas bubbles typically produced by cavitation or boiling. For these experiments a 57-line scan took 40 minutes, the speed being limited by signal to noise ratio. Recently Rousseau et al. [7] greatly increased the speed of AO imaging by using a high power pulsed laser source, which increased the optical intensity without exceeding the maximum permissible exposure. They were able to use AO imaging to depths of 6 cm.

We note that in addition to post-treatment imaging described here, continuous monitoring of lesion growth during HIFU is possible. In this case the acoustic field of the HIFU transducer would be used to excite the AO signal. Because HIFU uses long tone bursts rather than pulses the temporal resolution (vertical axis in Fig. 3) is forfeited. As the tissue starts to form a lesion, the increase in both the acoustic and the optical absorption will cause a decrease in the magnitude of the AOI signal, providing real time feedback on the formation of lesions in tissue.

ACKNOWLEDGMENTS

This work was supported in part by Gordon-CenSSIS, the Bernard M. Gordon Center for Subsurface Sensing and Imaging Systems, under the Engineering Research Centers Program of the National Science Foundation (Award Number EEC-9986821).

REFERENCES

1. T.D. Khokhlova, I.M. Pelivanov, O.A. Sapozhnikov, V.S. Solomatin, A.A. Karabutov. Opto-Acoustic Diagnostics Of The Thermal Action Of High-Intensity Focused Ultrasound On Biological Tissues:The Possibility Of Its Applications And Model Experiments. Quantum Electronics 36 (12) 1097-1102 (2006)
2. Bossy E, Sui L, Murray T, Roy R. Fusion Of Conventional Ultrasound Imaging and Acousto-Optic Sensing by Use of a Standard Pulsed-Ultrasound Scanner. Optics Letters 30 (7) p.774 (2005)
3. Dolfi D, Micheron F. Imaging process and system for transillumination with photon frequency marking, International Patent WO 89/00278, (1989)
4. Leveque S, Boccara A, Lebec M, Saint-Jalmes H. Ultrasonic tagging of photon paths in scattering media: parallel speckle modulation processing. Optics Letters 24 181-183 (1999)
5. Murray T, Sui L, Maguluri G, Roy R, Blonigen F, Nieva A, DiMarzio C. Detection of ultrasound modulated photons in diffuse media using the photorefractive effect Optics Letters 29 2509-2511 (2004).
6. F Ramaz, B Forget, M Atlan, A Boccara. Photorefractive Detection Of Tagged Photons In Ultrasound Modulated Optical Tomography Of Thick Biological Tissues Optics Express 12 5469 (2004)
7. Rousseau G, Blouin A, Monchalin J, Ultrasound-modulated Optical Imaging Using A Powerful Long Pulse Laser Optics Express 16(17) p.12577 (2008)

Optimization of Encoding Gradients for Magnetic Resonance Acoustic Radiation Force Imaging

Jing Chen[a,b], Ron Watkins[b] and Kim Butts Pauly[b]

[a]Department of Electrical Engineering
[b]Department of Radiology, Stanford University, Stanford, CA 94305, USA

Abstract. For HIFU treatments without significant heating, MR monitoring could be done by imaging the acoustic radiation force (MR-ARFI). MR-ARFI used motion-sensitizing gradients to encode the small displacement induced by the acoustic radiation force into the phase of the image. Unfortunately, large conventional gradients render the image sensitive to motion, and susceptible to artifacts, which are seen as a non-linear background phase and can be larger than the displacement-induced phase. In this work, MR-ARFI encoding gradients are optimized to minimize these problems. The proposed repeated bipolar gradients are robust against motion and eddy current, and the SNR is significantly enhanced at no cost of scan time or encoding sensitivity.

Keywords: magnetic resonance imaging, acoustic radiation force imaging
PACS: 87.50.yk, 87.61.Tg

INTRODUCTION

MR-guided high intensity focused ultrasound (HIFU) is promising for a variety of therapeutic applications including tumor ablation and targeted drug delivery (1). For tumor ablation, HIFU is used in "thermal mode" (high duty cycle). For targeted drug delivery, HIFU is used in "mechanical mode" with higher power pulses and a low duty cycle. This allows for a mechanical interaction with tissue, the blood brain barrier, or circulating liposomes, without significant tissue heating.

Instead of imaging tissue temperature, MR monitoring may be done by measuring displacements caused by the acoustic radiation force. This is referred to as MR acoustic radiation force imaging (MR-ARFI). MR-ARFI provides a way to monitor HIFU treatment in the mechanical mode, where temperature change is insignificant. For applications in the thermal mode, it is also potentially useful for tracking the focal spot before any heating damage.

However, conventional MR-ARFI uses a pair of Stejskal Tanner gradients to encode displacement into the phase of the image. Since the displacement is small (on the order of microns), it is necessary to use either averaging (2) or large motion sensitizing gradients (3). Unfortunately, large Stejskal Tanner gradients may render the image susceptible to eddy currents and signal loss from diffusion. The purpose of this work was to optimize the encoding gradient configurations to improve the accuracy and precision of MR-ARFI.

CP1113, *8th International Symposium on Therapeutic Ultrasound*, edited by E. S. Ebbini
© 2009 American Institute of Physics 978-0-7354-0650-6/09/$25.00

METHODS

Imaging was performed with a line scan (4) sequence (TR/TE=500/69 ms, FOV=24×3 cm, matrix size=256×31, slice thickness=5 mm, bandwidth=7.81 kHz, nex=5) on a 3T GE Signa MR scanner equipped with an MR-compatible HIFU system (InSightec, Israel). The Stejskal Tanner gradients will be referred to as the unipolars in this work, and compared to two new encoding gradient designs: the repeated bipolars and the inverted bipolars, and shown in Fig. 1. The maximum gradient amplitude (4G/cm) was used for all three sets.

The HIFU system was triggered by the MR sequence to emit ultrasound pulses (80W electrical power) synchronized with the encoding gradients, the timing of which is given by dotted lines in Fig. 1. For the unipolars, the sonication completely overlapped with one of the unipolars, such that the tissue will be at two different positions during the two unipolars due to the radiation force, and the difference can be recorded in the image phase. The sonication of the repeated bipolars was a little bit longer than the one of the unipolars, and for the inverted bipolars, the sonication was separated into two shots. But the total effective motion encoding time was kept to 18 ms, with the same encoding sensitivity for all three sets. The 1.0 MHz HIFU transducer array was focused at a depth of 12 cm in a gel phantom, with an ultrasound duty cycle of less than 5%. To obtain the baseline phase map, images were acquired without the application of the ultrasound.

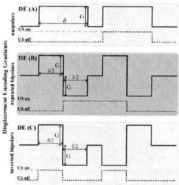

FIGURE 1. Three encoding gradient sets were compared, (A) conventional unipolars, (B) repeated bipolars and (C) inverted bipolars. Each of the bipolars was fully balanced by itself. The sonication was synchronized with the encoding gradients, with different timing for different sets. But the encoding sensitivity is the same for all three gradient sets.

To reconstruct the displacement map, images were scanned in pairs with identical sonication timing but opposite polarity of the encoding gradients. For each pair, the phase difference was calculated and then corrected by a two-step algorithm. In step one, a linear regression was performed outside the focal spot for each line along the readout direction, then the resulting constant and linear phase terms were removed from the whole line. In step two, the 3 baseline phase maps of gradient set (A), (B) and (C) were examined and subtracted from the corresponding step one output. After the two steps, the residual phase is proportional to the radiation force induced displacement with sensitivity of 2.6 µm/radian using the imaging parameters above.

RESULTS

The baseline phase maps acquired with the three gradient sets are shown in Fig. 2 (a). A nonlinear background phase was observed when the unipolar gradients were used, as shown in Fig.2 (a). This agrees with results from other groups (3), and was removed by step two of the reconstruction. This background phase was greatly reduced by replacing the unipolars with the bipolar gradients, especially with the repeated bipolars. As demonstrated in Fig.2 (a), a background phase correction was no longer required with the repeated bipolars.

For the fairness of the comparison, all three displacement maps in Fig.2 (b) were corrected for the background phase by reconstruction step two. The center of the focal spot was measured to have a displacement of ~0.4 µm by all 3 encoding gradients, but the bipolar gradients offered an enhanced signal to noise ratio (SNR) of the displacement map, as demonstrated in Fig.2 (b). This enhancement was contributed by the decreased diffusion-weighting of the bipolars. The b value of the unipolars was about 1200 s/mm^2, reduced to around 300 s/mm^2 by the bipolars. Since the repeated bipolars didn't need the background phase subtraction as in the reconstruction step two, the SNR could be further improved by $\sqrt{2}$.

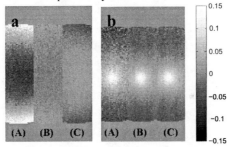

FIGURE 2. The baseline image (a) and the displacement map (b) acquired with the three encoding gradient sets, (A) conventional unipolars, (B) repeated bipolars and (C) inverted bipolars. The display range for both images is -0.15 to 0.15 radians, equal to -0.39 to 0.39 µm. The repeated bipolars significantly reduced the background phase distortion, and enhanced the SNR of the displacement map.

CONCLUSION AND DISCUSSION

In this work, the encoding gradient of MR-ARFI was optimized by using the repeated bipolars. The background phase was reduced, and the SNR of the measurement was significantly improved at no cost of scan time or displacement sensitivity.

One possible source of the background phase is high order eddy currents. The repeated bipolars placed the "on" and "off" of the gradient closer together, so the eddy currents generated could better cancel out each other. However, further breaking down the bipolars into multiple bipolars must take the system delay and tissue response time into account.

ACKNOWLEDGMENTS

The authors would like to thank Nathan McDannold, Ph.D., and Scott Hinks, PhD, for helpful discussions, and Yoav Medan, Ph.D., for technical support with the HIFU system. This work was supported by NIH RO1 CA111981, RO1 CA121163 and P41 RR009784.

REFERENCES

1. Mitragotri, *Nat Rev Drug Discov* **4(3)**, 255-260 (2005).
2. Yuan, *et al.*, *Phys Med Biol* **52(19)**,5909-5919 (2007).
3. N McDannold, SE Maier, *Med. Phys.* **35(8)**, 3748-3758 (2008).
4. H Gudbjartsson, *et al.*, Magn Reson Med **36(4)**, 509-519 (1996).

QUALITY ASSURANCE

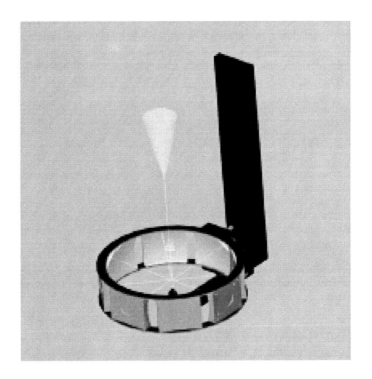

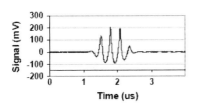

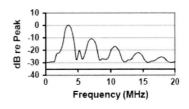

Agar-Silica-Gel Heating Phantom May Be Suitable for Long-Term Quality Assurance of MRgHIFU

Ari Partanen

Philips Healthcare, Äyritie 4, 01510, Vantaa, Finland

Abstract. In MRgHIFU, the purpose of frequent quality assurance is to detect changes in system performance to prevent adverse effects during treatments. Due to high ultrasound intensities in MRgHIFU, it is essential to assure that the procedure is safe and efficacious and that image-based guidance of the treatment is reliable. We aimed to develop a guideline for MRgHIFU QA by acquiring MR temperature maps during ultrasonic heating of an agar-silica-gel phantom over a four month-period using three separate MRgHIFU uterine leiomyoma treatment systems. From this data, the stability of the maximum temperature elevation, the targeting accuracy, and the dimensions of the heated volume were analyzed. Additionally, we studied the sensitivity of these parameters to reveal hypothetical decrease in HIFU performance. After calibration, the mean targeting offsets of the heated volume were observed to be less than 2 mm in the three orthogonal directions. The measured maximum temperature elevation and the length and the width of the heated volume remained consistent throughout the four-month period. Furthermore, it was found that the parameters under investigation were sensitive to reveal the decreased HIFU performance. We conclude that an agar-silica –based phantom is suitable for targeting accuracy and heating properties QA of MRgHIFU system even in long-term use. Moreover, this simple QA method may be used to reveal small changes in HIFU performance assuring consistent functionality and safety of the MRgHIFU system.

Keywords: Thermotherapy, Magnetic Resonance Imaging, High Intensity Focused Ultrasound, Tissue Mimicking Phantom, HIFU, MRgHIFU, Quality Assurance.
PACS: 43.80.Vj, 87.63.Hg, 87.61.-c

INTRODUCTION

In MRgHIFU, the purpose of quality assurance (QA) is to detect changes in system performance to prevent adverse effects related to positioning and heating. The use of MRI-based temperature images acquired during HIFU exposures (sonications) into a tissue-mimicking phantom allows for a rapid test of the functionality of a HIFU device [1, 2].

In this study, the aim was to develop a pre-treatment protocol for MRgHIFU QA by weekly acquiring MR temperature maps during ultrasonic heating of custom made agar-silica-gel phantoms over a four month-period. The protocol consisted of measurements that were conducted to validate the agar-silica phantom to be used for acceptance testing of clinical MRgHIFU equipment and to evaluate the safety, functionality, and performance of the device.

CP1113, *8th International Symposium on Therapeutic Ultrasound,* edited by E. S. Ebbini
© 2009 American Institute of Physics 978-0-7354-0650-6/09/$25.00

From the data, the stability of the temperature rise, the maximum temperature elevation, the targeting accuracy, and the dimensions of the heated volume were analyzed. Additionally, it was determined whether the quality of the manufactured phantoms was adequate and the studied parameters sensitive enough to reveal hypothetical decrease in HIFU performance.

MATERIALS AND METHODS

The study was performed with a Philips MRgHIFU treatment system that integrates an ultrasound transducer with MR-imaging and electromechanical transducer positioning system, delivering spatially and temporally controlled ultrasound energy. The thermometry to monitor local temperature elevations during sonications was accomplished using the known linear dependence of proton resonance frequency (PRF) as a function of temperature.

Custom made agar-silica-gel tissue-mimicking phantoms with known acoustic properties were used in the experiments. Phantoms were positioned on the patient table, and acoustic coupling was achieved using a gel-pad and degassed water. A dedicated pelvic MR coil was placed over the phantom and the table was subsequently advanced into the bore of the MR scanner. T2-weighted TSE images of the phantom were acquired as a 3D coronal stack and used for ultrasound exposure planning. A multi-shot T1-weighted FFE-EPI sequence was performed in near real-time (every 2.9 s) for five slices perpendicular to the beam-axis (three in the target region, one in both near- and far-field) and one slice along the beam-axis to monitor heating. Sonication parameters used in the experiments were: 4 mm diameter target cell, 20 s duration, 50 W acoustic power, and frequency of 1.2 MHz. Target cells were positioned onto a plane located 60 mm into the phantom (Fig. 1). An initial low-energy Test Shot sonication was done to calibrate and confirm the correct location of the heating.

Tests were repeated in phantoms from different manufactured batches to assess phantom dependence. A total of seven phantoms were used for this study. When not in use, the phantoms were stored in a refrigerator (~6°C). To include the day-to-day variations in the MRgHIFU table set-up, individual sets of sonications were performed over four months with three separate MRgHIFU systems.

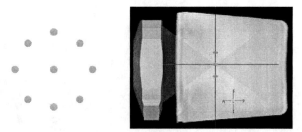

FIGURE 1. The cell pattern for the QA procedure, consisting of nine 4 mm diameter target cells prescribed over a 40 mm × 40 mm grid, and an MR-image of the phantom parallel to the beam-axis. Transducer and beam-path graphics are superimposed on the image.

As empirically demonstrated, the coronal scan plane is least affected by the partial volume effect [3]. Thus, the temporal behavior of temperature was measured in the scan plane perpendicular to the beam-axis. The targeting accuracy was measured as the distance between the center of the target cell and the center of mass of temperature rise. The diameter and length of the heated volume (temperature elevations above 2°C) were also measured. In addition, experiments were done with 10%, 20%, and 30% of the transducer's 256 elements disabled to simulate a condition of malfunctioning equipment. This was done to study if the measured parameters are sensitive and the quality of the phantoms is sufficient enough to detect such decrease in the performance of the system.

RESULTS

All parameters measured from the QA sonications (N = 306) fell well within acceptable limits (±3 SD). The mean values together with standard deviations and ranges are collected in Table 1. The temperatures reported are the maximum temperature elevations observed within the focal region. Fig. 2 shows typical heating patterns in a phantom at the end of a 20 s sonication. A sample offset, diameter, and length measurement is illustrated in Fig. 3.

The absolute magnitudes of the initial offsets in a Test Shot sonication were in the range of 0.06–1.80 mm, 0.08–3.65 mm, and 7.92–11.26 mm in the left-right, inferior-superior, and anterior-posterior directions, respectively. After Test Shot calibration, the mean spatial targeting accuracy in agar-silica-gel phantoms was well within the order of the dimension of a sub-pixel (<2.5 mm), with the used imaging resolution of 2.5 × 2.5 × 7.0 mm. The accuracy was best in the left-right direction, with absolute mean offsets of less than one millimeter, and worst in anterior-posterior direction, with absolute mean offsets still less than two millimeters. The spatial cross-sectional temperature profiles were used to estimate the stability of the size and shape of the heated volume. The diameters and lengths of the heating volume were stable in subsequent measurements and also over the whole period of study, the mean diameters and lengths being 12.8 ± 0.7 mm and 65.1 ± 4.3 mm, and 14.7 ± 0.7 mm and 69.8 ± 2.6 mm for the phantoms with 2% and 3% silica concentrations, respectively. Furthermore, the maximum temperature elevations and heating volume diameters and lengths from the three experiments with 10%, 20%, and 30% of the transducer's 256 elements manually disabled are collected in Table 2.

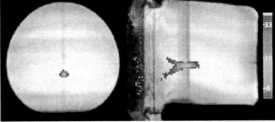

FIGURE 2. Temperature elevations in a phantom at the end of a 20 s sonication. Temperature maps both perpendicular (left) and parallel (right) to the direction of the ultrasound beam overlaid on a magnitude image are shown.

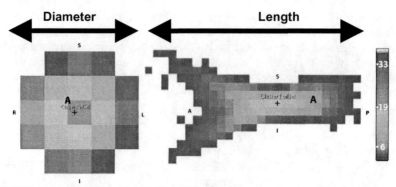

FIGURE 3. Temperature maps of a Test Shot calibration sonication, showing offset corrections in both scan planes. The center of the target cell is indicated in the image with an 'A'. The heating center of mass is marked with a black cross. The dimension of each pixel is 2.5 × 2.5 mm. Slice thickness was 7 mm. Example measurements of cross-sectional areas are also shown.

TABLE 1. The measured minimum, maximum, and mean values together with standard deviations of all sonications (N = 306) in agar-silica phantoms at a constant acoustic power of 50 W. The offsets reported are absolute distances.

	Agar-silica 2%			Agar-silica 3%		
	Mean	SD	Range	Mean	SD	Range
Maximum temperature elevation (°C)	20.9	1.7	17.5 – 24.4	33.2	2.3	29.5 – 37.7
Heating area diameter (mm)	12.8	0.7	11.7 – 14.1	14.7	0.7	13.5 – 15.9
Heating area length (mm)	65.1	4.3	52.5 – 70.0	69.8	2.6	62.5 – 72.5
Offset left-right (mm)	0.77	0.34	0.14 – 1.54	0.63	0.44	0.05 – 1.53
Offset inferior-superior (mm)	1.08	0.47	0.17 – 1.96	1.20	0.64	0.25 – 2.38
Offset anterior-posterior (mm)	1.40	0.52	0.22 – 2.64	1.46	0.63	0.23 – 2.25

TABLE 2. The measured mean values together with standard deviations of sonications (N = 24) into agar-silica 2% phantom from the three experiments with 10%, 20%, and 30% of the transducer's 256 elements disabled.

	Channels disabled					
	10%		20%		30%	
	Mean	SD	Mean	SD	Mean	SD
Maximum temperature elevation (°C)	17.4	1.2	15.1	0.8	12.5	0.5
Heating area diameter (mm)	12.4	0.7	11.7	0.8	11.1	0.7
Heating area length (mm)	58.9	5.0	55.8	7.3	53.2	7.6

DISCUSSION AND CONCLUSION

As opposed to the other directions, the offset in anterior-posterior direction prior to Test Shot sonication was comparatively large and attributable to deviating ultrasound propagation speeds in the coupling gel-pad, phantom, and degassed water. The initial calibration Test Shot practically guarantees high spatial targeting accuracy within 3 mm of the target in a homogeneous heating phantom.

Power loss, e.g. a drop in the number of active channels, has been shown to affect the measured parameters such that a deviation in the system performance can be identified. For example, by disabling 10%, 20%, and 30% of the transducer elements, respective deviations of 3.5°C, 5.8°C, and 8.4°C could be seen in the mean of maximum temperatures (Table 2). Unusual behavior of the mean of maximum temperatures alone would indicate that something is off the mark, and could be further verified by monitoring the other measured parameter values.

As a conclusion, an agar-silica –based phantom is suitable for targeting accuracy and heating properties QA of an MRgHIFU system even in long-term use. Furthermore, the measurements with agar-silica phantoms seem to be sensitive to changes in system parameters and adequate to detect deviations in the system performance. Thus, this simple QA method may be used to reveal small changes in HIFU performance, assuring consistent functionality and safety of the MRgHIFU system. In the future, instead of measuring just the maximum temperature and dimensions of the heated volume, the spatial distribution of the temperature in the focal point region could be determined and compared to a defined model. Additionally, diffusion and absorption coefficients could be determined based on the heating, and the results compared to known agar-silica heating phantom specific values to monitor phantom deterioration.

ACKNOWLEDGEMENTS

This study was carried out at Philips Medical Systems MR Finland. The author would like to thank Teuvo Vaara, Gösta Ehnholm, Julia Enholm, Max Köhler, Heikki Nieminen, and Jaakko Tölö for their advice and comments.

REFERENCES

1. T. Wu and J.P. Felmlee, *J. Appl. Clin. Med. Phys.* **3(2)**, 162–167 (2002).
2. N. McDannold and K. Hynynen, *Med. Phys.* **33(11)**, 4307–4313 (2006).
3. K.R. Gorny, N.J. Hangiandreou, G.K. Hesley, et al., *Phys. Med. Biol.* **51**, 3155–3173 (2006).

Temperature Measurements in Tissue-Mimicking Material during HIFU Exposure

Subha Maruvada, Yunbo Liu, Bruce A. Herman, and Gerald R. Harris

U.S. Food and Drug Administration, Center for Devices and Radiological Health, 10903 New Hampshire Ave., Silver Spring, MD, 20993

Abstract. Cavitation in high intensity focused ultrasound (HIFU) procedures can yield unpredictable results, particularly when the same location is targeted for more than several seconds. To study this effect, temperature rise was measured in tissue mimicking material (TMM) during HIFU exposures. A 50 um thin wire thermocouple (TC) was embedded in the center of a hydrogel-based TMM that was previously developed for HIFU applications. HIFU at 825 kHz was focused at the TC junction. Thirty second HIFU exposures of increasing pressure from 1-7 MPa were applied and the temperature rise and decay during and after sonication were recorded. B-mode imaging was used to monitor any cavitation activity during sonication. If cavitation was noted during the sonication, the sonication was repeated at the same pressure level two more times at 20 minute intervals in order to characterize the repeatability given that cavitation had occurred. The cavitation threshold of the TMM was determined to be approximately 3 MPa at 825 kHz. Temperature traces obtained at various pressure levels demonstrated a wide range of heating profiles in the TMM due to the occurrence of cavitation.

Keywords: HIFU, Cavitation, Tissue-mimicking material
PACS: 43.80.Ev, 43.80.Gx, 43.80.Vj

INTRODUCTION

Given the need for measurement guidelines and standards in high intensity focused ultrasound (HIFU), a reusable hydrogel-based tissue mimicking material (TMM) suited to the specific needs for HIFU has been developed [1]. The TMM has both thermal and acoustic properties close to that of soft tissue. In order to further characterize the TMM, experiments were done to sonicate the TMM at HIFU pressures and record the temperature rise at the focus using embedded thermocouples (TCs). Since pressures associated with HIFU levels often induce cavitation, B-mode imaging was employed to monitor and study the effects of cavitation on HIFU temperature measurements.

MATERIALS AND METHODS

System Setup

The setup of the experiment is shown in Fig. 1. The driving electronics consist of a function generator (Wavetek 81, Fluke Corp., Everett, WA) and power amplifier (ENI

CP1113, *8th International Symposium on Therapeutic Ultrasound*, edited by E. S. Ebbini
2009 American Institute of Physics 978-0-7354-0650-6/09/$25.00

2100L or ENI A-300, Rochester, NY). A 50 dB dual-directional coupler (Amplifier Research, Model DC2000, Souderton, PA), two power sensors (Model 8482A, Agilent Tech., Palo Alto, CA) and a power meter (Model E4419B, Agilent Tech., Palo Alto, CA) are placed between the amplifier and transducer to monitor the forward and reversed electrical power to the transducer. The presence of cavitation bubbles is also monitored with a Siemens Antares diagnostic imaging system (Siemens Medical Solutions, Malvern, PA). Imaging was done at 5.33 MHz using the VF7-3 linear array transducer.

An 8-cm diameter cylindrical mold was constructed with an opening for the imaging transducer. A 50-μm diameter Cu-Co bare wire TC (Omega Engineering Inc., Stamford, CT) was affixed through the center of the mold. The TMM mold with TC was then treated by boiling in degassed water with added surfactant for 20 minutes. Once the TMM was prepared, it was immediately poured into the mold with the TC and allowed to set within the mold. The TC recorded the temperature during the HIFU sonication via a computer controlled acquisition system (OMB-DAQ-3000, Omega Engineering Inc., Stamford, CT).

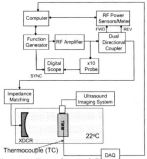

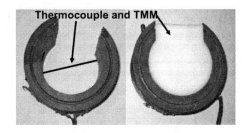

Figure 1. Experimental Setup highlighted on left by black line.

Figure 2. TMM Mold with embedded thermocouple,

Experimental Protocol

The TMM was sonicated for 30 s starting at pressure level 1 and the temperature rise was recorded before, during and after sonication. Images were taken during and after sonication. If cavitation was not observed in either the temperature trace (via an abnormal increase or decrease) or on the imager (via scattering pattern), sonication was continued at the next higher pressure amplitude after the temperature had returned to baseline. If cavitation was observed, then the sonication was repeated after 20 minutes at the same pressure level. This procedure was done twice after the initial sonication, giving a total of 3 sonications for cases of observed cavitation. The focal pressure range of the exposure levels was approximately from 1 to 7 MPa.

Calculation of Threshold Pressures

In order to obtain a more accurate assessment of the actual acoustic pressure at the focus within the TMM, simulations from a two-layer nonlinear propagation model based on the KZK equation were performed using the measured acoustic power and attenuation coefficient of the TMM [2]. The simulation yielded the axial pressure and intensity waveforms, the axial harmonic distribution and the pressure waveform on the axis at the location of peak positive pressure. For establishing the cavitation threshold, we used the pressure calculated from the obtained intensity.

Temperature Analysis

The temperature measured by the TC at the end of sonication (EOS) may be different than the actual temperature were the TC not present due to viscous heating of the TC, cavitation yielding enhanced or diminished heating at the TC, and other TC artifacts (thermal conduction due to the metal of the TC or distortion of the ultrasound beam due to the wire). In order to better determine the EOS temperature given these measurement artifacts, the thermal decay curve following the EOS was extrapolated back to the ultrasound "off" time. A similar technique has been reported previously for obtaining the EOS temperature in ultrasound hyperthermia and ultrasound characterization using small thermal sensors [3]. Specifically, a cubic fit was performed on a 10 second section of the temperature data from 2 s to 12 s after ultrasound exposure ceased to insure that the viscous and/or cavitation effects introduced by the TC sensor were avoided. We employ a cubic fit because this analytic form gives an excellent estimate of the EOS temperature rise, based on back extrapolation of theoretically derived temperature decay curves. Figure 3 shows an overlay of the fit curve on an example temperature curve. Effects due to very local TC perturbation decay quickly after the EOS, leaving a temperature decay curve indicative of mm (focal dimensions) rather than μm (TC dimensions) heated volume. Using different time windows produced very little variation in the extrapolated EOS temperature.

RESULTS

Figure 3 shows an example of various temperature rise curves at non-cavitating and cavitating pressure levels. The black dots indicate the extrapolated EOS temperature rise. The upper left plot is an example of expected temperature rise curves in one TMM sample. These are traces that do not have evidence of induced cavitation. A viscous heating artifact is present in the Level 2 trace, as evidenced by the difference between the final TC value and the extrapolated EOS temperature rise. The upper right plot is an example of induced cavitation on the first run, while the next two runs yielded expected temperature traces. However, the EOS temperatures for all three runs are nearly the same, indicating that cavitation was a very local (to the TC) event that did not affect the absorption of energy in most of the focal region within the TMM. The lower left plot is an example of induced cavitation in the first run only as well; however the EOS temperature is much higher than the EOS temperatures for the following two runs, which yielded expected temperature traces. This is an indication of cavitation enhanced heating of the TMM material surrounding the TC junction. The lower right plot show examples of both decreased temperature rise, possibly due to blocking of the focus by bubbles in the first run, and bubble enhanced heating in the following two runs.

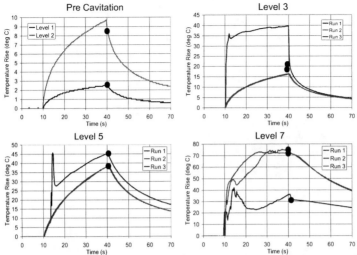

Figure 3. Example of various temperature curves at non-cavitating and cavitating pressure levels. Black dots are extrapolated EOS temperature rises.

The temperature traces can be grouped into three different categories: precavitation (normal temperature curves and no changes in TMM were seen in the ultrasound images), thermally insignificant cavitation (normal temperature curves with small local perturbations and no change seen in ultrasound images), and thermally significant cavitation (temperature curves showed enhanced or decreased heating and hyperechoic regions formed on the ultrasound image during sonication). Figure 4 shows an example of a temperature trace which shows evidence of bubble enhanced heating and the corresponding ultrasound images during the sonication. The formation of a bubble cloud is evident. The bright funnel pattern in the two images on the left, narrowest near the location of the HIFU focus, is possibly due to electrical saturation in the receiving electronics caused by large amplitude scattering [4].

Six TMMs without embedded TCs were also sonicated using the same exposure protocol. Ultrasound imaging was used to detect the onset of cavitation. The cavitation threshold for the TMMs with and without embedded TCs was 2.5 MPa and 4.1 MPa, respectively. Figure 5 shows the EOS temperature rise results for each TMM. The x-axis pressure values are those obtained from the modeled intensity. If cavitation occurred at a particular level, then the point on the plot is an average of the three sonications. All the points at greater than 2.5 MPa represent an average of three sonications since the cavitation threshold for the TMMs with a TC was 2.5 MPa.

DISCUSSION AND CONCLUSION

The cavitation thresholds for the HIFU TMM based on the temperature traces were in the range of 2-3 MPa at 825 kHz. Below the cavitation threshold the temperature traces were as expected, the only artifact noted being viscous heating. Up to 5 MPa, the EOS temperature rise increased monotonically with pressure, even if cavitation had occurred, as would be expected for a TMM whose properties do not change when exposed repeatedly to HIFU pressures. At the highest level, there was a slight decrease in EOS temperature rise. At this level, there was always a strong hyperechoic region that formed that could indicate a large bubble cloud that sometimes blocked the energy at the focus, resulting in lower EOS temperatures. When evidence of cavitation was seen in the TC measurement, the ultrasound image always contained a corresponding feature such as an echoic region. This region usually dissipated during the 20 minutes between repeat sonications. Conversely, the appearance of a bright funnel pattern in the image but without a distinct echoic region as noted in Fig. 4 nearly always coincided with anomalies in the temperature trace.

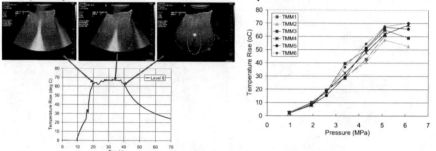

Figure 4. Example of temperature trace that exhibits evidence of bubble enhanced heating and the corresponding ultrasound images taken during the sonication

Figure 5. EOS temperature rise

As expected, this work shows that cavitation effects must be considered in temperature rise testing of HIFU devices. Once cavitation occurs, care must be taken in interpreting the results due to the possibility of both enhanced heating and shielding. We found that both monitoring the TC output and B-mode imaging were reliable methods for observing the onset of thermally significant cavitation. However, the cavitation threshold was found to be lower when a TC was present at the focus, even when measures were taken to clean the TC.

Note: The mention of commercial products, their sources, or their use in connection with material reported herein is not to be construed as either an actual or implied endorsement of such products by the Department of Health and Human Services. This research was supported by the Defense Advanced Research Projects Agency (DARPA) through IAG # 224-05-6016.

REFERENCES

1. R. L. King, B. A. Herman, S. Maruvada, K. A. Wear, G. R. Harris, "Development of a HIFU Phantom",Proceedings for International Society on Therapeutic Ultrasound, Oxford, UK, 2006.
2. J. Soneson, "A User-Friendly Software Package for HIFU Simulation", to be published in the Proceedings for International Society on Therapeutic Ultrasound, Minneapolis, MN, 2008.
3. K. J. Parker, "The thermal pulse decay technique for measuring ultrasonic absorption coefficients", J. Acoust. Soc. Am., 74 (5), November 1983, pp 1356 – 1361.
4. C-C Wu, C-N Chen, M-C Ho, W-S Chen, and P-H Lee, "Using the acoustic interference pattern to locate the focus of a high-intensity focused ultrasound (HIFU) transducer", Ultra. Med. Biol., 34 (1), 2008, pp. 137 – 146.

Temperature-dependent Physical Properties of a HIFU Blood Mimicking Fluid

Yunbo Liu[1], Subha Maruvada[1], Randy L. King[2], Bruce A. Herman[1], and Keith A. Wear[1]

[1]Center for Devices and Radiological Health, Food and Drug Administration, Silver Spring, MD 20993
[2]Department of Bioengineering, Stanford University, Stanford, CA, 94305

Abstract. A blood mimicking fluid (BMF) has been developed and characterized in a temperature dependent manner for high intensity focused ultrasound (HIFU) ablation devices. The BMF is based on a degassed and de-ionized water solution dispersed with low density polyethylene micro-spheres, nylon particles, gellan gum and glycerol. A broad range of physical parameters, including frequency dependent ultrasound attenuation, speed of sound, viscosity, thermal conductivity and diffusivity were characterized as a function of temperature (20°C to 70°C). The nonlinear parameter B/A and backscatter coefficient were also measured at room temperature. The attenuation coefficient is linearly proportional to the frequency (2 MHz – 8 MHz) with a slope of about 0.2 dB cm^{-1}MHz^{-1} in the 20°C to 70°C range as has been reported for human blood. All the other temperature dependent physical parameters are also close to the reported values in human blood. These properties make the BMF a useful HIFU research tool for developing standardized exposimetry techniques, validating numerical models, and determining the safety and efficacy of HIFU ablation devices.

Keywords: HIFU, blood mimicking fluid, ultrasound characterization, thermal ablation.
PACS: 43.80.Ev, 43.80.Cs, 43.80.Vj

INTRODUCTION

High Intensity Focus Ultrasound (HIFU) has been used for both benign and malignant cancer therapy, in which the primary physical mechanisms of action are coagulative thermal necrosis and cavitation damage [1]. New biomedical applications of this therapeutic method are also being developed, such as cauterization of deep bleeding vessels for non-invasive hemorrhage control [2] or arterial thermal occlusion in perfused tissue [3]. During all these HIFU applications, the perfusion of blood flow in the targeted area, especially in large vessels, can affect the required acoustic power, thermal deposition pattern and corresponding lesion formation process at the focus [1, 2]. In order to develop measurement techniques, validate theoretical models, and characterize specific HIFU ablation devices, a HIFU blood mimicking fluid (BMF) with well characterized physical properties needs to be developed. Relevant engineering testing can then be conducted before larger scale animal or clinical studies are performed.

The BMF devised in this work is a degassed water solution mainly dispersed with low density polyethylene and nylon micro-spheres. The temperature dependence of acoustic attenuation, speed of sound, thermal diffusivity, thermal conductivity, and

CP1113, *8th International Symposium on Therapeutic Ultrasound*, edited by E. S. Ebbini
© 2009 American Institute of Physics 978-0-7354-0650-6/09/$25.00

viscosity were systematically studied from 20^0C to 70^0C using established measurement methods. As another critical aspect for HIFU applications, the nonlinear parameter B/A and the ultrasound backscatter coefficient of the BMF were also characterized at room temperature.

MATERIALS AND METHODS

Blood Mimicking Fluid Production

Table I summarizes the specific additives and their corresponding function in the BMF recipe. In order to simulate the ultrasound attenuation of human blood, low density polyethylene (LDPE) micro-spheres (D = 6 µm, CL-1080, Sumitomo Seika, Japan) and nylon particles (D = 8-12 µm, SP-10, Kobo Product Inc, South Plainfield, NJ) are used as absorptive and scattering elements, respectively. Both the LDPE and nylon micro-spheres can be dispersed uniformly in the solution by adding a non-ionic, low-foam surfactant (Tergitol L64, Dow Chemical Co., Midland, Michigan). Glycerol (G7757, Sigma Co., St. Louis, MO) and gellan gum (Kelcogel CG-LA, CP Kelco, Atlanta, GA) are added to optimize the density (particles will stay dispersed for couple hours without stirring) and match the speed of sound, B/A, and viscosity with that of human blood. Gellan gum is an agar-like, nontoxic, polysaccharide powder produced from the bacterium *Pseudomonas elodea*. Density is optimized to make the LDPE and Nylon particle neutrally buoyant in the phantom solution. The BMF holders were two custom-designed cylindrical test chambers (inside diameter = 4 cm; thickness = 2 cm and 4 cm) with 25 µm LDPE membranes covering both ends.

Table I. Blood mimicking fluid recipe

Materials	Function	Content
Degassed H_2O	Solvent	100 ml
LDPE	Absorption	6 g (6 µm)
Nylon	Scattering	0.5 g (8-12 µm)
Gellan Gum	Viscosity	0.1 g
Glycerin	Viscosity / Density/(B/A)	10 ml
Low Foam Surfactant	LDPE/Nylon wetting	1 ml

Measurement of Physical Properties

In the current study, frequency (2 – 8 MHz) and temperature-dependent (20^0C - 70^0C) ultrasound attenuation and sound speed of the HIFU BMF were investigated using an ultrasonic time delay spectrometry (TDS) system in a temperature-regulated water bath [4]. The attenuation (insertion loss) was measured by subtracting the spectrum (in dB) transmitted through the 2-cm and 4-cm thick BMF samples in order to eliminate the reflection losses at the anterior and posterior interfaces. For nonlinear parameter B/A measurement, a recently developed method based upon the finite amplitude insert-substitution (FAIS) technique was employed. The second harmonic amplitudes following transmission of an unfocused tone burst having a fundamental frequency of 2.25 MHz through degassed water with and without a 2-cm BMF sample were measured [5]. The ratio of these second harmonic amplitudes yields the B/A of the samples given the known B/A value for water. An advantage of this technique is that neither absolute pressure amplitude measurements nor diffraction corrections are required. The ultrasound backscatter coefficient ($cm^{-1}Sr^{-1}$) was measured based on a broadband pulse-echo reference phantom technique [6]. The thermal properties of targeted tissues, e.g. conductivity and diffusivity, play an important role in the development of the *in situ* temperature distribution and corresponding therapeutic effects. Therefore, the thermal conductivity and diffusivity of the BMF were quantified with a thermal property analyzer (KD-2, Decagon Devices Inc, Pullman, WA) from 20°C to 70°C. The non-Newtonian behavior of the BMF viscosity was first evaluated using a computer-controlled rotational rheometer (AR-G2, TA Instruments, New Castle, DE) across a wide range of flow shear rates. Then the temperature dependent dynamic viscosity of the BMF was quantified with another rotational DV-E viscometer (Brookfield Inc, Middleboro, MA). Finally, the fluid density of the BMF was measured at room temperature using a digital density_meter (DMA35, Anton Paar K.G., Austria).

RESULTS

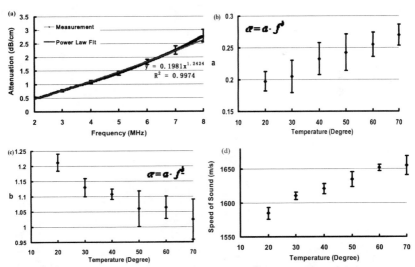

FIGURE 1. (a) Ultrasound attenuation of the BMF at 20°C (b) Coefficient *a* as a function of temperature (c) Coefficient *b* as a function of temperature (d) Temperature dependent sound speed

The frequency-dependent attenuation coefficient was characterized through power law ($\alpha = a \cdot f^b$) regression (R > 0.95) from 2 – 8 MHz based upon experimental results to yield the specific coefficients a and b. Figure 1a is the ultrasound attenuation of the BMF at 20 °C. The corresponding power law regression was found to be $0.2f^{1.24}$ dB·cm^{-1}, which is very close to the reported attenuation in human blood [7]. Figure 1b and 1c present the corresponding coefficient a and b as a function of temperature from 20°C to 70°C. Sound speed (Fig. 1d) increases from 1585 m·s^{-1} at 20°C to 1621 at 40°C to 1655 at 70°C. This trend is comparable with that typically observed in biological tissues [7]. At room temperature (20°C), the B/A of the BMF was measured to be 5.6±0.6 and its density is 1.021±0.0008 g/cm^3.

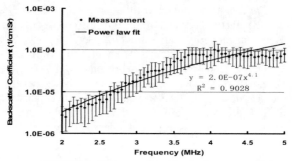

FIGURE 2. Frequency-dependent backscatter coefficient

Figure 2 depicts the backscatter coefficient as a function of frequency from 2 to 5 MHz at room temperature. Within this frequency range, the BMF has comparable backscatter coefficient levels with human blood. For instance, the averaged backscatter coefficient of the BMF is 5.3±2.6 x 10^{-5} cm^{-1}Sr^{-1} at 3.5 MHz, while that of human blood is about 2~5 x 10^{-5} cm^{-1}Sr^{-1} at this frequency [7].

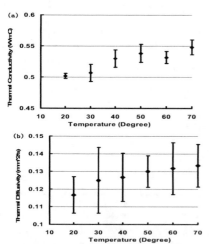

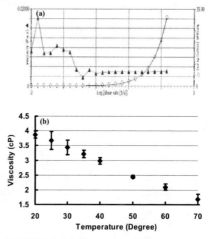

FIGURE 3. Temperature dependent (a) thermal conductivity and (b) thermal diffusivity

FIGURE 4. (a) Shear rate and (b) temperature dependent dynamic viscosity

The measurement results in Fig. 3 indicate that the BMF has very close thermal properties to human blood [7]. Both of the thermal parameters increased slightly (8% for thermal conductivity and 18% for thermal diffusivity) from 20^0C to 70^0C. Figure 4a reveals an initial decreasing viscosity at extremely low shear rate ($< 1/s$) and a plateau viscosity level (3.8 cp) over the entire shear rate range of 1-100/s. This result is different from the non-Newtonian behavior observed in the human blood and therefore the current BMF should be considered as a Newtonian fluid. As the temperature increases, the viscosity demonstrates a steady decrease from 3.8 cp to 3 cp to 1.7 cp at 20^0C, 40^0C and 70^0C, respectively (Fig. 4b).

DISCUSSION AND CONCLUSIONS

In summary, this blood mimicking fluid developed for HIFU applications is a degassed water solution dispersed with LDPE, nylon, gellan gum and glycerol. The temperature dependence of the acoustical, thermal and mechanical properties were studied form 20^0C to 70^0C based upon established methods. The ultrasound attenuation and backscatter coefficients of the BMF were found to be largely dictated by the two primary additives, LDPE and nylon micro-spheres. The density, nonlinear parameter B/A, thermal properties and viscosity are mainly dependent upon the content ratio of water, glycerol and gellan gum powder. A synergistic combination of multiple controllable additives provides an effective and flexible method for engineering BMFs with variable physical properties for any specific application. With similar physical properties to human blood, this BMF provides a potential tool for developing standardized exposimetry techniques, validating numerical models, and determining the safety and efficacy of HIFU ablation devices.

ACKNOWLEDGMENTS

This research was supported by the Defense Advanced Research Projects Agency (DARPA) through IAG # 224-05-6016. Note: The mention of commercial products, their sources, or their use in connection with material reported herein is not to be construed as either an actual or implied endorsement of such products by the Department of Health and Human Services.

REFERENCES

1. Bailey, M.R., Khokhlova, V.A., Sapozhnikov, O.A., Kargl, S.G., and Crum, L.A. *Acoustical Physics* **49**, 437-464 (2003).
2. Vaezy, S., and Zderic, V. *Int. J. Hyperthermia*. **23**, 203-11 (2007).
3. Ichihara, M., Sasaki, K., Umemura, S., Kushima, M., Okai, T. *Ultrasound Med Biol*. **33**, 452-9 (2007).
4. Gammell P.M., Maruvada S., and Harris G.R. *IEEE Trans. Ultrason., Ferroelect., Freq. Contr.*, **54**, 2007, pp.1036-1044.
5. Harris, G.R., Liu, Y., Maruvada, S., and Gammell, P.M. *IEEE Ultrasonics Symposium Proc.* pp. 2072-2074 (2007).
6. Wear, K.A. *J. Acoust. Soc. Am.* **106**, 3659-64 (1999).
7. Duck, F. A. "Physical properties of tissue: A complete reference book" Academic Press, London, 1990.

Feasibility of Agar-Silica Phantoms in Quality Assurance of MRgHIFU

Ari Partanen[a], Charles Mougenot[b,c], Teuvo Vaara[a]

[a]Philips Healthcare, Äyritie 4, 01510, Vantaa, Finland
[b]Philips Healthcare, 33 rue de Verdun, 92156 Suresnes, France
[c]Laboratory for Molecular and Functional Imaging, 146, rue Léo Saignat, 33076 Bordeaux, France

Abstract. Although many phantom types for magnetic resonance guided high intensity focused ultrasound (MRgHIFU) exist, the number of reusable phantoms for quality assurance (QA) purposes is limited. For reliability, the phantom should be structurally and compositionally uniform, and acoustically isotropic. It should also be cheap and easy to produce, and maintain its physical and chemical properties even in long-term use. Various authors have used water, agar, and silicon-dioxide (silica) to produce phantoms with ultrasound attenuation coefficient in a range typical of soft tissues. However, their applicability in MRgHIFU use has not been investigated systematically or verified in previous studies. In this study, agar-gel-based tissue-mimicking heating phantom material is optimized and its MRgHIFU-usability is tested and verified. Acoustic properties of the phantom material with different concentrations of silica were determined experimentally. The ultrasound attenuation coefficient was found to be linearly and positively proportional to the silica concentration. It was observed that phantom material with 2% and 3% mass concentrations of agar and silica, respectively, adequately mimics soft tissues with the following physical properties: ultrasound attenuation coefficient = 0.58 ± 0.06 dB/cm (@1MHz), ultrasound speed = 1490 ± 10 m/s, density = 1.03 ± 0.01 g/cm^3, and acoustic impedance = $1.54 \pm 0.01 \times 10^6$ kg/(m^{2}s). By varying the silica concentration, ultrasound attenuation can be controlled without affecting ultrasound speed. To conclude, we have systematically established and verified a protocol to produce cheap, easy-to-make, reusable, and MR-compatible agar-silica-gel phantom material with tissue-mimicking ultrasound properties for potential use in MRgHIFU QA.

Keywords: Thermotherapy, Magnetic Resonance Imaging, High Intensity Focused Ultrasound, Tissue Mimicking Phantom, HIFU, MRgHIFU, Quality Assurance.
PACS: 43.80.Vj, 87.63.Hg, 87.61.-c

INTRODUCTION

Due to the high powers used during MRgHIFU, it is essential to assure that the treatment procedure is safe and that reliable image guidance can be provided, before a patient can be treated with MRgHIFU ablation method. Thus, there is a need for simple and reliable QA phantom to ensure system stability and quality of the treatment. Ideally, MRgHIFU QA phantom should acoustically mimic soft tissue in terms of ultrasound propagation speed, attenuation, density, and acoustic impedance.

CP1113, *8th International Symposium on Therapeutic Ultrasound*, edited by E. S. Ebbini
© 2009 American Institute of Physics 978-0-7354-0650-6/09/$25.00

However, there is a scarcity of acceptable reusable QA phantoms for MRgHIFU use. In this study, solid, simple, reliable, and reusable tissue-mimicking (TM) heating phantom material to be used in repetitive daily QA tests was manufactured and tested.

The acoustic properties were determined by transmission measurements of ultrasound waves at room temperature under controlled conditions. Moreover, the phantom material's applicability in MRgHIFU use was tested and verified.

MATERIALS AND METHODS

The MRgHIFU heating phantom material should be easy to produce, structurally and compositionally uniform, acoustically isotropic, and chemically and physically stable to ensure reliable results from day to day and so that it could be used as a quality assurance method. Additional desirable characteristics include a simple and inexpensive fabrication process.

Many materials have been used as HIFU tissue-mimicking phantoms in the literature. Some of these are based on aqueous solutions that work well also with MRI: pure gels of gelatin, agar, polyvinyl alcohol, silicone, or polyacrylamide.

Commonly used microbiological culture medium agar has been widely used by researchers as an acceptable base for tissue-mimicking material, since its acoustic characteristics can be easily controlled in the manufacturing process. While agar-gel provides the necessary matrix for the tissue-mimicking material, it is acoustically transparent and prone to bacterial contamination. Thus, other ingredients need to be added to help maintain the stability, and to alter the acoustic properties of the gel.

N-propanol, sodium benzoate, thimerosal, formaldehyde, and p-methylbenzoic acid are commonly used to protect the gel from contamination by bacteria growth, while ultrasound scatterers and absorbers in form of Intralipid®, evaporated milk, glass beads, graphite, BSA, etc. are used to adjust the acoustic properties.

Some authors have used silicon dioxide (silica) as an additive in agar-gel to match the ultrasound acoustical attenuation coefficient of the tissue-mimicking material to the range observed in soft tissues (Table 1) [1]. Silicon dioxide is inert and harmless white powdery substance, having a density of 2.2 g/cm^3 and a melting point of 1650°C. It is insoluble in water and is manufactured in particle sizes of 0.5-50 μm.

TABLE 1. Minimum and maximum values for acoustic properties of soft tissues usually reported in the literature [2], along with proposed optimal values for Tissue-Mimicking MRgHIFU phantom material.

	Minimum	Maximum	"Optimal" TM phantom
Ultrasound propagation speed ($\frac{m}{s}$)	1450	1610	1540
Attenuation coefficient ($\frac{dB}{cm \cdot MHz}$)	0.3	2.0	0.3-0.7
Density ($\frac{g}{cm^3}$)	0.92	1.07	1.04
Acoustic impedance ($\frac{10^6 kg}{m^2 s}$)	1.35	1.72	1.6

Purified agar in granulated form (Merck, Germany) was dissolved in 1.0 l of distilled water. For conservation purposes, to eliminate deterioration by bacteria, 5 ml of sodium benzoate (Vitabalans, Finland) was added. The mixture was heated to 90°C for the agar to melt. Scatterers in form of 0.5-10 μm silica particles (Sigma-Aldrich, Germany) were added to the agar-gel base material with the intention of producing phantom samples with a fixed concentration of silica suspensions in a solid matrix of agar and distilled water. After stirring for 30 minutes, the mixture was poured into square (8×8×2cm) frames and left to harden. Phantom samples of pure agar-gel without any added scattering material as well as agar-gel with various concentrations of silica particles were produced.

Phantom material samples were mounted in a frame and submerged in a degassed and distilled water bath. The function of the water was to act as a coupling medium, and as a reference path for the measurements. A non-focused piston transducer with a diameter of 15mm and center frequency of 1.35MHz was used both as an ultrasound source and a receiving element. The transducer was aligned with a 120mm thick aluminum block and the phantom sample was placed in between.

Measurements of ultrasound propagation speed and attenuation coefficient were made using a known through-transmission pulse technique. The signal was received after near-total reflection from the aluminum block and two-way transmission through the sample. The frequency response and time shift of tone burst, with displacement of water by the sample, were measured. This allowed computation of the time delay Δt it took for the ultrasound to travel back and forth in the material. With the thickness d of the material known, the speed of sound c in the material could thus be calculated. The attenuation coefficient α was calculated from the ratio of the received signal with and without the submerged sample. Attenuation at different frequencies was obtained from the frequency response curve.

By using a precision weight balance, the density of the phantom samples was measured by the standard procedure of weighing a sample first in air, then submerged in a liquid of known density such as distilled water. Acoustic impedance was now calculable by multiplying density with propagation speed.

In addition, the MR-compatibility of the material was also tested. A sagittal image of the phantom setup in an MR-scanner is shown in Fig 1.

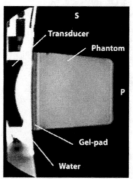

FIGURE 1. A sagittal image of the phantom setup.

RESULTS

The mean acoustic properties of all the tested materials are presented in Table 2. Uncertainties are according to the error calculations or standard deviations, whichever are larger. In addition to agar-silica phantom samples, the acoustic properties together with the density of an extracted piece of porcine thigh muscle (Meat) were measured as well, primarily to act as a reality check.

TABLE 2. The mean acoustic properties together with uncertainties for all the tested samples and Meat. Attenuation coefficient is listed only at 1 MHz.

Name	Propagation speed ($\frac{m}{s}$)	Attenuation coefficient (@ 1 MHz) ($\frac{dB}{cm}$)	Density ($\frac{g}{cm^3}$)	Acoustic impedance ($\frac{10^6 kg}{m^2 s}$)
Silica 0%	1492 ± 10	-	1.004 ± 0.001	1.50 ± 0.01
Silica 1%	1493 ± 10	0.15 ± 0.02	1.012 ± 0.001	1.51 ± 0.01
Silica 2%	1491 ± 10	0.38 ± 0.04	1.019 ± 0.002	1.52 ± 0.01
Silica 3%	1492 ± 10	0.58 ± 0.06	1.029 ± 0.002	1.54 ± 0.01
Silica 4%	1491 ± 10	0.72 ± 0.07	1.037 ± 0.001	1.55 ± 0.01
Meat	1600 ± 20	0.98 ± 0.10	1.049 ± 0.022	1.68 ± 0.04

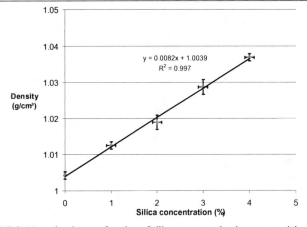

FIGURE 2. Mean density as a function of silica concentration in test material samples.

The silica concentration was linearly proportional to density, as expected (Fig 2). In addition, it is reasonable to assume that also the attenuation coefficient is linearly proportional to the concentration of silica (Fig 3). Test sample of pure agar-gel void of silica content was found to have no measurable attenuation. It is noticeable that the ultrasound propagation speed in the agar-silica-gel phantom samples was consistent and calculated to 1492 ± 10 m/s. Clearly, these concentrations of silica have no noticeable effect to the propagation speed. As the speed remains constant for all samples, density alone affects the values of acoustic impedance. The acoustic properties for meat were fully comparable to those reported in the literature (Table 1). This acts to validate the measurements for the material samples.

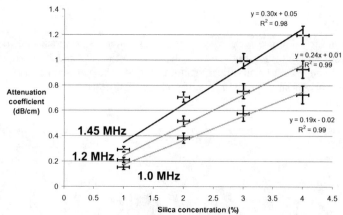

FIGURE 3. Attenuation as a function of silica concentration with three different frequencies.

DISCUSSION AND CONCLUSION

The successful use of agar and silica in forming a solid matrix with suspended particles has been demonstrated. Moreover, it has been found that using these materials, a long-lasting and reusable gel adequately mimicking the acoustic properties of soft tissues can be easily manufactured. Based on the results, gels with mass concentrations of 2% agar and 2%-3% of silica seem to have the most comparable acoustic properties with soft tissues. The material was found to be fully compatible with MRI yielding a good contrast in typical T1 and T2 weighted anatomical scans.

One key finding was that by varying the silica concentration, ultrasound attenuation can be controlled without affecting ultrasound speed. The tissue-mimicking properties could be further enhanced by adding a propagation speed modifying component into the agar-silica-gel. N-propanol has been used for this purpose, and it could well be considered in this application also [3].

To conclude, we have systematically established and verified a protocol to produce cheap, easy-to-make, reusable, and MR-compatible agar-silica-gel phantom material with tissue-mimicking ultrasound properties for use in MRgHIFU QA.

ACKNOWLEDGEMENTS

This study was carried out at Philips Medical Systems MR Finland. The authors would like to thank Matti Tillander and Matti Lindström for their advice.

REFERENCES

1. C. Mougenot, "L'asservissement par IRM d'un réseau matriciel ultrasonore et ses applications thérapeutiques,", Ph.D. Thesis, University of Bordeaux, France (2005).
2. F.A. Duck, A.C. Baker, and H.C. Starritt, Ultrasound in Medicine, London: Institute of Physics Publishing, Medical Science Series, 1998.
3. M.M. Burlew, E.L. Madsen, J.A. Zagzebski, et al., *Radiology* **134**, 517–520 (1980).

Development of a High Intensity Focused Ultrasound (HIFU) Hydrophone System

Mark E. Schafer[1] and James Gessert[2]

[1]Sonic Tech, Inc., Ambler, PA 19002 USA
[2]Sonora Medical Systems, Longmont CO 80503

Abstract. The growing clinical use of High Intensity Focused Ultrasound (HIFU) has driven a need for reliable, reproducible measurements of HIFU acoustic fields. We have previously presented data on a reflective scatterer approach, incorporating several novel features for improved bandwidth, reliability, and reproducibility [Proc. 2005 IEEE Ultrasonics Symposium, 1739-1742]. We now report on several design improvements which have increase the signal to noise ratio of the system, and potentially reduced the cost of implementation. For the scattering element, we now use an artificial sapphire material to provide a more uniform radiating surface. The receiver is a segmented, truncated spherical structure with a 10cm radius; the scattering element is positioned at the center of the sphere. The receiver is made from 25 micron thick, biaxially stretched PVDF, with a Pt-Au electrode on the front surface. In the new design, a specialized backing material provides the stiffness required to maintain structural stability, while at the same time providing both electrical shielding and ultrasonic absorption. Compared with the previous version, the new receiver design has improved the noise performance by 8-12dB; the new scattering sphere has reduced the scattering loss by another 14dB, producing an effective sensitivity of -298 dB re 1 microVolt/Pa. The design trade-off still involves receiver sensitivity with effective spot size, and signal distortion from the scatter structure. However, the reduced cost and improved repeatability of the new scatter approach makes the overall design more robust for routine waveform measurements of HIFU systems.

Keywords: HIFU; PVdF; dosimetry
PACS: 43.25.Zx, 43.35.Yb, 43.58.-e, 43.80.Vj

INTRODUCTION

High Intensity Focused Ultrasound (HIFU) is a novel technology for the destruction of cancerous tumors or other tissue structures within the body using ultrasound. The ultrasound is focused so that this destructive energy is directed only at a specific region (volume) within the patient. The principal problem with the measurement of HIFU fields is that the ultrasound field is of sufficient intensity that it can destroy or significantly alter the properties of the measurement device.

The general requirements for sensors to be used in high energy ultrasound fields were presented by Schafer and Lewin [1]. One approach uses a disposable piezopolymer film, which is designed to be self-monitoring [2,3]. However, in a HIFU field, there is both cavitation and heating, causing the piezopolymer to be destroyed within the first few seconds of exposure. Any design which places the piezopolymer film directly in the high intensity field is subject to rapid deterioration from the intense cavitation and thermal effects present in HIFU. Therefore another approach [4] uses a small reflective scatterer to reflect the ultrasound energy in a

CP1113, 8th International Symposium on Therapeutic Ultrasound, edited by E. S. Ebbini
© 2009 American Institute of Physics 978-0-7354-0650-6/09/$25.00

controlled manner. The reflected signal is detected by a separate PZT receiver. This approach removes the actual detector from the region of high energy (and thereby, from the region of potential destruction).

In our previously presented work [6], we combined the attributes of these different concepts, and developed a reflective scatterer approach as proposed by Kaczkowski et al [4], incorporating several novel features which improve the hydrophone's bandwidth, reliability, and reproducibility. Instead of a single, circular receiver element, we proposed an array of spherically shaped PVdF receivers oriented about a single reflector, in the shape of a truncated sphere. Figure 1 below is an illustration of the concept.

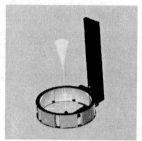

FIGURE 1. Schematic Diagram of HIFU Hydrophone Concept.

The prototype consisted of a single concave receiver made from 25 micron thick, bi-axially stretched PVdF, with a Pt-Au electrode on the front surface. The backing surface was anodized aluminum, which also served as a ground plane.

Evaluation of the prototype indicated several design issues. First, producing an assembly with multiple spherical segments would be cost prohibitive, and raised extreme challenges with regard to alignment. The small non-spherical scattering surface of the glass fibers resulted in low sensitivity (-318 dB re 1 mV/Pa) and the physical stability of the small fibers was questionable. The aluminum backing material caused internal reflections, and when a plastic backing was substituted, electrical interference became an issue.

MATERIALS AND METHODS

To address the problems identified, the following design changes were evaluated. First, a single truncated spherical segment with a 10 cm radius was used to minimize cost and alignment complexity. Second, a conductive, heavily loaded expoxide backing material provided both electrical shielding and ultrasonic absorption. The reflector/scatterer was changed to an artificial ruby sphere (0.5 and 4 mm diameters were evaluated). Finally, a lower cost option of using a uni-axially stretched 100u film with Ni-Cr coating was evaluated in comparison with the orginal 25u bi-axially stretched film with Pt-Au coating . A prototype assembly mounted in the AMS system with the acoustic source is shown in figure 2.

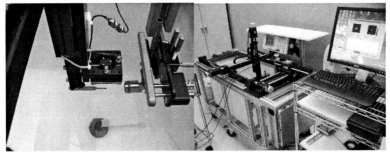

FIGURE 2. Pictures of prototype assembly in measurement tank

The modifications were evaluated by measuring a 3.5 MHz, 2.54 cm diameter, 5 cm focus acoustic source with both 3 and 70 cycle excitation driven by an ENI350L power amplifier at 300 Vp-p. Prototype measurements were compared to measurements made with a bilaminar membrane hydrophone, Sonora model S5, with effective spot size of 0.4 mm calibrated from 1-40 MHz. All measurements were made using the Sonora AMS acoustic measurements system and software shown in figure 2.

Measurements consisted of a Z-scan search to determine the location of the spatial peak along the beam axis, cross axis beam scans and a waveform capture with spatial averaging correction [7].

RESULTS

Figures 4 and 5 illustrate the comparative results for a short pulse between the reference bilaminar memberane hydrophone and the prototype HIFU hydrophone with 25 micron PVDF film and a 0.5 mm ruby ball. Figures 6 and 7 illustrate the comparative results for a long pulse used to simulate a CW measurement without damage to the bilaminar membrane hydrophone.

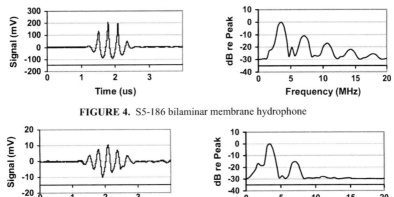

FIGURE 4. S5-186 bilaminar membrane hydrophone

FIGURE 5. HIFU hydrophone, 25 micron PVDF, 0.5 mm ball

303

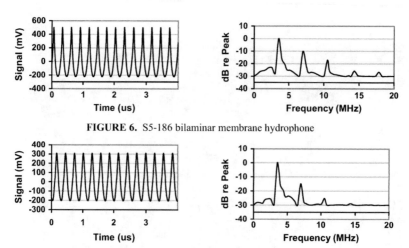

FIGURE 6. S5-186 bilaminar membrane hydrophone

FIGURE 7. HIFU hydrophone, 25 micron PVDF, 4 mm ball

The bandwidth of the HIFU hydrophone prototype measurements is less than that of the bilaminar membrane hydrophone but evidence of non-linear propagation is clearly shown by the harmonic content of the frequency spectrum. The reduction in bandwidth does not appear to be due to scattering. Figure 8 compares pulses from the bilaminar and HIFU hydrophone and the pulses are quite similar.

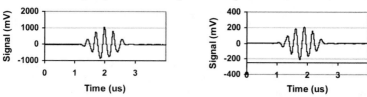

FIGURE 8. Bilaminar pulse (left) versus HIFU hydrophone pulse (right)

A comparison of the short pulse beam patterns is shown in figure 9.

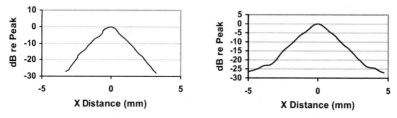

FIGURE 9. Bilaminar pulse beam pattern (left) versus HIFU hydrophone (right)

Table 1 summarizes the results from comparative sensitivity measurements. The reference sensitivity is -265.85 dB re 1V/uPa. The use of the larger scattering balls greatly increased the sensitivity from our previous work. Also note the 5-7 dB shift between CW and pulsed measurements which is due to the integrated effect of the bandwidth differences between the reference hydrophone and the backed PVDF elements.

Relative Sensitivity	Long Pulse dB	Short Pulse dB
Hydrophone S5-186	0.0	0.0
0.5 mm ball Silver Film	-40.5	-35.2
0.5 mm ball Gold Film	-30.2	-23.3
4 mm ball Silver Film	-7.5	-2.0
4 mm ball Gold Film	-2.3	3.4

TABLE 1. Sensitivity comparison

Table 2 contains a comparison of the measured beam dimensions between the reference bilaminar hydrophone and the HIFU hydrophone prototype. Measured beam dimensions were quite dependent on how well the HIFU hydrophone was aligned. Sub-optimal alignment tended to reduce measured beam size.

Beam comparison	X beam cm	Y beam cm
Hydrophone S5-186	0.159	0.151
0.5 mm ball Silver Film	0.133	0.104
0.5 mm ball Gold Film	0.118	0.119
4 mm ball Silver Film	0.146	0.150
4 mm ball Gold Film	0.122	0.126

TABLE 2. Measured beam dimension comparison

DISCUSSION AND CONCLUSIONS

Based on the measurements taken the following conclusions were reached: sensitivity was significantly improved, reverberation issues were reduced and electrical interference was controlled. Results were promising but work remains to: improve the frequency response, investigate and improve alignment and optimize scattering ball size.

REFERENCES

1. P.A. Lewin and M.E. Schafer, "Shock Wave Sensors: I. Requirements and Design," J. Lithotripsy and Stone Disease, 3(1), 3-17, 1991.
2. M.E. Schafer and T.L. Kraynak, "Shock Wave Hydrophone with Self-Monitoring Feature," U.S. Patent # 5,072,426.
3. M.E. Schafer, "Cost-Effective Shock Wave Hydrophones," J. Stone Disease, 5(2), 101-105, 1993.
4. P. Kaczkowski, B. Cunitz, V.Khokhlova, and O. Sapozhnikov, "High Resolution Mapping Of Nonlinear Mhz Ultrasonic Fields Using A Scanned Scatterer" Proc. 2003 IEEE Ultrasonics Symposium, 982-985, 2003.
5. M.E. Schafer, J. Gessert and W. Moore, "Development of a High Intensity Focused Ultrasound (HIFU) Hydrophone system" Proc. 2005 IEEE Ultrasonics Symposium, 2005
6. R.C. Preston, D.R. Bacon, and R.A. Smith, "Calibration of Medical Ultrasound Equipment: Procedures and Accuracy Assessment," IEEE Transactions on Ultrasonics, Ferroelectrics, and Frequency Control, Vol. UFFC-35(2), pp. 110-121, 1988.

THERAPEUTIC DEVICES

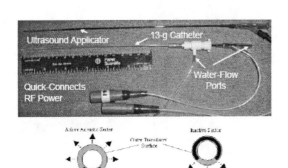

Ultrasound Applicator — 13-g Catheter — Water-Flow Ports — Quick-Connects RF Power

Active Acoustic Sector — Outer Transducer Surface — Inactive Sector — Inactive Sector — Active Acoustic Sector

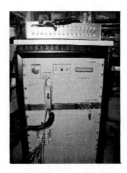

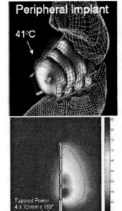

Peripheral Implant

41°C

Tapered Power
4 x 10 mm x 180°
q=0.5 kg m⁻³ s⁻¹
16 min

1 cm

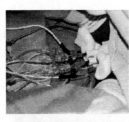

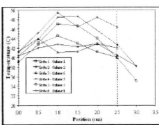

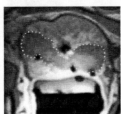

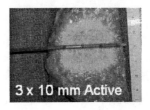

3 x 10 mm Active

Three-Dimensional Thermal Therapy using Multiple Planar Ultrasound Transducers with Real-time MR Temperature Feedback in Gel Phantoms

Kee Tang[a], Matthew Asselin[a], Mathieu Burtnyk[a,b], Rajiv Chopra[a,b], and Michael Bronskill[a,b]

[a]Sunnybrook Health Sciences Centre, 2075 Bayview Ave., Toronto, ON, Canada, M4N 3M5.
[b]Department of Medical Biophysics, University of Toronto

Abstract. High intensity ultrasound delivered transurethrally is a promising approach for the treatment of localized prostate cancer. The use of multiple planar ultrasound transducers mounted on an MR-compatible applicator with rotational capability can provide precise control over the spatial deposition of energy within the gland. Using MR thermometry for adaptive temperature feedback, accurately shaped three-dimensional heating patterns can potentially be achieved. The goal of this study was to evaluate the feasibility of simultaneously controlling multiple elements with real-time MR temperature feedback in gel phantoms in a 1.5T MR imager. Numerical simulations were used initially to determine treatment delivery strategies and appropriate tuning of the temperature feedback control algorithm. Two typical prostate shapes were then treated in tissue-mimicking polyacrylamide gel phantoms using a prototype system to demonstrate conformity of the thermal damage patterns to the target boundaries. Five planar gradient-echo MRI slices with a spatial resolution of 1.7x3.4x5mm and a temporal resolution of 5s were obtained. Each slice was centered on a transducer element which had a length of 9mm operating at 7.7MHz. Results showed high correlation between the desired target boundary and the 55°C isotherm with an average error of 1.0 ± 1.5mm (n=5) for shape # 1 and 1.0 ± 1.2mm (n=5) for shape # 2 across five slices with target volumes of approximately 53cm^3 and 58cm^3 respectively. The feasibility of MRI-guided active feedback for accurate, 3D, multi-planar treatments has been demonstrated and further investigation *in vivo* will be done.

Keywords: MRI-guided, Prostate, Thermal Therapy, Active Feedback, Transurethral.
PACS: 87.55.-x, 87.50.yt, 87.50.yk, 87.57.qp, 87.61.-c.

INTRODUCTION

Although existing treatments for localized prostate cancer are able to achieve effective disease control, they are often associated with significant long-term complications to urinary, rectal and sexual function [1]. One promising technique that aims to reduce these complication rates is MRI-guided transurethral ultrasound thermal therapy [2, 3]. This technique is gaining clinical interest as a minimally invasive means to treat primary tumours, or as a palliative treatment for late stage or metastatic disease in patients ineligible for other types of treatments [4]. A significant challenge in prostate cancer therapy, however, is the necessity to achieve adequate

CP1113, *8th International Symposium on Therapeutic Ultrasound*, edited by E. S. Ebbini
© 2009 American Institute of Physics 978-0-7354-0650-6/09/$25.00

treatment of the entire gland while minimizing any damage to surrounding tissues leading to undesirable side effects. By using real-time MRI thermometry information for guidance as well as for control, adaptability to changing tissue properties and accurate shaping of the thermal damage pattern to the prostate gland can be achieved.

In a previous study with a single ultrasound transducer, 2D thermal damage patterns contoured in gel phantoms and *ex-vivo* tissues demonstrated excellent agreement between the desired target region and the actual 55°C isotherm boundary [5]. However, moving towards a 3D treatment with multiple ultrasound transducers poses many challenges: independent modulation of transducer power while limited to a single rotational rate for the entire device, heat conduction from neighbouring elements, achieving proper balance between element size and its output power, and the trade-offs between acquiring more MRI slices and acquisition time. In this study, the feasibility of a three-dimensional control algorithm was investigated through experiments conducted in gel phantoms using two typical human prostate shapes. Numerical simulations were used to evaluate the most effective tuning parameters to achieve proper control in selecting powers and rotation rates [6].

METHODS & MATERIALS

All experiments were performed in a closed-bore, 1.5T, clinical MR imager (Signa, GE Healthcare) using a prototype treatment system developed in-house consisting of radio-frequency electronics, MRI-compatible motors and heating applicator [3]. A schematic of the apparatus as used in these experiments is shown in Figure 1.

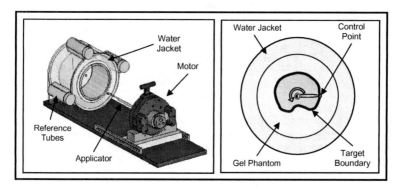

FIGURE 1: (left) Experimental apparatus for the gel phantom experiments; (right) An axial view of the chosen target boundary, the gel phantom and the water jacket.

The phantoms used for this study were tissue-mimicking polyacrylamide gels designed in-house with ultrasound absorption properties similar to tissue [7]. The gel sample was placed in a cylindrical acrylic container, which was then inserted inside a water jacket containing doped water at 37°C (Figure 1). This water jacket was used to ensure that the gel phantom maintained a constant baseline temperature comparable to human core body temperature. Three reference tubes containing mineral oil were placed around the water jacket to monitor phase stability in the magnet. A prototype, multiple-element ultrasound heating applicator was then inserted into the center of the gel phantom, which simulated the urethra position within the target boundary. The entire apparatus was placed in a standard GE birdcage head coil, and the applicator was aligned with the main magnetic field of the MR imager. All images were acquired transverse to the heating applicator at the centers of the transducers, in an axial plane.

To evaluate the control algorithm, two prostate shapes were selected from a patient database and each shape was treated five times. The prostate shapes (PS1 & PS2) had a boundary ranging from 10.0 – 23.4 mm from the urethra center. The prostate volumes were 53cm^3 and 58cm^3 for PS1 and PS2 respectively.

Heating Applicator and Treatment Delivery System

A prototype multi-element transurethral heating applicator was used for all experiments. The applicator consisted of five planar ultrasound transducers (9mm long x 3.5mm wide) operating at 7.7MHz with approximately 60% efficiency. Water at 37°C was circulated through the device at a flow rate of ~300 ml/min to cool the transducer and for coupling of ultrasound energy into the surrounding gel through a thin plastic window (12 μm). Each planar transducer produced a directional ultrasound beam, which generated a localized region of heating extending radially from the device.

Temperature Calculations and Control Algorithm

Temperature maps were derived from MR phase images acquired with a fast spoiled-gradient (FSPGR) sequence: TE/TR = 10/69.2 ms, slice thickness = 5 mm, spacing between slices = 4mm, FOV = 22 cm, flip angle = 30°, NEX = 1, and matrix size = 128x64. Changes in phase were determined by calculating the phase difference between the current phase map and a reference baseline image (average of the first five images). This phase difference was then converted to an absolute temperature using the following relationship based on the PRF shift method:

$$T = T_{base} + \frac{\Delta\varphi}{2\pi \cdot \alpha \cdot \gamma \cdot B_o \cdot TE} \tag{1}$$

where T_{base} is the baseline temperature of the reference phase image, $\Delta\varphi$ is the calculated phase difference, α is the proton resonance frequency temperature coefficient [ppm/°C], γ is the gyromagnetic ratio [42.58 x 10^6 MHz/T], B_o is the strength of the main magnetic field [T], and TE is the echo time [s] of the imaging sequence.

Implementation of real-time active feedback control involved interfacing the MR scanner, the treatment delivery monitoring interface (designed in C++) and the hardware interface application designed in Labview (National Instruments). The entire process from the end of image acquisition to the calculation of updated device parameters took less than 1 second. Image acquisition took place every 5 seconds until a complete treatment was achieved (~365° rotation) in approximately 12 minutes total. Rotation rates were set to 32dpm for target radii greater than 15mm and to 50dpm for target radii less than 15mm. These rotation rates were selected to approximate tuning curves obtained using simulation models. Power values were modulated by multiplying the ΔTr_i values measured at the target boundary for each slice with a proportional gain constant (K_p) (Figure 2). K_p was set to 1 for radii less than 15mm and set to 2 otherwise.

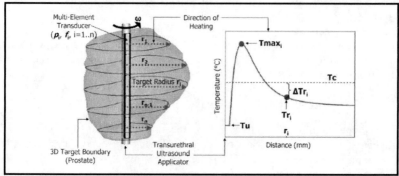

FIGURE 2: Illustration of a multi-element applicator with a 3D target boundary. The control algorithm obtains a temperature profile along the heating direction for each element and adjusts power based on the difference in temperatures at the target boundary (ΔTr_i) and the desired 55°C temperature (Tc). Tu represents the temperature near the applicator which is typically much lower due to urethral device cooling. Maximum temperatures ($Tmax_i$) along the heating direction were capped at 90°C to prevent boiling.

RESULTS

In the five gel phantom experiments for PS1, the average distance error between the intended target boundary and the measured 55°C isotherm was found to be 1.0 ± 1.5 mm (ranging from -2.5 to 5.5mm), as shown in Figure 3. The error bars represent the standard deviation in radius achieved at each angle across the five experiments. Similarly, in the five gel experiments for PS2, the average difference in radial distance between the two boundaries was measured to be 1.0 ± 1.2 mm (ranging from -2.2 to 3.4 mm).

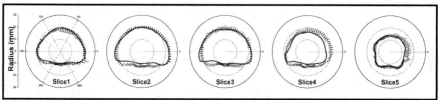

FIGURE 3: Polar plots showing the errors between the target boundary and the average 55°C isotherm for the gel phantoms for each slice for PS1 (solid line represents target boundary, error bars represent standard deviation of 55°C isotherm). The average of all distance errors was found to be 1.0 +/- 1.5mm and 1.0 +/- 1.2mm for PS1 and PS2 respectively.

Results from the heating experiments performed in the gel phantoms produced maximum temperatures that did not exceed 90°C. Temperature uncertainty, or noise, measured in unheated regions was approximately 1°C for these experimental conditions.

DISCUSSION & CONCLUSIONS

The results from these experiments demonstrate that excellent spatial control in producing three-dimensional prostate-shaped thermal damage patterns using active feedback with MRI thermometry measurements can be achieved. For both prostate shapes the average radial discrepancy between the two boundaries was approximately 1 mm. A slight increase in error was seen near the posterior side of the target boundaries where, in addition to rapid changes in radii, the target boundaries were found to be shorter. This could be alleviated through better tuning of the control algorithm and with implementation of a dual-frequency transducer design.

Although there are many issues associated with accurate MR thermometry, the results from these experiments show that an adaptive three-dimensional, closed-loop, MRI-guided feedback system can achieve good results under conditions which mimic ultrasound therapy of the entire human prostate. *In-vivo* experiments will be conducted based on the foundations presented here with future work aimed at improving the control algorithm for energy deposition.

ACKNOWLEDGMENTS

Support for this study was provided by the Terry Fox Foundation, the Ontario Research & Development Challenge Fund, and the Canadian Institutes of Health Research.

REFERENCES

1. L. Potosky, W. W. Davis, R. M. Hoffman, J. L. Stanford, R. A. Stephenson, D. F. Penson, and L. C. Harlan. (2004) *"Five-year outcomes after prostatectomy or radiotherapy for prostate cancer: the prostate cancer outcomes study."* J Nat Cancer Inst, 96 (18): 1358-1367.

2. C. Mougenot, R. Salomir, J. Palussiere, N. Grenier, C. T. Moonen. (2004) *"Automatic spatial and temporal temperature control for MR-guided focused ultrasound using fast 3D MR thermometry and multispiral trajectory of the focal point."* Magn Reson Med, 52 (5): 1005-15.

3. R. Chopra, N. Baker, V. Choy, A. Boyes, K. Tang, D. Bradwell, and M.J. Bronskill. (2008) *"MRI-compatible transurethral ultrasound system for the treatment of localized prostate cancer using rotational control."* Med Phys, 35 (4): 1346-1357.

4. M. W. Dewhirst, L. Prosnitz, D. Thrall, D. Prescott, S. Clegg, C. Charles, J. MacFall, G. Rosner, T. Samulski, E. Gillette, and S. LaRue. (1997) *"Hyperthermic treatment of malignant diseases: current status and a view toward the future."* Semin Oncol, 24 (6): 616-25.

5. K. Tang, V. Choy, R. Chopra, and M.J. Bronskill. (2007) *"Conformal thermal therapy using planar ultrasound transducers and adaptive closed-loop MR temperature control: demonstration in gel phantoms and ex vivo tissues."* Phys Med Biol, 52: 2905-2919.

6. R. Chopra, J. Wachsmuth, M. Burtnyk, M. A. Haider, and M. J. Bronskill. (2006) *"Analysis of factors important for transurethral ultrasound prostate heating using MR temperature feedback."* Phys Med Biol, 51: 1-17.

7. M. McDonald, S. Lochhead, R. Chopra, and M. J. Bronskill. (2004) *"Multi-modality tissue-mimicking phantom for thermal therapy."* Phys Med Biol, 49: 2767-2778.

Treatment Control and Device Optimization of Transurethral Curvilinear Applicators for Prostate Thermal Therapy

Mallika Sridhar[a], Jeffery H. Wootton[a], Titania Juang[a] and Chris J. Diederich[a]

[a]Thermal Therapy Research Group, Department of Radiation Oncology,
University of California, San Francisco,
1600 Divisadero Street, San Francisco, CA 94115

Abstract. Transurethral ultrasound catheter devices in curvilinear configurations are being optimized for improved treatment control and accuracy, reduced treatment times and minimizing surrounding heating of thermally sensitive structures beyond the prostate. A transient acoustic and biothermal model was used to estimate prostate temperature distributions, treatment times and rectal heating for various device configurations and control strategies while accommodating sweeping of curvilinear applicators, power modulation, outer target boundary pilot-point temperature control (sequential rotation) and changes in attenuation with lethal thermal dose. Large prostates can be treated in clinically reasonable times (20-40 min) with low rectal heating if the curvilinear device radius of curvature are increased to 25 mm, device frequency is kept low between 5-6.5MHz and large device dimensions are chosen (5 X 20 mm) with high maximum allowable temperatures along device length. Pilot-point temperature feedback treatment control can be enhanced with decreased rectal thermal dose by using variable boundary temperatures at the posterior prostate near rectum.

Keywords: Transurethral ultrasound devices, Pilot-point feedback control, Thermal therapy
PACS: 80

INTRODUCTION

Transurethral ultrasound devices are under development by our group and others to perform thermal therapy on the prostate as a minimally invasive option for treating benign prostatic hyperplasia (BPH) and localized prostate cancer [1-8]. As example, catheter-based transurethral applicators (Figure 1) have been constructed with independently powered transducer segments operating at 6.5 MHz and measuring 3.5 mm X 10 mm in either a curvilinear (slightly focused) with a 15 mm radius of curvature or planar configuration (unfocussed). These devices have previously been successful in producing spatially selective regions of thermal destruction in the prostate of in-vivo animals [4,5]; where MR thermal imaging and thermal dose maps through the target volume were used to control therapy delivery (rotation, power levels, duration) [1]. Specific applicator configurations and corresponding energy penetration must be carefully considered in order to properly target specific treatment zones, reduce treatment duration, and avoid the accumulation of thermal dose in sensitive structures beyond the prostate. The curvilinear devices can produce more narrow yet equally penetrating heating zones compared to planar devices, and may

CP1113, 8th International Symposium on Therapeutic Ultrasound, edited by E. S. Ebbini
© 2009 American Institute of Physics 978-0-7354-0650-6/09/$25.00

provide an advantage for controllable contouring of target boundaries in specific situations.

The objective of this study is to explore methods of control and transducer parameters associated with curvilinear transurethral devices as a means to improve treatment accuracy, possibly reduce treatment times, and minimize heating of surrounding structures such as rectum.

Planar & Curvilinear Transurethral Applicators

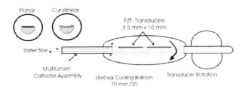

FIGURE 1. Transurethral ultrasound applicator showing planar and curvilinear configurations.

BIOTHERMAL SIMULATIONS AND TESTING

A transient acoustic and biothermal model that uses a simplified anatomical depiction of the prostate with pre-assigned thermal properties was used [8]. The model employs finite difference methods to solve for prostate temperature distributions using the Pennes bioheat transfer equation and Rayleigh–Sommerfield diffraction integral for acoustic pressure distributions. Radial grid spacing of 0.1 mm and finite difference time step of 0.2 s was used to ensure a convergent solution. The model accommodates sweeping of the planar and curvilinear applicators with dual control of both maximum temperature (power modulation) and outer target boundary pilot-point temperature control (sequential rotation). The model also accounts for dynamic changes in perfusion and a two-fold increase in attenuation with lethal thermal dose and assumes the ultrasonic energy is completely absorbed by the tissue.

Various simulations were run for different device configurations. The device was placed in the urethra in the simulation and a 270° sector around the prostate was chosen as the treatment zone (Figure 4c), which included the posterior margin of the gland adjacent to the rectum. The aim of treatment was to achieve a temperature of 52°C or lethal thermal dose (t_{43}>240 min) at the prostate boundary in order to ensure thermal destruction. The applicators were chosen to successively rotate at 20° when the prostate boundary reached 52°C for most cases. Applied power was modulated to control maximum temperature (PID maximum temperature control), and pilot point control was applied at the outer target boundary for sequencing rotation step. Prostate cross-section sizes between 3-5 cm were simulated. Other critical parameters varied were: maximum temperature threshold within the prostate (70-90°), applied power (7-20 W with an efficiency of 50%), frequency (5-8 MHz), ROC: radius of curvature (10-35 mm) and transducer dimensions (3.5-5 mm width: 10-20 mm length) to assess treatment times (time to treat the lower 180° of the prostate), rectal heating and associate thermal dose. Based on clinical treatment times and associated rectal heating, recommendations were made for different prostate sizes. Pilot point control was also investigated where rotation step size and boundary temperature was decreased from boundary temperature of 52° to 48° and step size of 20° to 5° in a region adjacent to the rectum (See Figure 4) to determine if such strategies could spare the rectum additional thermal dose yet keeping treatment accuracy.

RESULTS AND DISCUSSION

As a guideline, the best device ROC should be chosen according to the prostate radius and is most applicable to treating well-defined regions of focal disease (See Figure 2). Low frequency devices allow for deeper penetration and shorter treatment times with 5 cm prostates, however increased rectal heating (up to 43°, $t_{43}<5$ min) can result. Effect of frequency becomes less and less prominent with small prostate sizes. The maximum allowable temperature in the prostate has a large impact on treatment time. Lowering this threshold causes extremely long treatment times (See Figure 3a). Due to temperature controller, increasing the power from 10W to 20W decreased the treatment time only by a few minutes. Device Dimensions alters treatment time between 5-10 mins. Increase in ROC significantly decreases treatment time especially in 5 cm prostates. Choice of a wider device helps in construction of the catheter, lower rectal heating (See Figure 3b) and reasonable treatment times (See Figure 3a). Proper selection of maximum temperature and target boundary set point at each rotation angle can be used to tailor treatment control and therapeutic margin to the target zone (Figure 4). Lower temperatures and smaller rotation angles can be used to improve safety margin but increase treatment time.

SUMMARY

In conclusion the posterior peripheral zone of large prostates can be treated in reasonable times (20-40 min) with low rectal heating if the ROC of the ultrasound transducers are increased, frequency chosen between 5-6.5MHz, large device dimensions are chosen and average power and high maximum allowable temperatures is applied. Variable boundary temperature and maximum temperature can be used to enhance control margin at posterior prostate near rectum.

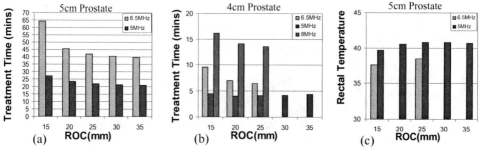

FIGURE 2. : Simulation results showing (a-b) treatment time (min) and (c) rectal temperature (°C) for curvilinear devices when ROC and device frequency were varied. Simulation Parameters: Power: 15W, device size = 5X20mm, Max Temp: 90° (5cm) and 85° (4cm).

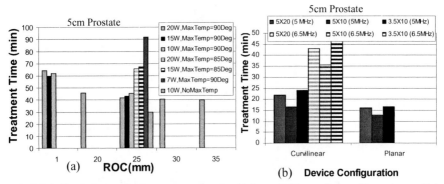

FIGURE 3. Simulation results for treatment time for (a) 5 mm X 20 mm devices for varying applied power and maximum allowable temperature (b) for varying device dimension for both curvilinear and planar devices.

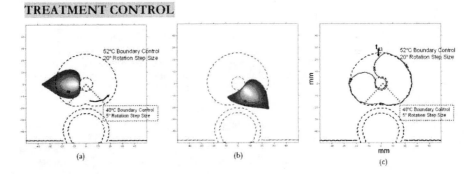

FIGURE 4. Simulation results showing pilot point boundary control around a 270° treatment region in a 5cm prostate, device frequency=6.5MHz and ROC=25mm. The edge temperature and step size of rotation was controlled around a 90° sector around the rectum as indicated. These parameters were changed from 52° boundary temperature and 20° step size to 48° boundary temperature and 5° step size.

ACKNOWLEDGMENTS

This work was supported by NIH R01CA111981 & NIH R01CA122276

REFERENCES

1. KB Pauly et.al, *Topics Magnetic Resonance Imaging*, **17**(3), 195-207 (2006).
2. CJ Diederich et.al. *Medical Physics*, **31**(2), 405-413 (2004).
3. R Chopra et.al. *Physics Medicine Biology*, **51**(4), 827-44 (2006).
4. AB Ross et.al. *Physics Medicine Biology*, **49**(1), 189-204 (2004).
5. AB Ross et.al, *Medical Physics*, **32**(6), 1555-1565 (2005).
6. AM Kinsey et.al, *Medical Physics*, **35**(5), 2081-2093 (2008).
7. R Chopra et.al, *Medical Physics*, **35**(4), 1346-1357 (2008).
8. JH Wootton et.al, *Int. J. Hyperthermia*, **23**(8), 609-622 (2007).

Catheter-Based Ultrasound for 3D Control of Thermal Therapy

Chris Diederich[1], Xin Chen[1], Jeffery Wootton[1], Titania Juang[1],
Will H. Nau[1], Adam Kinsey[1], I-Chow Hsu[1], Viola Rieke[2],
Kim Butts Pauly[2], Graham Sommer[2], Donna Bouley[2]

[1]Thermal Therapy Research Group,
Radiation Oncology Department, University of California San Francisco
[2] Department of Radiology, Stanford University

Abstract. Catheter-based ultrasound applicators have been investigated for delivering hyperthermia and thermal ablation for the treatment of cancer and benign diseases. Technology includes an intrauterine applicator integrated with an HDR ring applicator, interstitial applicators for hyperthermia delivery during brachytherapy, interstitial applicators for tumor ablation, and transurethral devices for conformal prostate ablation. Arrays of multiple sectored tubular transducers have been fabricated for interstitial and intrauterine hyperthermia applicators. High-power interstitial versions have been evaluated for percutaneous implantation with directional or dynamic angular control of thermal ablation. Transurethral applicators include curvilinear transducers with rotational sweeping of narrow heating patterns, and multi-sectored tubular devices capable of dynamic angular control without applicator movement. Performance was evaluated in phantom, excised tissue, *in vivo* experiments in canine prostate under MR temperature monitoring, clinical hyperthermia, and 3D-biothermal simulations with patient anatomy. Interstitial and intrauterine devices can tailor hyperthermia to large treatment volumes, with multisectored control useful to limit exposure to rectum and bladder. Curvilinear transurethral devices with sequential rotation produce target conforming coagulation zones that can cover either the whole gland or defined focal regions. Multi-sectored transurethral applicators can dynamically control the angular heating profile and target large regions of the prostate without applicator manipulation. High-power interstitial implants with directional devices can be used to effectively ablate defined target regions while avoiding sensitive tissues. MR temperature monitoring can effectively define the extent of thermal damage and provided a means for real-time control of the applicators. In summary, these catheter-based ultrasound devices allow for dynamic control of heating profiles along the length and angular expanse of the applicator during therapy delivery, are amenable to MR monitoring, and provide a minimally-invasive technique for true 3D control of hyperthermia and thermal ablation.

Keywords: Ultrasound, Hyperthermia, Thermal Therapy, Thermal Coagulation, Prostate, Interstitial, Transurethral, Minimally-Invasive Therapy.
PACS: 43., 44.

INTRODUCTION

Compelling biological and clinical evidence (Phase I/II, Phase III studies) strongly demonstrate that combining hyperthermia (40-45°C) and radiation therapy for treating locally advanced or recurrent cancer can significantly improve response and

CP1113, *8th International Symposium on Therapeutic Ultrasound,* edited by E. S. Ebbini
© 2009 American Institute of Physics 978-0-7354-0650-6/09/$25.00

survival[1,2]. The heating techniques used in many of these studies do not effectively localize a prescribed temperature distribution nor provide a means of verifying delivery of adequate thermal dose.   High-dose rate (HDR) brachytherapy, implemented with advanced image-based treatment planning techniques, can deliver highly-conformable radiation dose distributions using implanted plastic catheters, and is part of the standard regimen for applying radiation to sites in the pelvis, breast, head&neck, and bulky tumors. High-temperature thermal therapy (typically >50°C, t_{43}>240 min) is currently being implemented as a minimally-invasive alternative to traditional surgery in the treatment of disease and cancer[3]. Many different types of energy sources are applied, including laser, RF current, microwave, ultrasound and thermal conduction based devices. Heating energy can be applied by external means or internally via interstitial, intraluminal, or intracavitary approaches.

Investigations of interstitial and endocavity ultrasound devices, consisting of arrays of miniature transducers, have demonstrated performance characteristics ideal for delivering hyperthermia and thermal ablative therapy to localized tissue regions. These catheter-based ultrasound devices are a novel technology that has potential to deliver highly-controllable and penetrating therapeutic heating to implanted target regions. The purpose of this paper is to review advances of this technology by our research group; in particular, interstitial and intrauterine devices for hyperthermia in conjunction with HDR brachytherapy; interstitial for ablation of soft tissue sites such as liver, prostate and myomas; and transurethral for ablation of prostate tissue.

DEVICES & EVALUATION

Interstitial and Endocavity Applicators

The interstitial ultrasound applicators (Fig. 1) utilize arrays of small tubular ultrasound radiators, designed to be inserted within plastic implant catheters[4,5] . Water-flow is used during power application to couple the ultrasound and improve thermal penetration. The multiple tubular segments, with separate power control and frequency selection, allow the power deposition or heating pattern to be adjusted along the applicator axis. The angular or rotational heating pattern can be modified to produce angularly selective heating patterns (i.e., 90°, 180°, or 360°)[6,7]. The orientation of these directional applicators within a catheter can be used to protect critical normal tissue or dynamically rotated and power adjusted to more carefully tailor the regions of heating, as used for clinical hyperthermia (Fig. 2). These devices and driving hardware are also compatible with MRI and MR thermal imaging[8,9] Larger diameter devices of similar design are being developed for intrauterine treatment of cervical cancer (as described in Wootton et al. ISTU 2008). Operating at high power levels, single or multiple applicators can generate substantial size thermal lesions up to 20 mm radial distance within 5 min treatment times, while maintaining axial and angular control of lesion shape (Fig. 2).

319

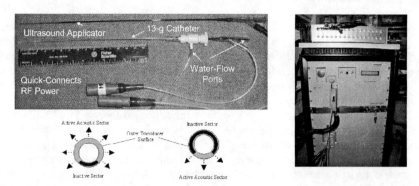

FIGURE 1. (a) Interstitial ultrasound applicators designed for hyperthermia or thermal ablation from within plastic catheters. Separate control of multiple transducer sections with (b) 32 channel amplifier, ability to sector or direct energy, and favorable energy penetration make these the most controllable interstitial heating technology.

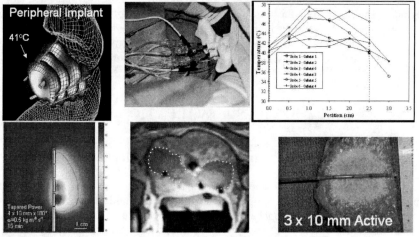

FIGURE 2. Interstitial performance: Top – 3D treatment plan & clinical prostate hyperthermia with temperature profile; Bottom – simulated shaped thermal ablation, multiple directional applicators ablating canine prostate and avoiding rectum (T1 w/contrast MRI), and large shaped lesion in extricated human uterine fibroid with TTC stain.

Transurethral Applicators

Transurethral applicators (Fig. 3) devised by our group have been using arrays of tubular, planar, or curvilinear transducers[10-14]. Sectored tubular, with directional heating patterns, and the planar and curvilinear configurations produce selective or narrow heating patterns that can be rotated in real-time using MR temperature imaging and compatible motors to sweep out or contour target regions. Each applicator configuration consists of transducer sections (6- 10 mm long, 6.5-8 MHz), mounted on a 4 mm delivery catheter with an inflatable 10 mm urethral cooling balloon and bladder positioning balloon. A water-cooling jacket integrated with an endorectal coil for MR imaging can provide cooling of the rectum. Devices have been evaluated using in vivo canine prostate model. The curvilinear transurethral applicator produces a narrow heating pattern (~20 sector, 15-20 mm penetration), and can be finely controlled with MRTI to tightly conform the thermal ablation to the outer prostate boundary (Fig. 4). Multi-sectored tubular transurethral applicators (three separately controllable 120° sectors on each transducer) allow for electronic control of the angular heating pattern without the need for rotation, with relatively fast (10-15 min) coagulation of large volumes possible. Coronal, sagittal, or axial imaging planes can be used to tightly control the heating distribution to the targeted boundary with these devices (Fig. 4).

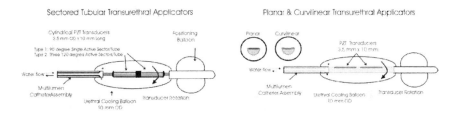

FIGURE 3. General schematics of transurethral applicators devised by our group for image guided thermal ablation of prostate tissue.

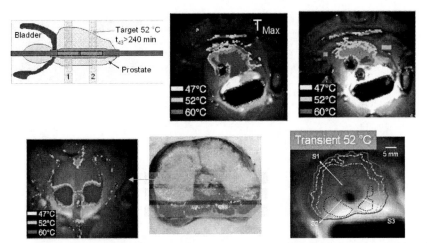

FIGURE 4. Transurethral performance in canine prostate with MR guidance: Top – multiple slice MRI used to monitor 52°C contour around each transducer and rotate curvilinear applicator to sweep out therapy zone in prostate; Bottom – multisectored device with coronal imaging slice to monitor and localize heating in prostate, resultant thermal damage from two sector activation directing energy away from rectum to outer prostate capsule, and transient progression of temperature for three sector control.

ACKNOWLEDGMENTS

This work was supported by NIH R01CA122276 & NIH R01CA111981.

REFERENCES

1. Wust, P. et al. Hyperthermia in combined treatment of cancer. *Lancet Oncol* **3**, 487-97 (2002).
2. van der Zee, J. Heating the patient: a promising approach? *Ann Oncol* **13**, 1173-84 (2002).
3. Diederich, C. J. Thermal ablation and high-temperature thermal therapy: overview of technology and clinical implementation. *Int J Hyperthermia* **21**, 745-53 (2005).
4. Diederich, C. J. Ultrasound applicators with integrated catheter-cooling for interstitial hyperthermia: theory and preliminary experiments. *International Journal of Hyperthermia* **12**, 279-297 (1996).
5. Nau, W. H., Diederich, C. J. & Burdette, E. C. Evaluation of multielement catheter-cooled interstitial ultrasound applicators for high-temperature thermal therapy. *Medical Physics* **28**, 1525-34 (2001).
6. Deardorff, D. L. & Diederich, C. J. Angular directivity of thermal coagulation using air-cooled direct-coupled interstitial ultrasound applicators. *Ultrasound in Medicine and Biology* **25**, 609-22 (1999).
7. Nau, W. H., Diederich, C. J. & Stauffer, P. R. Directional power deposition from direct-coupled and catheter-cooled interstitial ultrasound applicators. *International Journal of Hyperthermia* **16**, 129-44 (2000).
8. Diederich, C. J. et al. Catheter-based ultrasound applicators for selective thermal ablation: progress towards MRI-guided applications in prostate. *International Journal of Hyperthermia* **20**, 739-56 (2004).
9. Nau, W. H. et al. MRI-guided interstitial ultrasound thermal therapy of the prostate: a feasibility study in the canine model. *Med Phys* **32**, 733-43 (2005).
10. Diederich, C. J. et al. Transurethral ultrasound applicators with directional heating patterns for prostate thermal therapy: in vivo evaluation using magnetic resonance thermometry. *Medical Physics* **31**, 405-413 (2004).
11. Ross, A. B. et al. Highly Directional Transurethral Ultrasound Applicators with Rotational Control for MRI Guided Prostatic Thermal Therapy. *Physics in Medicine and Biology* **49**, 189-204 (2004).
12. Ross, A. B. et al. Curvilinear transurethral ultrasound applicator for selective prostate thermal therapy. *Med Phys* **32**, 1555-65 (2005).
13. Kinsey, A. M. et al. Transurethral ultrasound applicators with dynamic multi-sector control for prostate thermal therapy: in vivo evaluation under MR guidance. *Med Phys* **35**, 2081-93 (2008).
14. Diederich, C. J. & Burdette, E. C. Transurethral ultrasound array for prostate thermal therapy: initial studies. *IEEE Transactions on Ultrasonics, Ferroelectrics and Frequency Control* **43**, 1011-22 (1996).

322

Therapeutic Ultrasound Research And Development From An Industrial And Commercial Perspective

Ralf Seip

Philips Research, 345 Scarborough Road, Briarcliff Manor, NY 10510

Abstract. The objective of this paper is to share the challenges and opportunities as viewed from an industrial and commercial perspective that one encounters when performing therapeutic ultrasound research, development, manufacturing, and sales activities. Research in therapeutic ultrasound has become an active field in the last decade, spurred by technological advances in the areas of transducer materials, control electronics, treatment monitoring techniques, an ever increasing number of clinical applications, and private and governmental funding opportunities. The development of devices and methods utilizing therapeutic ultrasound to cure or manage disease is being pursued by startup companies and large established companies alike, driven by the promise of profiting at many levels from this new and disruptive technology. Widespread penetration within the clinical community remains elusive, with current approaches focusing on very specific applications and niche markets. Challenges include difficulties in securing capital to develop the technology and undertake costly clinical trials, a regulatory landscape that varies from country to country, resistance from established practitioners, and difficulties in assembling a team with the right mix of technological savvy and business expertise. Success is possible and increasing, however, as evidenced by several companies, initiatives, and products with measurable benefits to the patient, clinician, and companies alike.

Keywords: Challenges, Opportunities, Therapeutic Ultrasound.
PACS: 43.10.Qs, 43.15.+s, 43.80.Sh, 43.80.Vj.

INTRODUCTION

During the early stages, performing therapeutic ultrasound research and development activities within an industrial or commercial framework is very similar to work that would occur within an academic environment. The basic and fundamental interactions between the ultrasound exposure and tissue need to be investigated and understood, prior to being able to explore potential applications of this technology. At these stages, initial seed funding in the form of a government grant or institution budget, a basic ultrasound laboratory (outfitted with watertanks, hydrophones, measurement equipment, computers, and electronics and mechanical instrument manufacturing capability), transducer expertise, and a small and focused team are necessary and sufficient to make good progress. Once an application has been defined, collaboration with clinical staff for subsequent validation of the technology in an *in-vivo* pre-clinical setting is paramount. Around this stage, development activities in the field of therapeutic ultrasound from a commercial perspective typically deviate from those from the academic environment.

CP1113, *8th International Symposium on Therapeutic Ultrasound*, edited by E. S. Ebbini
© 2009 American Institute of Physics 978-0-7354-0650-6/09/$25.00

CHALLENGES

The largest challenge facing companies in the therapeutic ultrasound field (after having shown that the fundamental science is on solid footing and a viable commercial application of the technology has been identified), is to secure and maintain a funding level capable of seeing the development effort all the way through the clinical approval process, first sales, and beyond. An equal and important challenge is to be able to maintain the project focused and the enthusiasm high for the technology at the employee, management, board, investor, and end-user level (clinician and/or patient) through constant updates and progress to overcome rough patches along the way. With development activities in this field taking between 2-4 years, verification in *in-vitro* and pre-clinical models taking between 1-2 years, and the approval processes in this field typically taking between 4-6 years, perseverance, commitment, and patience are necessary attributes. Companies and groups must also prepare for a regulatory landscape that is changing, learning, and in some cases needs guidance from the technology developers themselves as this disruptive therapeutic ultrasound technology is maturing.

Therapeutic ultrasound device development should also be undertaken within a quality system framework, which is typically not in place in academic setting or a research institution. Such a framework can be provided by ISO 13485 (Medical devices – Quality management systems – Requirements for regulatory purposes) or ISO 9001 (Quality management systems – Requirements), and should conform to additional requirements, such as those listed in MDD 93/42/EEC (Directive concerning medical devices), if the device will be marketed in Europe, for example. Development and manufacturing within an established quality system significantly simplifies the regulatory and approval process, which in the United States typically follows one of the following two routes: PMA (Premarket approval process) or 510(k) (Premarket submission process – substantial equivalency), depending on the nature of the therapeutic ultrasound device itself. Other countries impose similar or additional requirements on the device manufacturer prior to granting approval for sale and usage of the device.

Differences in performing these activities in large vs. small companies tend to be minor, overshadowed mostly by the effort required in the development and approval process of the device or ultrasound technology itself.

A final significant challenge is related to the adoption of this technology by users. Therapeutic ultrasound solutions tend to be disruptive, often blurring the lines between established specialties such as surgery and radiology, merging aspects from both and creating non-invasive image-guided therapeutic procedures. This requires change and a different way to approach these procedures by the clinical community, which can take time to implement. The most important steps one can take is to work with and involve luminary physicians early in the development process, and to keep in mind that for this new technology to be successful, it needs not only to bring about the desired therapeutic effect safely to the patient, but be easy to use, and be designed to appeal to the research clinician and to the general practitioner, as these users will ultimately determine the commercial success of the application.

OPPORTUNITIES

Regardless of these challenges, progress in the development and clinical use of therapeutic ultrasound devices and procedures is increasing. Most commercial approaches are currently focusing on using ultrasound to bring about a therapeutic effect thermally via tissue ablation. Many companies are now offering procedures that utilize a custom therapeutic ultrasound applicator with image guidance for treatment planning and monitoring. Some devices have already been approved for clinical use, others are undergoing clinical trials, while still others are in the product development stage. Academia and industry are investigating other applications for therapeutic ultrasound as well, including therapies that exploit non-thermal therapeutic effects brought about by the ultrasound energy, such as mechanical tissue fractioning, drug and gene delivery, sonoporation, acoustic hemostasis, etc. Commercialization of these devices and procedures provide additional opportunities for the clinical application of this technology.

Future therapeutic ultrasound devices and procedures benefit from the early successes, as regulatory pathways become more established and mainstream for these applications, and new devices can piggy-back off of already approved devices via the substantial equivalence approval process. The market entry threshold is also further reduced, as awareness of the benefits of therapeutic ultrasound technologies takes hold.

CONCLUSIONS

The field of therapeutic ultrasound is very active and growing, as evidenced by the:

- increasing number of presentations and publications at international acoustics and ultrasound conferences and journals,
- emergence of therapeutic ultrasound-specific organizations,
- increasing emergence of startup companies offering clinical devices and services in the field of therapeutic ultrasound,
- growing involvement of larger and established medical device companies, and
- increasing support, recognition, and involvement of government and regulatory agencies.

Experience has shown that good and resourceful people are the key for commercial success, especially due to the interdisciplinary nature of therapeutic ultrasound: an engineering, clinical, regulatory, and business development/marketing savvy team is a must. Long timelines for development and regulatory approval require extensive financial investments on the order of $20M to $50M or more, and success is not guaranteed. Government small-business research grants and other assistance are essential in the early research and development phases of a therapeutic ultrasound application, and can provide needed seed funds to launch the endeavor. Additional funding in the form of venture capital, partnerships, company research commitments, etc. are required in the later stages of the process. A fine balance between publishing early results and intellectual property is required as well: the former increases visibility of the research and development activities, while the latter provides some protection from competitors and creates tangible value. Finally, these issues are faced equally by both large and startup companies, as the requirements for resources and expertise are similar in both cases.

ACKNOWLEDGEMENTS

I would like to thank all of my friends, coworkers and colleagues in industry, government, and academia who continue to push the therapeutic ultrasound envelope to help ensure that the promise of non-invasive, low-morbidity, and high-efficacy treatments that therapeutic ultrasound can offer is being realized today.

REFERENCES

1. International Society of Therapeutic Ultrasound, http://www.istu2008.org
2. Focused Ultrasound Surgery Foundation, http://www.fusfoundation.org
3. IEEE Ultrasonics Symposium, http://ewh.ieee.org/conf/ius_2008
4. Ultrasonic Industry Association, http://www.ultrasonics.org
5. Acoustical Society of America, http://asa.aip.org
6. FDA PMA Process Overview, http://www.fda.gov/cdrh/devadvice/pma
7. FDA 510(k) Process Overview, http://www.fda.gov/cdrh/devadvice/314.html
8. ISO Standards, http://www.iso.org/iso/iso_catalogue.htm

Progress in Development of HIFU CMUTs for use under MR-guidance

Serena H. Wong*, Ronald D. Watkins[†], Mario Kupnik*, Kim Butts Pauly[†], and B.T. Khuri-Yakub*[¶]

Stanford University
450 Via Palou,
Stanford, CA 94305, USA
* Department of Electrical Engineering, Ginzton Laboratories
†Department of Radiology, Lucas Center

Abstract. High intensity focused ultrasound (HIFU) guided by magnetic resonance imaging (MRI) is a noninvasive treatment that potentially reduces patient morbidity, lowers costs, and increases treatment accessibility. Traditionally, piezoelectric transducers are used for HIFU, but capacitive micromachined ultrasonic transducers (CMUTs) have many advantages, including fabrication flexibility, low loss, and efficient transmission. We designed, fabricated, and tested HIFU CMUTs for use under MRI guidance and have demonstrated continuous wave (CW) focusing. In this paper, we demonstrate that CMUTs can be designed for therapeutic ultrasound. First, we demonstrate successful unfocused heating of a HIFU phantom to 18.6°C, which was successfully monitored under MR guidance. Second, we demonstrated a focused CMUT array whose beam profile matched with simulation. In the future, we will expand the array and system for upper abdominal cancer therapy.

Keywords: MR-guided HIFU, CMUT.

INTRODUCTION

Minimally invasive, therapeutic ultrasound treatments of cancers have become popular in recent years because they reduce morbidity, mortality, and recovery time. Traditionally, piezoelectric transducers have been used for medical applications, but recently CMUTs have shown competitive advantages including the ease and flexibility in fabrication, integration with electronics, and competitive performance [1,2]. CMUTs are fabricated using silicon micro-machining methods that provide uniformity and sub-micron accuracy, so shapes and geometries can be optimized for performance.

In previous years, we presented finite element models (FEM) and optimization of the transducer array and CMUT membrane designs for external HIFU ablation of upper abdominal cancers [3]. Transducers were designed for low frequency operation from 1-4 MHz and surface output pressure of 1-2 MPa peak to peak. Based on FEM, we fabricated single-element test transducers and sub-costal annular arrays for ablation of liver cancers. These transducers were tested with special regard to high power CW operation. This year, we successfully demonstrated MR-temperature maps of the heating produced by an unfocused CMUT. With this successful demonstration, we continued to design, fabricate, and test a focused 8-element annular array for noninvasive HIFU therapy.

CP1113, *8th International Symposium on Therapeutic Ultrasound*, edited by E. S. Ebbini
© 2009 American Institute of Physics 978-0-7354-0650-6/09/$25.00

CMUT MEMBRANE FABRICATION

Circular CMUTs cells with center frequency of 3 MHz and 1 MPa peak to peak output pressure, were patterned into 2.5 mm by 2.5 mm test transducers and 3 cm, 8-element, concentric ring arrays (Fig. 1). Cells were fabricated using the silicon wafer bonding process [4] that utilizes a low resistivity silicon membrane, which acts as the top electrode. The low resistivity silicon improves electrical contact resistance [5], series parasitic capacitance, and problems associated with electromigration [6].

CMUT designs for HIFU

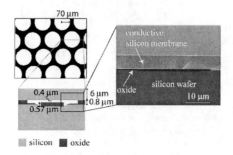

FIGURE 1. Simplified schematics and SEM images of the cross-section of part of a single CMUT cell.

EXPERIMENTAL SETUP

We measured the static and dynamic responses of the design before testing in noncontact heating situations. We mounted the test transducers on a printed circuit board (PCB) using silver epoxy and connected the pads with gold wire bonds. For dynamic response, such as frequency response as well as CW and tone-burst pressure measurements, the CMUTs were immersed in soybean oil, which provides electrical insulation and has acoustic properties like liver tissue [1]. A hydrophone (Onda Corporation, Sunnyvale, CA) was positioned 2 cm from the surface to measure the output pressure. The data was corrected for the hydrophone's frequency response [7] and sound attenuation and diffraction [8] to calculate the surface pressure. For dynamic response, DC biases were swept from 50-90% of the collapse voltage and a 2.5 MHz, 30-cycle burst with amplitudes from 0-300 Vpp was applied. Based on the pressures measured from these voltage sweeps, we chose to operate at a DC voltage that was 70% of the collapse voltage and an AC voltage of 250 Vpp.

We monitored heating from CW operation of a test transducer using a 3.0 T GE MRI scanner (Wakesha, WI). We placed the test CMUT on the bench top and isolated it electrically from a gel phantom by covering it with soybean oil and a sheet of polyethylene. An ultrasonic gel (MediChoice, Mechanicsville, VA) coupled sound into the HIFU phantom (Insightec, Haifu, Israel). The CMUT, which was matched to 50 Ω with an air-core inductor, was operated in CW mode for five minutes. The temperature in the phantom was measured in the sagittal plane using a fast gradient echo sequence with TR/TE (Repetition Time/Echo Time) of 28.7/19.1 seconds; one hundred images were captured over 12 minutes. Temperature change was detected by a shift in the proton resonance frequency and the change in phase. We calculated this phase changes by subtracting the phase images of successive frames [9].

Temperature Measurement Setup

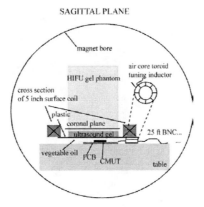

FIGURE 2. Schematic of the setup used to measure unfocused heating in a HIFU phantom.

Finally, the equal-area, concentric ring array was fabricated from the CMUT cells and driven by the focusing electronics. The electronics consisted of digital synthesizers and amplifiers with variable gain and phase. Only four channels were used to reduce the complexity of the electronics and also because of the yield of the array, as we will explain later. The phase was calculated for a focus at 35 mm from the transducer's surface. A hydrophone was then scanned in this plane to measure the beam profile and the results were compared to a simulation [10].

RESULTS AND DISCUSSION

We first measured the artefacts of the HIFU CMUT using the same MR sequence used to collect the temperature information. This artefact extended less than 1 mm into the phantom, which indicates that temperature measurements should be accurate and unaffected by the transducer even at distances very close to the transducer. An unfocused HIFU CMUT was then used to heat a HIFU phantom and monitored the temperature rise in the 3.0 T MRI scanner. We found that the transducer was 68% efficient and the phantom reached a maximum temperature change of 18.6°C over 5 min. (Fig. 3), which is adequate for HIFU applications [11].

With this success, we tested a larger focused transducer. The beam profile matches the expected profile calculated using Huygen's principle. The beam width is comparable, but the side lobe energy is increased because of the dispersive guided wave (Fig. 4). The agreement with the model is promising for further HIFU transducer development. However, the array design needs to be changed to improve the yield; because each ring was near 1 cm^2 in size, it was difficult to achieve a perfectly defect free area. To improve this, we will use a segmented 2-D array design, with switches in the backside electronics that remove the elements with defects.

HIFU heating by unfocused transducer

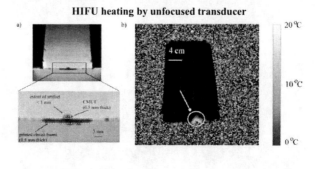

FIGURE 3. An unfocused CMUT demonstrated minimal artifact (a) in the MR scanner. MR temperature maps were able to monitor the unfocused heating a HIFU phantom (b).

Annular array beam profile

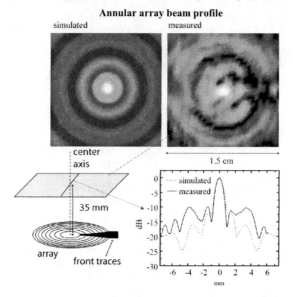

FIGURE 4. Comparison of simulated and measured beam profile.

CONCLUSION

CMUT membranes designed for non-invasive HIFU have been fabricated and tested. We have demonstrated MR temperature mapping of the therapy applied by an unfocused HIFU CMUT. Even an unfocused transducer was efficient enough to heat the phantom by 18.6°C in 5 min. With focusing, the heating will be faster and the treated region will be greater. We have also demonstrated focusing of 4-elements concentric ring array. In the future, we plan to build full-scale ring arrays that are more robust to small fabrication defects and demonstrate liver cancer ablation.

ACKNOWLEDGMENTS

This research was supported by NIH R01 CA77677, R01 CA 121163, F31 EB007170.

REFERENCES

1. O. Oralkan, A.S. Ergun, C. Cheng, J.A. Johnson, M. Karaman, T. Lee, B.T. Khuri-Yakub, "Volumetric Ultrasound Imaging Using 2-D CMUT Arrays," IEEE Transactions on Ultrasonics, 50(11), pp. 1581–1594.

2. D.M. Mills and L.S. Smith, "Real Time In-vivo with Capacitive Micromachined Ultrasound Transducer (cMUT) Linear Arrays," in Proceeings of IEEE Ultrason. Symp., 2003, pp.568-571.

3. S.H. Wong , M. Kupnik, K. Butts Pauly, B.T. Khuri-Yakub, "Design of HIFU CMUT Arrays for Treatment of Liver and Renal Cancers," in Proceeding of the International Symposium of Therapeutic Ultrasound, 2006.

4. Huang, Y.L., et al., "Fabricating capacitive micromachined ultrasonic transducers with wafer-bonding technology, " Journal of Microelectromechanical Systems, 12(2), pp. 128-137.

5. R.F. Pierret, Semiconductor Device Fundamnetals, Reading, Massachussets: Addison-Wesley, 1996.

6. K. Jhachaturyan, "Mechnical fatigue in thin films induced by piezoelectric strains as a cause of ferroelectric fatigue," J. Apply Phys. 77(12), pp.6449-6455.

7. http://www.ondacorp.com

8. G. Kino, Acoustics Waves:Devices,Imaging, and Analog Signal Processing, Englewood Cliffs, New Jersey: Prentice-Hall, 1987.

9. H.E. Cline, K. Hynynen, C.J. Hardy, R.D. Watkins, J.F. Schenck, and J.F. Jolesz. Mr temperature mapping of focused ultrasound surgery. Magnetic Resonance in Medicine, 31(6):628–636, 1994.

10. E. B. Hutchinson, M. T. Buchanan, and K. Hynynen, "Design and optimization of an aperiodic ultrasound phased array for intracavitary prostate thermal therapies," Med. Phys., vol. 23, no. 5, pp. 767–776, 1996.

11. S. H. Wong, R. D. Watkins, M. Kupnik, K. Butts Pauly, and B. T. Khuri-Yakub, "Feasibility of MR-Temperature Mapping of Ultrasonic Heating from a CMUT," Ultrasonics, Ferroelectrics and Frequency Control, IEEE Transactions on, vol. 55, no. 4, pp. 811-818, April 2008.

In Vitro Validation of a Sector-Switching HIFU Device for Accelerated Treatment

Lorena Petrusca[a], Lucie Brasset[b], Francois Cotton[c], Rares Salomir[a], Jean-Yves Chapelon[a]

[a]Inserm U556, 151, cours Albert Thomas, 69424 LYON Cedex 03, France
[b]EDAP-TMS, 4, Rue du Dauphiné, 69120 VAULX EN VELIN, France
[c]Radiology, RMN Unit, CHU Lyon Sud, Pierre-Bénite, France

Abstract. A sector-switching method that increases the HIFU sequence duty-cycle and reduces the equivalent treatment time was tested in vitro. The MR-compatible HIFU device used consisted of 2 symmetric sectors arranged on a truncated spherical cap (focus = 45mm, long diameter = 57.5mm, short diameter = 35mm). A MR-compatible, 2D positioning system provided 0.5 mm accuracy. Two sonication sequences were considered, each with the same pattern for the focal point trajectory and with identical on-state power. First, both sectors radiated simultaneously, with a power duty cycle of 60%. Second, the sectors radiated separately with balanced temporally-interleaved sonication and a power duty cycle of 87.5%. Numerical simulations were performed to predict the shape of the lesion for a given set of sequence parameters, according to a theoretical model. Fast MR thermometry (voxel size: 0.85x0.85x4.25 mm3; temporal resolution: 2 sec) was performed in two orthogonal planes (sagittal and transverse) while the 2D sonication pattern was contained in the coronal plane. Fresh samples of degassed porcine liver were used, and the macroscopic lesions were measured after HIFU. The 14400 s equivalent thermal dose isolevel was compared respectively for the two sonication sequences, both with numerical simulations and experimental MR data. No susceptibility or RF artifacts could be detected on MR data. The lesion's size ratio between reference versus the sector-switched sequence was 1.12 from simulations and 1.25 (±3.2%) from MRI derived TD. Switching the device sectors reduced the treatment time by 20% while the shape and size of the lesions were maintained. In vivo studies are required for pre-clinical validation.

Keywords: cancer therapy, sector-switching, MRI monitoring
PACS: D87.54.Br, D87.54.Hk

INTRODUCTION

Different treatments for localized cancer are proposed, but minimally invasive methods are preferred. Thermal therapy is an approach under continuous development which is gaining more and more popularity. It is a good alternative to other existing treatments and consists of thermal coagulation of the heated zone in order to destroy the affected volume. Radiofrequency, laser, thermal conduction or microwaves are energy sources that have been studied in view of cancer treatments. An ultrasound heating applicator was investigated using MR thermometry for temperature feedback (Chopra, 2006). Chapelon (1999) described a High Intensity Focused Ultrasound (HIFU) transducer coupled with ultrasound imaging guidance and the results of this

CP1113, *8th International Symposium on Therapeutic Ultrasound*, edited by E. S. Ebbini
© 2009 American Institute of Physics 978-0-7354-0650-6/09/$25.00

type of treatment in patients were also studied (Poissonnier, 2007). Ultrasound therapy involves the delivery of energy to affected zones. It is as minimally invasive as possible and represents a promising therapy for cancer treatment (Murat, 2007).

HIFU therapy consists in sonication of a given point using a high-intensity ultrasound beam that produces local elevation of temperature. This can cause necroses of the tissue in a localized volume. MRI guidance offers information about quantitative thermometry during sonication and also about the shape of the treated volume.

The study described here proposes HIFU therapy under MR guidance, using a 2 sectors MR compatible HIFU device. A new sector-switching method was tested in vitro using fresh liver samples. The performance of this sequence was compared with the reference sequence, in order to determine the advantage. Time saving is considerable using the same power.

MATERIALS AND METHODS

The dedicated device for this proposed method is MRI-compatible and consists of 2 symmetrical sectors arranged on a truncated spherical cap (Fig. 1). The long diameter of the transducer is 57.5 mm, the short diameter is 35 mm, and the focal point is at a distance of 45 mm. The 2 sectors are characterized by identical surface and geometry and independent activation. The frequency of the transducer was set at 3MHz.

A MR compatible 2D mechanical system (Fig. 2) was used to move the probe on 2 axes. The system has an accuracy of less than 0.5mm and it is controlled using an ESP 300 Microcontrole Unit. A plastic holder between the system and the device was added, which allows the probe and the system to follow the same trajectory. All the in vitro fresh liver samples were degassed before and set in physiological serum. The C3 standard Philips coil was used.

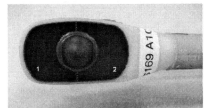 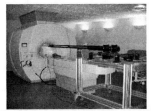

FIGURE 1. The HIFU MR compatible device with 2 sectors 1 and 2.   FIGURE 2. The MR compatible XY mechanical system

The electronic commutation card can command the probe at a distance using a sequence defined by the user. The commutation system permits activation or inhibition of the 2 sectors, independently of each other.

The numerical simulations made with a fast version of the HIFU simulation program permitted us to identify a sector-switching sequence that permits reduction of the treatment time without compromising efficiency or patient safety, reported at the performances obtained with the reference sequence. The optimal shot parameters were obtained for in vivo numerical simulations, but the comparison was between in vitro simulations and in vitro experiments. For the reference sequence the 2 sectors of the probe are activated simultaneously with a duty cycle of 10 seconds: 6 seconds active shot (both sectors) + 4 seconds pause (Fig 3a). The duty-cycle of sector-switching sequence contains 3.5 seconds active shot (first sector), then 3.5 seconds active shot (the second sector) and then 1 second of pause after the 2 shots (Fig. 3b). The power applied to the 2 sectors was the same. By activating the sectors in an alternative mode it is possible to keep a continuous sonication in the focal point for a longer period of time. The 2 types of lesions, obtained with the reference sequence and with the sector-switching sequence were compared to determine the advantages.

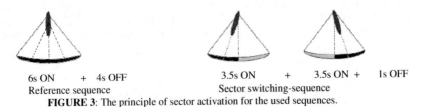

6s ON   +   4s OFF   3.5s ON   +   3.5s ON +   1s OFF
Reference sequence   Sector switching-sequence
FIGURE 3: The principle of sector activation for the used sequences.

RESULTS

The theoretical model considers in vitro samples with the simulated applied power of 50% from the optimal value (to conform to the experimental model). Figure 4 shows the numerical simulation results obtained with the reference sequence for XZ and YZ planes in the central section of the lesions, and the 3D lesion surface. The same parameters were utilized for the second sequence simulations. In Figure 5 are shown the XZ and YZ planes in the central section of the lesion and the 3D lesion surface for sector-switching sequence.

a   b   c

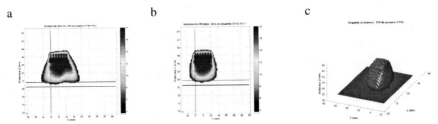

FIGURE 4. The reference sequence numerical simulations results obtained in (a) XZ plane, central section, (b) YZ plane, central section and (c) 3D lesion surface.

a   b   c

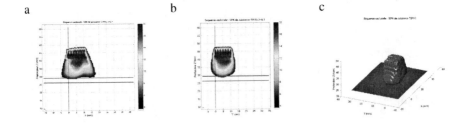

FIGURE 5. The sector-switching sequence numerical simulation results obtained in (a) XZ plane, central section, (b) YZ plane, central section and (c) 3D lesion surface.

Using the same set of sequence parameters, in vitro experiments on pig liver were conducted. Only 50% power was used because during high power heating and for a temperature >100°C, the MR signal drops and we can't correctly record the temperature. T1w images with a short TR were made before HIFU (Fig. 6a) and inversion-recuperation sequences with a long TR were made after HIFU (Fig. 6b). The images were made in axial plane with a voxel size of 0.5x0.5x4mm.

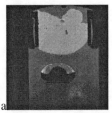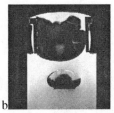

FIGURE 6. (a) T1w image before HIFU, (b) Inversion-recuperation, after HIFU

Fast MR thermometry using the proton resonance frequency method was performed in 2 orthogonal planes: axial and sagittal. The voxel size was the same as for the numerical simulations: 0.85x0.85x4.25 mm^3, while the temporal resolution was 2 seconds and the temperature accuracy was 0.5°C. Figure 7 shows the temperature (T) and the thermal dose (TD) images obtained with the reference sequence (a,c) and with the sector-switched sequence (b,c) in 2 orthogonal planes. The images for every set of figures are taken before the shot (the first image of every set), during the active shot (the second, the 3rd, the 4th and the 5th image) and after the shot, during the cooling period (the 6th image).

Reference sequence   Sector-switching sequence

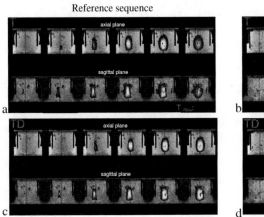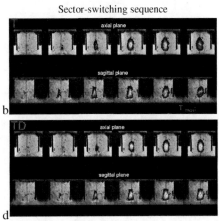

FIGURE 7. The temperature and the thermal dose images, for reference and sector-switching sequences in axial and sagittal plane.

The 14400 s equivalent thermal dose isolevel was compared respectively for the two sonication sequences both with numerical simulations and experimental MR data.

The lesion's size ratio between reference versus the sector-switched sequence was 1.12 from simulations and 1.25 (±3.2%) from MRI derived TD. Macroscopic lesions (Figure 8) were also measured after HIFU and the size ratio between the reference and the sector-switched sequences are similar.

Reference sequence

Sector-switching sequence

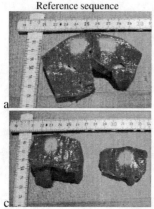 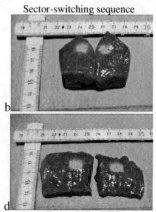

FIGURE 8. Macroscopical pictures after HIFU in (a), (b) sagittal plane (c), (d) axial plane

CONCLUSION

Switching the device sectors reduces the treatment time by 20% while the shape and size of the lesions were maintained. In vivo studies are required for pre-clinical validation.

ACKNOWLEDGMENTS

This work is supported by ANR Grant RNTS / SUTI with technological support from Edap-Tms.

REFERENCES

1. R. Chopra, *Phys. Med. Biol.* **51,** 827-844 (2006).
2. J. Y. Chapelon, *European Journal of Ultrasound* **9,** 31-38 (1999).
3. L. Poissonnier, *European Urology* **51,** 381-387 (2007),
4. F. J. Murat, *Cancer Control* **14,** no 3, 244-249 (2007).

Effect of Beam Size on Stone Comminution in Shock Wave Lithotripsy

Jun Qin[a,b], W. Neal Simmons[a], Georgy Sankin[a], and Pei Zhong[a]

[a]Department of Mechanical Engineering and Materials Science, Duke University,
P.O.Box 90300, Durham, NC 27708, USA
[b]Biomedical Engineering Program, College of Engineering, Southern Illinois University Carbondale,
Engineering D - Mail Code 6603, 1230 Lincoln Drive, Carbondale, IL, 62901, USA

Abstract. The effect of beam size on stone comminution in the Dornier HM-3 lithotripter were investigated using a modified reflector (MR), which was developed to produce an acoustic field with higher peak pressure and smaller beam size compared to the original reflector (OR) of the HM-3. The acoustic fields produced at 20 kV by the MR in the focal plane, and by the OR in the focal and pre-focal plane (z = -15 mm) were characterized using a light spot hydrophone. The efficiencies of stone comminution in a mesh holder were similar, but the corresponding values produced by using the MR in a membrane holder were significantly lower than those produced by the OR in the focal and pre-focal planes. These results suggest that a broad beam size could increase stone comminution efficiency when fragments are spreading out or moving due to respiratory motion in a large area during SWL. In contrast, when stone fragments are confined and well aligned to lithotripter focus the beam size may not influence significantly the treatment outcome.

Keywords: Shock wave lithotripsy, Beam size, Stone comminution.
PACS: 43.80.Vj

INTRODUCTION

Since its introduction in the early 1980s, shock wave lithotripsy (SWL) has rapidly emerged as the primary treatment modality for most urinary tract calculi world-widely [1]. Up to now, more than 30 different models of the 2nd- and 3rd- generation lithotripters have been designed and marketed [2]. Compared to the original Dornier HM-3 lithotripter, however, a growing number of clinical studies have demonstrated that these newer generation lithotripters are often less effective in stone comminution and yet have higher propensity for tissue injury and increased stone recurrent rate [3, 4]. A major change in the design of the newer generation lithotripters is the increased peak pressure with concomitantly reduced beam size [5]. In this study, we developed a method to modify the reflector geometry of the HM-3 to produce a lithotripter field with narrow beam size and high peak pressure so that the effect of beam size on stone comminution can be compared using the same energy source. The characteristics of acoustic fields produced by the modified and original reflectors were investigated and compared. Stone fragmentation experiments *in vitro* were carried out in different types of stone holders to evaluate the effect of beam size on stone comminution.

CP1113, *8th International Symposium on Therapeutic Ultrasound*, edited by E. S. Ebbini
© 2009 American Institute of Physics 978-0-7354-0650-6/09/$25.00

METHODS

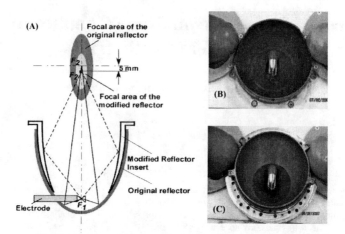

FIGURE 1: (A) A schematic diagram of the original and modified reflector configurations in an HM-3 lithotripter, and photographs of the (B) original and (C) modified reflectors.

The experiments were carried out in an HM-3 lithotripter, which uses an 80-nF capacitor and truncated ellipsoidal brass reflector with a semimajor axis a=138 mm, a semiminor axis b=77.5 mm, and a half-focal length c=114 mm. To generate an acoustic field with higher peak positive pressure and smaller beam size, a reflector insert (a'=134.4 mm, b'=75 mm and c'=111.5 mm) was fabricated and combined with the original HM3 reflector (Figure 1).

The acoustic fields produced by the modified reflector (MR) in the focal plane, and the original reflector (OR) in the focal and pre-focal planes (z = -15 mm) were characterized using a light spot hydrophone. Stone comminution was evaluated in three different types of holders: 1) a 15-mm mesh holder, 2) a 30-mm membrane holder and 3) a 30-mm matrix holder. (Figure 2)

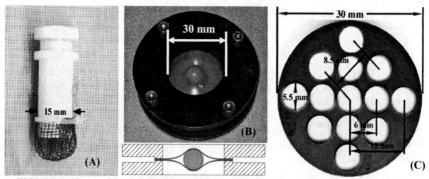

FIGURE 2: Photos of three different types of stone holders: (A) a mesh holder, (B) a membrane holder, and (C) a matrix holder insert.

338

RESULTS AND DISCUSSION

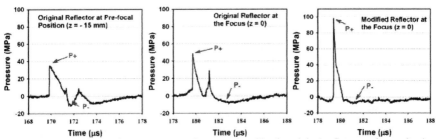

FIGURE 3: Representative pressure waveforms produced by the original reflector at the pre-focal
position (left) and F_2 (middle), and the modified reflector at F_2 (right)

The typical pressure waveforms produced by at 20 kV using the OR at the pre-focal position ($z = -15$ mm) and the focus (F_2) and the MR at F_2 of the HM-3 lithotripter are shown in figure 3. For the OR, a typical LSW arrives at F_2 in about 180 μs after the spark discharge, and the LSW consists of a leading compressive wave with dual-peak structure, followed by a tensile wave. This dual-peak structure is presumably caused by the truncation in the lateral sides of the ellipsoidal reflector to facilitate the bi-planar fluoroscopic imaging for stone localization [6]. In comparison, the shock wave measured at the pre-focal position arrives at the central axis in about 170 μs. The waveform also shows a dual-peak structure in the compressive phase, followed by a trailing tensile component. Interestingly, the trench between the dual peaks of the LSW at the pre-focal position is deeper, and it may be caused by the stronger edge wave at the pre-focal position [7]. On the other hand, using the MR, the pressure waveform at F_2 has a very strong single peak in the leading compressive wave.

TABLE 1. Characteristics of Acoustic Fields

	Original Reflector at $z = -15$ mm	Original Reflector at $z = 0$ mm	Modified Reflector at $z = 0$ mm
Peak Positive Pressure (MPa)	32.6 ± 5.2	48.9 ± 1.3	86.9 ± 3.8
Peak Negative Pressure (MPa)	-9.8 ± 2.7	-10.7 ± 0.4	-10.6 ± 0.6
-6 dB Beam Size, x-axis (mm)	19.9	12.5	3.4
-6 dB Beam Size, y-axis (mm)	16.8	9.3	4.4
Acoustic Pulse Energy (mJ)	115.9	121.7	116.1

Note: x-axis: foot to head direction, and y-axis: left to right direction.

The characteristics of the lithotripter fields are summarized in Table 1. The peak positive pressure produced at F_2 using the MR was measured to be 86.9 MPa, which is significantly higher than the corresponding value of the OR (48.9 MPa), and both are higher than the 32.6 MPa produced in the pro-focal position ($z = -15$ mm). However, the peak tensile pressures were found to be similar, -10.6 MPa for the MR in the focal plane, -10.7 MPa in the focal plane and -9.8 MPa in the pre-focal plane for the OR, respectively. Furthermore, the MR was found to have the narrowest -6 dB beam size

(3.4 mm on x-axis and 4.4 mm on y-axis), while the OR produced a broader beam size in the focal plane (12.5 mm on x-axis and 9.3 mm on y-axis), and the broadest beam size in the pre-focal plane ($z = -15$ mm) with 19.9 mm on x-axis and 16.8 mm on y-axis. Importantly, the derived acoustic pulse energy under these three aforementioned field focal conditions (i.e., 115.9 mJ, 121.7 mJ and 116.1 mJ) was found to be comparable in the 28-mm diameter cross-sectional area, which covers essentially the inner area of the membrane holder.

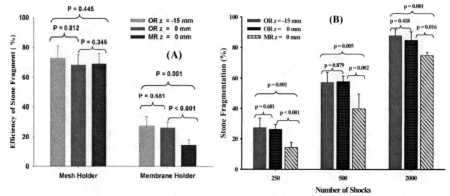

FIGURE 4: (A) Stone fragmentations in the mesh and membrane holders after 250 shocks, and (B) dose-dependence of stone fragmentations in the membrane holder.

The results of stone comminution in the mesh and membrane holders after 250 shocks are shown in figure 4A. In the mesh holder, there is no statistical difference in stone fragmentation among the OR in the focal and pre-focal planes, and the MR in the focal plane. However, in the membrane holder, the efficiency of stone fragmentation produced by using the MR in the focal plane was found to be significantly lower than the corresponding values of the OR both in the focal and pre-focal planes. In addition, the efficiencies of stone fragmentation in the membrane holder are much lower than the corresponding values in the mesh holder. This is mainly caused by the accumulation and lateral spreading of stone fragments during lithotripsy. Since the 30-mm diameter of the membrane holder is significantly larger than the beam size of acoustic fields in the HM-3, these results suggest that the wide beam size in the original HM-3 may increase stone comminution efficiency when stone fragments are spreading out to a large area during SWL. In contrast, when the fragments are confined during lithotripsy, the beam size may not influence significantly the outcome of the treatment.

Figure 4B shows the dose-dependency of stone comminution in the membrane holder. From 250 to 2000 shocks, the efficiencies of stone comminution produced by the original reflector both in the focal and pre-focal planes were found to be significantly higher than those produced by the modified reflector in the focal plane. However, no statistically significant difference was observed in stone fragmentation between the OR in the focal and pre-focal planes.

340

The distribution of stone comminution in the matrix holder is shown in figure 5. At the center of the matrix holder, the stone comminution produced by both the OR in the pre-focal plane and by the MR in the focal plane were found to be higher than that produced by the OR in the focal plane. In comparison, at a radial distance between 6 mm and 8.5 mm, the OR in both the focal and pre-focal planes produces higher comminution results than the MR in the focal plane. Therefore, the effective areas of stone comminution for the OR both in the focal and pre-focal planes are larger than that of the MR in the focal plane.

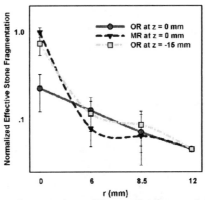

FIGURE 5: Variation of stone fragmentation at different radial distances from the lithotripter axis in the matrix holder after 500 shocks produced by the HM-3 at 20kV.

ACKNOWLEDGMETS

This work was supported in part by NIH through grant # R01-DK05298.

REFERENCES

1. Chaussy, C. and G.J. Fuchs, *Current state and future developments of noninvasive treatment of human urinary stones with extracorporeal shock wave lithotripsy.* J. Urol., 1989. **141**: p. 782-792.
2. Lingeman, J.E. and F.S. Zafar, *Lithotripsy systems.* Smith's Textbook of Endourology, 1996: p. 553-589.
3. Kohrmann, K.U., et al., *THE CLINICAL INTRODUCTION OF A 3RD GENERATION LITHOTRIPTOR - MODULITH SL-20.* Journal of Urology, 1995. **153**(5): p. 1379-1383.
4. Graber, S.F., et al., *A prospective randomized trial comparing 2 lithotriptors for stone disintegration and induced renal trauma.* J. Urol., 2003. **169**(1): p. 54-57.
5. Lingeman, J.E., et al., *Shockwave lithotripsy: Anecdotes and insights.* Journal of Endourology, 2003. **17**(9): p. 687-693.
6. Zhou, Y.F. and P. Zhong, *Suppression of large intraluminal bubble expansion in shock wave lithotripsy without compromising stone comminution: Refinement of reflector geometry.* Journal of the Acoustical Society of America, 2003. **113**(1): p. 586-597.
7. Hamilton, M.F., *Transient axial solution for the reflection of a spherical wave from a concave ellipsoidal mirror.* Journal of the Acoustical Society of America, 1993. **93**(3): p. 1256-1266.

Intracranial Catheter for Integrated 3D Ultrasound Imaging & Hyperthermia: Feasibility Study

Carl D. Herickhoff[a], Edward D. Light[a], Kristin Frinkley Bing[a], Srinivasan Mukundan[b], Gerald A. Grant[c], Patrick D. Wolf[a], Ellen Dixon-Tulloch[a], Timothy Shih[a], Stephen J. Hsu[a], Stephen W. Smith

[a]*Department of Biomedical Engineering, Duke University, Durham, NC 27708, USA*
[b]*Department of Radiology, Brigham and Women's Hospital, Boston, MA 02115, USA*
[c]*Division of Neurosurgery, Duke University Medical Center, Durham, NC 27708, USA*

Abstract. In this study, we investigated the feasibility of an intracranial catheter transducer capable of real-time 3D (RT3D) imaging and ultrasound hyperthermia, for application in the visualization and treatment of tumors in the brain. We designed and constructed a 12 Fr, integrated matrix and linear array catheter transducer prototype for combined RT3D imaging and heating capability. This dual-mode catheter incorporated 153 matrix array elements and 11 linear array elements, on a 0.2 mm pitch, with a total aperture size of 8.4 mm × 2.3 mm. This array achieved a 3.5°C *in vitro* temperature rise at a 2 cm focal distance in tissue-mimicking material. The dual-mode catheter prototype was compared with a Siemens 10 Fr AcuNav™ catheter as a gold standard in experiments assessing image quality and therapeutic potential, and both probes were used in a canine brain model to image anatomical structures and color Doppler blood flow and to attempt *in vivo* heating.

Keywords: Catheter transducer, real-time 3D imaging, hyperthermia, dual-mode array
PACS: 87.50.yt

INTRODUCTION

In 2008, an estimated 13,070 people will die (>2% of all cancer deaths) from a primary malignant brain and central nervous system (CNS) tumor and 21,810 new cases will be diagnosed in the U.S.[1] Malignant gliomas account for 81% of all malignant primary brain/CNS tumors, and 51% of gliomas are WHO grade IV subtype glioblastoma multiforme (GBM), the most common intracranial neoplasm.[2,3]

The goal of this project is to extend real-time 3D (RT3D) ultrasound to minimally invasive catheters for intracranial imaging of the brain combined with ultrasound hyperthermia for neuro-oncology. This dual-mode technology could be used to visualize a tumor target in 3D and then trigger the release of chemotherapeutic drugs contained within microbubble or liposomal agents molecularly targeted to regions of tumor angiogenesis. The catheter will be designed to be thin and flexible enough to be manipulated through the internal jugular vein into the dural venous sinuses (see Fig. 1), which provide minimally invasive access to virtually the entire brain volume. Here

CP1113, *8th International Symposium on Therapeutic Ultrasound*, edited by E. S. Ebbini
© 2009 American Institute of Physics 978-0-7354-0650-6/09/$25.00

we describe an initial dual-mode prototype catheter to demonstrate the feasibility of our long term goal.

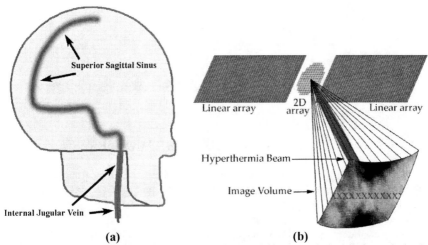

FIGURE 1. (a) Intended catheter pathway affording intracranial access to the brain volume via dural venous sinuses. (b) Integrated 2D matrix & linear array. The centered 2D array scans a pyramidal volume in real-time, and adjacent linear arrays generate a hyperthermia beam, steerable in azimuth.

DUAL-MODE CATHETER DESIGN & FABRICATION

We designed a prototype catheter device integrating a matrix array and a linear array on a custom 10 Fr multi-layer flexible circuit by Microconnex (Snoqualmie, WA, USA). The flex circuit could accommodate an array with 198 matrix elements and 18 linear elements, diced on a 0.2 mm pitch, for a total aperture size of 8.4 mm × 2.3 mm. The beam pattern of this array was simulated and compared with that of a Siemens 10 Fr AcuNav[TM] catheter probe (as a gold standard) using Field II[4]. Each computation included a 0.5 dB/cm/MHz attenuation factor to simulate brain tissue[5].

A piece of 0.35-mm-thick PZT-5H was bonded to the flex circuit with silver epoxy, and diced on a 0.2 mm pitch both vertically and horizontally to create the matrix array. The linear array was then built in the adjacent spaces: a piece of PZT-5H was bonded to each side and diced (0.2 mm pitch), and MicroFlat cables from W.L. Gore & Associates, Inc. (Newark, DE, USA) were soldered with appropriate spacing to the exposed border contact. Double-sided metallized liquid crystal polymer (LCP) was attached to the face of the transducer for a front grounding contact and overall electronic shielding; there was no acoustic matching layer. An acoustic backing was attached before bending the flex circuit into a side-viewing configuration and packaging the transducer into the catheter lumen. The dual-mode RT3D/hyperthermia catheter prototype construction yielded 153 matrix array elements (77% yield) and 11 linear array elements (61% yield).

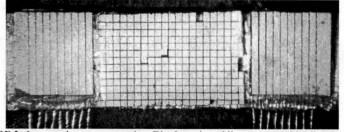

FIGURE 2. Integrated array construction: Diced matrix and linear arrays with MicroFlat cables soldered to linear array contacts. Total aperture size: 8.4 mm × 2.3 mm.

IN VITRO IMAGING & THERMAL TESTS

The dual-mode catheter was compared with a Siemens 10 Fr AcuNav as a gold standard to assess imaging capability and therapeutic potential. Various wire, tumor, and cyst phantoms were imaged with each probe; the dual-mode catheter performed comparably to the AcuNav in terms of lateral and axial resolution.

To assess therapy potential of each probe, the maximum I_{SPTA} was measured. At a 2 cm transmit focus, our RT3D scanner delivered an I_{SPTA} = 2.43 W/cm^2 using a 12-cycle, 3.64 MHz pulse at 6.6 kHz PRF with the dual-mode catheter. With the same settings, the dual-mode catheter created a temperature rise of 3.5°C at a 2 cm depth in tissue-mimicking material[6]. The AcuNav's projected maximum settings were a 10-cycle, 5.33 MHz pulse at 6.6 kHz PRF and 55% system voltage. To avoid self-heating, I_{SPTA} measurements were taken for lower voltage settings and we extrapolated to an estimate of I_{SPTA} = 4.10 W/cm^2. No *in vitro* hyperthermia measurement was attempted.

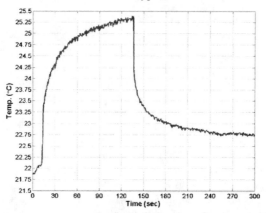

FIGURE 3. Dual-mode catheter: 3.5°C temperature rise in tissue-mimicking material at 2 cm depth.

IN VIVO CANINE BRAIN MODEL

In accordance with a large animal protocol approved by the Duke University IACUC, each ultrasound catheter was placed in the superior sagittal sinus of a canine

344

via a 1 cm burr hole in the skull. For hyperthermia trials, a hypodermic needle thermocouple was inserted into the cerebrum exposed by an adjacent burr hole.

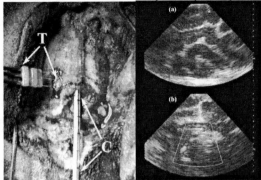

FIGURE 4. *In vivo* canine model: the dual-mode catheter (C) was placed in the superior sagittal sinus through a burr hole created in the skull, and a thermocouple(T) was inserted into the cerebrum through the dura mater exposed by a second burr hole, for hyperthermia. (a) AcuNav Echo image showing various gyri and sulci of the cerebrum. (b) Color Doppler image showing the internal carotid artery.

Both echo and Doppler images were acquired with each probe. The AcuNav produced clear delineation of cerebral gyri and sulci, as well as color Doppler images of the internal carotid artery, without the use of contrast.

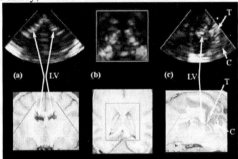

FIGURE 5. Dual-mode prototype in *in vivo* canine model. (a,b,c) Intracranial RT3D echo images in coronal, axial, and sagittal planes, respectively, compared to corresponding anatomical images (Courtesy T.F. Fletcher). The lateral ventricles (LV) are clearly seen in (a) and (b). The tentorium (T) and cerebellum (C), as well as a posterior horn of the lateral ventricle, are visible in (c).

The dual-mode catheter prototype acquired RT3D images of a pyramidal volume extending from the transducer face toward the base of the cranial cavity. The Volumetrics scanner simultaneously displayed two perpendicular B-mode sectors and two C-scans (parallel to the transducer face), which can be inclined at any desired angle. The coronal plane was key to orienting the transducer's field of view, enabling the operator to identify structures more quickly, with greater confidence and accuracy.

For 3D color Doppler imaging, a bolus of agitated saline was delivered into the left internal carotid artery for contrast, and vessels comprising the Circle of Willis became clearly visible. The color Doppler look-up table was modified because of aliasing, thus eliminating directional information.

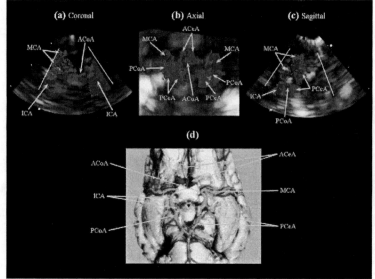

FIGURE 6. (a,b,c) Intracranial RT3D color Doppler images in coronal, axial, and sagittal planes, respectively. (d) Latex-injected sheep brain vasculature for anatomical reference (Courtesy R.R. Miselis). The internal carotid arteries (ICA), left middle cerebral artery (MCA), and anterior communicating artery (ACoA) are visible in (a). The Circle of Willis is seen in (b).

For heating trials, the thermocouple was located and aligned by imaging, and high power pulse sequences were initiated. The AcuNav achieved a 4.5°C temperature rise, but this was due to self-heating and conduction, which damaged the probe. The dual-mode catheter achieved a temperature rise just over 0.85°C, but it was found later that the transmit efficiency of the elements had been considerably weakened before and/or during the experiment.

Our results lead us to conclude that the development of an intracranial ultrasound catheter combining RT3D imaging and hyperthermia capability is feasible.

REFERENCES

1. ACS. Cancer Facts & Figures 2008. Atlanta: American Cancer Society, 2008. p. 4.
2. CBTRUS. Statistical Report: Primary Brain Tumors in the United States, 2000-2004: Central Brain Tumor Registry of the United States, 2008. pp. 10, 17-18.
3. Kleihues P, Cavenee WK, International Agency for Research on Cancer., International Society of Neuropathology., International Academy of Pathology., Preuss Foundation for Brain Tumor Research. Pathology and genetics of tumours of the nervous system. Lyon: IARC Press, 2000.
4. Jensen JA, Svendsen NB, Calculation of Pressure Fields from Arbitrarily Shaped, Apodized, and Excited Ultrasound Transducers. IEEE Trans. Ultrason. Ferroelectr. Freq. Control 1992;39:262-267.
5. Goss SA, Johnston RL, Dunn F, Comprehensive Compilation of Empirical Ultrasonic Properties of Mammalian-Tissues. Journal of the Acoustical Society of America 1978;64:423-457.
6. Bacon DR, Shaw A, Experimental Validation of Predicted Temperature Rises in Tissue-Mimicking Materials. Physics in Medicine and Biology 1993;38:1647-1659.

Dual-mode 5-element transducer for image-guided interstitial ultrasound therapy: In vitro evaluation

N.R. Owen[a], G. Bouchoux[a], A. Murillo-Rincon[a], S. Merouche[a], A. Birer[a], J.Y. Chapelon[a], R. Berriet[b], G. Fleury[b], and C. Lafon[a]

[a]Inserm, U556, Lyon, F-69003, France ; Université de Lyon, Lyon, F-69003, France
[b]IMASONIC, 70190 Voray sur l'Ognon, France

Abstract. Interstitial probes with dual-mode transducers are effective devices to guide and monitor with ultrasound imaging the application of ultrasound therapy. Here, a dual-mode 5-element transducer, with oscillatory motion for sector imaging and directive therapy, was characterized and evaluated in vitro with porcine liver. The transducer had 3.8x3.0-mm^2 elements, a 20x3.0-mm^2 aperture, and was cylindrically focused to 14-mm. In therapy mode, elements were maximally efficient, 72±4% (ave±std), at 5.6-MHz. In imaging mode, the pulse-echo impulse response for each electrically-matched element was 160±16 ns long at -6 dB, and insertion loss was minimally 9.8±0.5 dB at 5.2-MHz. Electrical crosstalk was less than -57 dB at 5.6-MHz. Lateral resolution, measured by scanning a wire of 0.1-mm diameter wire though the focal plane, was 1.0-mm at -6 dB. During experiment, an initial B-mode image was formed over a 140° sector. Then, therapy was applied for 90 s, with 18-W/cm^2 transducer surface intensity, at each of 5 angles (Δθ=20°) to form volumes of composite protein denaturization. Pulse-echo data were collected periodically to monitor therapy with real-time M-mode imaging. After therapy, another B-mode image was formed, and the depth of protein denaturization was measured by gross histology. B-mode images adequately represented the liver structure. Analysis of M-mode images was consistent with gross histology.

Keywords: dual-mode, transducer, ultrasound, therapy
PACS: 43.80.Sh, 43.80.Jz

INTRODUCTION

Miniaturized ultrasound transducers have been used to deliver minimally invasive thermal therapy in laboratory and clinical settings [1-4]. Image guidance assists the placement of the probe in close proximity to or in contact with the targeted tissue, and imaging may also assist the assessment of therapy during or after treatment. The use of dual-mode transducers for ultrasound imaging and therapy aims to improve guidance proximal to the probe, as well as enable treatment monitoring [5,6].

Here we report the *in vitro* evaluation of an oscillating dual-mode interstitial probe that was piloted by a prototype imaging/therapy system. The transducer was subjected to many standard tests to characterize its electrical and acoustical properties in imaging and therapy modes. Then, during evaluation in porcine liver, the probe and imaging/therapy system were used to form B-mode images, apply high intensity ultrasound at several angles, and form M-mode images during therapy.

CP1113, *8th International Symposium on Therapeutic Ultrasound*, edited by E. S. Ebbini
© 2009 American Institute of Physics 978-0-7354-0650-6/09/$25.00

METHODS AND MATERIALS

Figure 1 shows the interstitial probe and the dual-mode transducer. A digital servomotor (ERG-VZ, Sanwa, Japan) in the base of the probe was used to control the position of the transducer for sector imaging and directive therapy. The 5-element piezocomposite transducer (IMASONIC, Voray sur l'Ognon, France) had an aperture of 3.0 x 20 mm² and was cylindrically focused to 14 mm. Each element was 3.8 mm in height and the spacing between elements was 0.250 mm. Imaging mode was driven by a single pulser/receiver (USBox, Lecoeur Electronique, France) that was multiplexed between the transducer elements using a network of broadband relays. In therapy mode, the elements were driven in parallel by a signal generator (AFG3102, Tektronix Inc., Beaverton, OR) and a power amplifier. A circuit of chilled, degassed water ran continuously across the surface of the transducer. The outer diameter of the probe tip was 4 mm.

Electrical and acoustical properties of the dual-mode transducer were measured using several standard methods including radiation force balance, pulse/echo from a planar reflector at the focus, and pulse/echo from a point scatterer. Once characterized, the probe was evaluated *in vitro* using degassed porcine liver samples that were submerged in water at room temperature. Experiments were performed to the following sequence. 1) The probe was implanted in the liver to allow each transducer approximately 40 mm of propagation. 2) Each transducer element was used to form a B-mode image over a 140° sector. RF lines were taken at 1° increments. Echo data were band pass filtered from 2 MHz to 8 MHz, envelope detected, log compressed, and mapped to Cartesian coordinates. 3) High intensity ultrasound treatment was applied at 18 W/cm² for 90 s at each angle: -40°, -20°, 0°, 20°, and 40°. RF lines were taken with a preselected transducer element every 125 ms during treatment to update an M-mode image. 4) Step 2 was repeated. 5) Gross histology was preformed to measure the depth of protein denaturization in the liver.

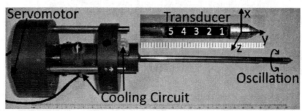

FIGURE 1. Oscillating interstitial probe and dual-mode transducer for ultrasound imaging and therapy. The probe was designed to perform sector imaging and directive thermal therapy.

RESULTS

Table 1 summarizes the characterization data measured in therapy and imaging modes. The transducer was maximally efficient at 5.6 MHz, which was chosen as the working frequency. Acoustic output was tested up to a surface intensity of 30 W/cm². Axial resolution was calculated at 0.48 mm using the average impulse response length and a propagation speed of 1500 m/s.

Figure 2 shows B-mode images that were formed before and after treatment at the five angles. Imaging resolution was highest proximal to the transducer and decreased linearly with distance. Quantitatively, lateral resolution at -6 dB was 0.5 mm at z = 7 mm, 1.0 mm at z = 14 mm, and 1.8 mm at z = 25 mm, as calculated using pulse/echo data from a 0.1 mm-diameter wire. Figure 3 shows M-mode images that were taken during treatment at -40°, 0°, and 40°. The observation of distortion on the images was consistent with the measurement of protein denaturization during gross histology, and presumably indicates temperature rise in the tissue samples. A similar effect was reported by Bouchoux *et al.* [5]. Figure 4 shows a cross section of protein denaturization that was measured during gross histology. The radius of protein denaturization, traced in black, was about 15 mm. Its depth was 14.9 ± 2.4 mm (average ± standard deviation) for the 17 experiments that were performed.

TABLE 1. Electrical and acoustical properties of the dual-mode transducer. (*Average ± standard deviation of data measured for the 5 elements.)

Property	Value
Working Frequency	5.6 MHz
Electro-acoustic Efficiency at 5.6 MHz	72 ± 4%*
Pulse-echo Insertion Loss at 5.2 MHz	9.8 ± 0.4 dB*
Pulse-echo Impulse Response Length at -6 dB	160 ± 16 ns*
Fractional Bandwidth at -6 dB	53 ± 2%*
Lateral Resolution in the Focal Plane at -6 dB	1.0 mm
Electrical Crosstalk in Air at -6 dB	≤ - 57 dB

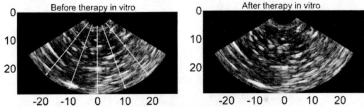

FIGURE 2. B-mode sector images taken before and after treatment using transducer element 1. White lines indicate the five treatment angles. The image scale is in mm, and the 8-bit image was log-compressed into a dynamic range of 40 dB.

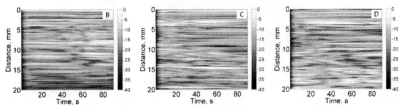

FIGURE 3. M-mode images formed during treatment at (B) -40°, (C) 0°, and (D) 40°. Observation of distortion beginning at 40 s in (B) and at 10 s in (C) and (D) was consistent with the measurement of protein denaturization during gross histology.

DISCUSSION AND CONCLUSIONS

An interstitial probe with a dual-mode transducer for ultrasound imaging and therapy was characterized by standard methods and then evaluated *in vitro* using porcine liver. The system was used to form B-mode images, apply high intensity ultrasound to induce protein denaturization, and form M-mode images. The transducer performed well in therapy and imaging modes, indicated by efficiency above 70% and fractional bandwidth above 50%. For miniaturized probes, high efficiency is necessary to reduce transducer self heating during treatment. B-mode images provided an adequate visualization of the liver structure and could assist placement of the probe. A hyperechoic region, which can indicate protein denaturization, was not observed in this work. However, it is known that protein denaturization can be induced without observing hyperecho and, further, the transducer is sensitive and broadband enough to detect hyperecho if boiling or cavitation occurs.

The appearance of distortion on M-mode images was a qualitative indicator of protein denaturization and presumably the visualization of temperature rise in the liver as a result of the absorption of ultrasound energy. Underlying phenomena were most likely changes in the speed of sound in the liver and thermal expansion. The times at which distortion appeared, 40 s on image (B) and 10 s on images (C) and (D), were consistent with the effects of adjacent heating, which were used here to treat a large volume of tissue (between 5 cm^3 and 7 cm^3) in short time (about 450 s). Though not tested here, because the goal of this work was only to evaluate the probe, further processing of echo data taken during treatment may reveal an estimate for the depth of protein denaturization as a function of time.

Continuation of this work includes an evaluation of the probe and imaging/therapy system *in vivo*.

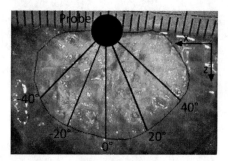

FIGURE 4. Photograph of protein denaturization induced by high intensity ultrasound. The photograph was taken in the xz-plane at the half height of the transducer. Black lines trace the radius, about 15 mm, and indicate the 5 treatment angles.

ACKNOWLEDGMENTS

This work was supported by ANR-05-RNTS-01101 and an Inserm Post-Doctoral Fellowship.

REFERENCES

1. C. Lafon, Y. C. Chapelon, F. Prat, F. Gorry, J. Margonari, Y. Theillère, and D. Cathignol, *Ultrasound in Med. & Biol.* **24**, 113-122(1998).
2. D. Melodelima, C. Lafon, F. Prat, Y. Theillère, A. Arefiev, and D. Cathignol, *Ultrasound in Med. & Biol.* **29**, 285-291 (2003).
3. I. R. S. Makin, T. D. Mast, W. Faidi, M. M. Runk, P. G. Barthe, and M. H. Slayton, *Ultrasound in Med. & Biol.* **31**, 1539-1550 (2005).
4. D. Deardorff and C. J. Diederich, *IEEE Trans. Biomedical Eng.* **47**, 1356-1365 (2000).
5. G. Bouchoux, C. Lafon, R. Berriet, J.Y. Chapelon, G. Fleury, and D. Cathignol, *Ultrasound in Med. & Biol.* **34**, 607-616 (2008).
6. S. E. Ebbini, H. Yao, and A. Shrestha, *Ultrasonic Imag.* **28**, 65-82 (2006).

New design for an endo-esophageal probe intended for the ablation of cardiac muscle in the left-atrium: A parametric simulation study

Samuel Pichardo* and Kullervo Hynynen†

*Thunder Bay Regional Research Institute 980 Oliver Rd. Thunder Bay, ON, CANADA, P7B 6V4
Email: pichards@tbh.net
†Research Imaging Sunnybrook Health Sciences Centre University of Toronto
2075 Bayview Ave. Toronto, ON, CANADA, M4N 3M5

Abstract. A parametric simulation study was carried out to establish optimal dimensions of endo-esophageal devices intended to treat the atrial fibrillation (AF). The devices are spherical-surface sections truncated at 15mm (depth of 4mm) and cut in concentric-rings each composed of independently driven sectors. The number of independent elements (N) was minimized for different values of ratio of amplitude of secondary lobe over main lobe (E) of 0.35, 0.4, 0.45 and 0.5 and for a volume of interest (VOI) of $24 \times 27 \times 28mm^3$ (located at 23.5mm from the center of the device), which is large enough to contain all the targets identified in the Visible Human Project Male specimen. Operating at 1MHz, E and N were calculated in function of the element size and focal length (F). After keeping values of F and normalized dimensions of the independent elements in terms of wavelength, higher frequencies were considered: 1.25 and 1.5MHz. Lesion formation in the heart chamber showed that the twelve configurations were able to produce the typical lesion used to treat the AF while preserving surrounding structures. For an exposure of 5s and maximal temperature of 70°C, the average (s.d.) acoustical intensity at transducer surface varied from 22.3(5.8)W/cm² for a device with F=98mm at 1MHz to 9.2(2.1)W/cm² for a device with F=186mm at 1.5MHz, while requiring 319 and 1158 elements, respectively, and achieving values of E of 0.5 and 0.41, respectively.

Keywords: ultrasound; treatment; atrial fibrillation; simulation
PACS: 43.80.Sh, 43.35.Yb, 87.85.Ox, 43.38.+n

1. INTRODUCTION

Atrial fibrillation (AF) is the most frequently sustained cardiac arrhythmia affecting humans. It concerns 2% of unrelated adult population and is associated with an increase of mortality rate in both women and men [1]. A minimal invasive transesophageal cardiac thermal ablation technique has been proposed in earlier studies where focused ultrasound is used to ablate the cardiac tissue [2, 3]. Pulmonary-vein isolation with ultrasound has been proposed using a transvenous catheter [4] and endo-esophageal access [2, 5]. The esophageal duct is located just behind the posterior wall of the LA, allowing a favourable acoustic window of the region of the heart.

In an earlier numerical study [3], the feasibility of inducing lesions in the cardiac muscle was established under realistic anatomical conditions for a planar 2-D phased array ($60 \times 10mm^2$, 2280 elements, 1 MHz). From the segmentation of histological

CP1113, *8th International Symposium on Therapeutic Ultrasound*, edited by E. S. Ebbini
© 2009 American Institute of Physics 978-0-7354-0650-6/09/$25.00

images of the thorax, the cardiac muscle and the blood-filled cavities in the heart were identified and considered in the sound propagation and thermal models. The 2-D planar array used in the earlier study, which had a large number of elements, was able to produce the circumferential lesions surrounding the PVs that are typically required to treat the AF. In the present work, a parametric study was executed to design a device with a minimal number of elements that renders the device fabrication feasible while keeping the circumferential lesions around the PVs.

2. MATERIAL AND METHODS

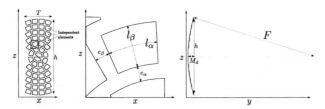

FIGURE 1. Scheme of endo-esophageal, multi-element device for the treatment of the atrial fibrillation. Left: Frontal view (xz). Center: Close-up of one element of the device where l_α is the arc of an azymuthal angle in relation to y and l_β is the arc of a polar angle on the xz plane. Right: Lateral view (yz)

A truncated surface section of sphere was used as array geometry to fit the device in the esophagus (FIGURE 1). The Cartesian $+x$, $+y$ and $+z$ directions were oriented in relation to human anatomy, respectively, from left to right, from posterior to anterior, and from caudal to cranial. The origin was set on the center of the device. The surface of the device was cut in concentric rings of equal width where each ring was composed of angular-sector elements. Each element is characterized by the arc lengths l_α and l_β, which were kept constant for all elements in the device. The truncation of the probe (T) and the maximal depth (M_d) were set constant to 15 and 4 mm, respectively.

Our goal was to study device configurations that would be able to induce a localized tissue coagulation in the LA wall while keeping a minimal number of independent elements. A simple parametric function was used to select several candidates of optimal configuration. This function evaluates the degree of focusing combined with the number of elements. A setup for lesion prediction in the LA chamber was used for the chosen configurations and an analysis of lesion volume, safety, and required power was done.

A volume of interest (VOI) was chosen from the results shown in [3] where the largest absolute values of the coordinates of the targets location were identified. For the ablation of the PVs with RF, these targets are found in the incipient tubular formation of the PVs in the LA [6]. The target locations in the PVs of the Male specimen were used to define the VOI because the centered position of his esophagus. The VOI was modeled by the prism enclosed by the coordinates $(-12, 10, -9,)$ mm and $(12, 37, 9)$ mm, which was large enough to contain all the target locations in the PVs identified in the Male specimen.

The parameters of the device chosen to be varied were the focal length F and the normalized arc lengths $\lambda_\alpha = l_\alpha/\lambda$ and $\lambda_\beta = l_\beta/\lambda$, where λ is the wavelength under water conditions. The space between elements, which are denoted by e_α and e_β, was set to $1/20$ of λ. The height of the device (h) was limited indirectly by the maximal depth of the device M_d and the focal length F (FIGURE 1c). Each configuration was identified by the notation $\kappa(f,F,\lambda_\alpha,\lambda_\beta)$. Parameters λ_α and λ_β were varied from 0.5 to 2 with a stepping of 0.1. The focal length F was varied from 70 mm to 220 mm with a stepping of 2 mm.

The degree of focusing $E = \frac{|q_2|}{|q_1|}$ was used to quantify the ratio between the amplitude of the first secondary lobe q_2 and the main lobe of the acoustic field q_1. The lower was the value of E the more focused was the resulting acoustic field.

For each κ, the 3-D pressure distribution was calculated for three focal locations (x,y,z) of the VOI: p_1, p_2, and p_3. p_1 was located at $(-12,10,-9)$ mm, p_2 at $(0,23.5,0)$ mm and p_3 at $(12,37,9)$ mm. The degree of focusing E_i was calculated for each focal point p_i. The parametric cost function $E_{par}(\kappa) = \max\{E_1,E_2,E_3\}$ allowed choosing for the optimization of the worst case of focusing of each configuration κ found between the close, medium and far conditions.

For a given value of f, the optimal device was found by the configuration κ showing a small value of E_{par} and a small number of independent elements N_e. Optimal configurations were found for several ranges of goal values for E_{par}, where the optimal device was obtained by the configuration κ showing the minimal value of N_e. After preliminary results, it was found that the smallest possible value of E_{par} was close to 0.35. The selected value ranges of E_{par} for optimal configurations were $(0..0.35]$, $(0.35..0.4]$, $(0.4..0.45]$ and $(0.45..0.5]$.

The acoustic field was calculated using a multilayer transmission model between the transducer and the muscle [7]. A muscle medium located 6 mm from the device was used for the testing, with water acting as coupling medium. The tissue was modeled with dimensions 10 mm larger than the dimensions of the device on the x and z directions and with a value of y 10 mm larger than the focal point tested. The spatial resolution of the Cartesian medium was set to $\lambda/2$ in all directions. The parametric study was executed in its totality for a value of f of 1 MHz. Higher values of f were considered for the selected cases resulting from the study of the degree of focusing. The values of f considered were 1.25 MHz and 1.5 MHz. For a given optimal configuration κ at 1 MHz, the values of λ_α, λ_β and F were retained while the frequency f was varied.

Once a group of configurations was chosen, the effectiveness of inducing the required circumferential lesion formation in the LA chamber was evaluated. The required power was calculated and the safety of surrounding tissues was established. For this purpose, the setup described in [3] was used. Predictions were done for peak temperatures of 70°C and 80°C and ultrasound exposures of 5 s and 10 s. Scenarios are denoted as $t_{us}\uparrow T_p$ where t_{us} is the length of the ultrasound exposure and T_p the peak temperature. Physical constants used in the present study and details of the numerical implementation can be find in [3].

3. RESULTS

Results showed that a more effective degree of feasibility to focus ultrasound was obtained as the focal length F increased. Devices with small F were not able to focus the ultrasound as desired in any of the three locations of the VOI. Devices with large values of F were able to produce an effective focusing but at the expense of a large number of elements. Devices with short focal lengths ($F < 86$ mm) did not show any suitable device capable of focusing as desired in all the three desired locations of the VOI. The most demanding goal ranges, with the lowest values, required larger values of F before showing a suitable configuration.

Optimal devices for each range of E_{par} were selected and higher frequencies were considered by up-scaling the frequency while keeping the same values of F, λ_α and λ_β (both parameters scaled with the wavelength). Table 1 shows the configuration of all the devices, 12 in total, that were selected for the step of lesion formation. The process of up-scaling the operating frequency kept for the most the desired degree of focusing E_{par}.

Table 1 also shows both the average and standard deviation of the lesion volume and the required acoustic intensity at the transducer surface (I_{ac}) observed for each device and exposure conditions. No secondary lesions were observed for any combination of device, target location, exposure length, and maximal temperature. In average, and with all devices considered, the lesions obtained with an operating frequency of 1.25 MHz and 1.5 MHz had a lesion volume of 70% and 56% the lesion volume obtained at 1 MHz. A very similar situation was observed with the acoustic intensity that showed practically the same percentages when compared to the intensity required at 1 MHz.

TABLE 1. Dimensions and average($\pm$ std.) of the lesion volume and acoustic intensity induced with the selected devices for different exposure conditions.

						Lesion Volume (mm³)				Intensity at device surface (W/cm²)			
						Exposure conditions (Temp./Length)				Exposure conditions (Temp./Length)			
						70°C		80°C		70°C		80°C	
			N_e	Height	Active surface								
F (mm)	λ_α	λ_β	f (MHz)	(mm)	area (cm²)	E_{par}	5s	10s	5s	10s	5s	10s	5s	10s
			1	319	51	6	0.5	12(±4.6)	19.8(±6.4)	25.5(±8.9)	40.9(±14.1)	22.3(±5.8)	16.5(±4.1)	28.3(±6)	21.5(±5.4)
98	0.6	1.4	1.25	552	55	6.6	0.46	7.7(±2.6)	13.2(±4.3)	16.6(±5.6)	28(±9.2)	15.5(±4.1)	12.2(±3.5)	20.1(±5.2)	15.9(±4.5)
			1.5	807	54	6.7	0.47	6(±2.1)	10.6(±3.5)	13.2(±4.4)	22.4(±7.2)	11(±2.9)	8.9(±2.6)	14.2(±3.7)	11.6(±3.4)
			1	380	56	6.6	0.45	10.9(±4.1)	17.9(±5.9)	23(±8.1)	37.1(±12.7)	22.1(±5.6)	17(±4.9)	28.8(±7.1)	22.1(±6.2)
114	0.6	1.3	1.25	626	58	7	0.42	7.4(±2.6)	12.8(±4.2)	16(±5.4)	27.2(±8.8)	14.5(±3.7)	11.5(±3.3)	18.8(±4.7)	14.9(±4.2)
			1.5	941	59	7.4	0.41	5.7(±2)	10.1(±3.4)	12.5(±4.1)	21.4(±7)	10.5(±2.7)	8.5(±2.5)	13.7(±3.5)	11.1(±3.2)
			1	473	74	8.9	0.4	9.6(±3.2)	16.1(±4.9)	20.6(±6.7)	33.8(±10.3)	18.5(±4.6)	14.2(±4)	24(±5.9)	18.5(±5.2)
186	0.7	1.2	1.25	776	74	9.3	0.42	6.7(±2.2)	11.7(±3.7)	14.7(±4.6)	25.2(±7.7)	11.9(±2.8)	9.5(±2.5)	15.5(±3.6)	12.3(±3.2)
			1.5	1158	74	9.7	0.42	5.2(±1.7)	9.4(±3)	11.7(±3.6)	20.1(±6.1)	9.2(±2.1)	7.5(±1.9)	11.9(±2.7)	9.7(±2.5)
			1	763	81	10.2	0.35	9.7(±3.3)	16.9(±5.1)	21.2(±7.1)	36.3(±13)	18.8(±4.7)	14.5(±4.2)	24.4(±6)	18.9(±5.4)
220	0.5	1.2	1.25	1199	83	10.3	0.36	6.6(±2.2)	12(±3.7)	14.9(±4.8)	26.1(±8)	13.5(±3.2)	10.8(±2.9)	17.5(±4.1)	14(±3.8)
			1.5	1698	82	10.1	0.37	5.7(±2.1)	10.6(±4.5)	12.8(±4.9)	23.1(±11)	11.1(±3)	9.1(±2.8)	14.5(±3.9)	11.8(±3.6)

4. DISCUSSION

The range of parameters used in the present study allowed finding configurations with a minimal number of elements while keeping a low ratio between the amplitudes of the secondary lobe and the main lobe. Optimal devices were found for devices accomplishing a ratio E_{par} between $(0.45..0.5]$, $(0.4..0.45]$ and $(0.35..0.4]$. For the range of $E_{par} \in (0..0.35]$, the population of candidate devices was limited to two. Not a single secondary lesion outside of the focal volume was observed for any of combination of device, target and exposure conditions. This result suggests that a criterion of degree of focusing E_{par} of 0.5 is enough to preserve the surrounding structures such as the esophagus.

It is worth noting that, for the intended VOI, devices used in the present study with a criterion of $E_{par} \leq 0.5$ produces more focused acoustic fields than the fields produced with the device used in earlier studies [2, 3]. For that device ($60 \times 10mm^2$, 2280 elements, 1 MHz), the values of E_1, E_2 and E_3 are, respectively, 0.41, 0.39, and 0.55, which translate to a value of E_{par} of 0.55.

The use of higher frequencies certainly allowed reducing the required power on the elements and the same trend was observed for lesion volume (Table 1). This implies that higher frequencies allowed a more precise lesion formation that translates in a better preservation of surrounding structures. However, smaller individual lesions imply that more HIFU exposures are required to create a full circumferential lesion around a PV and this will result in longer treatments.

5. CONCLUSIONS

New endo-esophageal devices intended for the treatment of the atrial fibrillation were presented. The main interest for using an endo-esophageal approach is that it is a less invasive technique. The new multi-element devices were optimized for a lesion formation in the pulmonary veins of the left atrium of the heart. The devices are truncated sections of sphere and are composed of angular-sector elements arranged in rings. A parametric study was executed with the purpose of finding devices configurations that allow a high degree of focusing in the intended volume of interest while keeping a minimal number of independent elements. Results showed that it is feasible to use devices that imply fewer elements than planar 2D-arrays, while requiring a fraction of the power and producing more focusing fields and more precise lesions.

ACKNOWLEDGMENTS

This work was supported by grant No. R01 HL077606 from the National Health Institute and the CRC program.

REFERENCES

1. S. K. S. Huang, and M. A. Wood, *Catheter ablation for cardiac arrhythmias*, W.B. Saunders, Philadelphia, USA, 2006, chap. 15. Pulmonary Vein Isolation for Atrial Fibrillation, pp. 269–2888, ISBN 1416003126.
2. X. Yin, L. M. Epstein, and K. Hynynen **53**, 1138–1149 (2006).
3. S. Pichardo, and K. Hynynen, *Phys Med Biol* **52**, 4923–4942 (2007).
4. G. R. Meininger, H. Calkins, L. Lickfett, P. Lopath, T. Fjield, R. Pacheco, P. Harhen, E. R. Rodriguez, R. Berger, H. Halperin, and S. B. Solomon, *J. Intervent. Cardiac Electrophysiol.* **8**, 141–148 (2003).
5. S. W. Smith, W. Lee, K. L. Gentry, E. C. Pua, and E. D. Light, "Integrated Interventional Devices For Real Time 3D Ultrasound Imaging and Therapy," in *Proc 5th Int. Symp. Therapeutic Ultrasound. 27-29 October 2005, Boston, MA*, 2006, pp. 375–379.
6. A. Verma, N. F. Marrouche, and A. Natale, *J. Cardiovasc. Electrophysiol.* **15**, 1335–1340 (2004).
7. J. Sun, and K. Hynynen, *J. Acoust. Soc. Am.* **104**, 1705–1715 (1998).

New Approach to Design of Therapeutic Focused Phased Arrays

Leonid Kushkuley[a], Vladimir Goland[a], Alex Kamenichin[a], and Yehuda Zadok[b]

[a]UltraShape Ltd, New Industrial Park, POB 80, Yokneam, 20692, Israel;
[b]Department of Biomedical Engineering, Tel Aviv University, POB 39040, Tel Aviv, 69978, Israel

Abstract. For therapeutic treatment of adipose tissues it is necessary to dynamically focus acoustic energy at depths from 5 to 40 mm under the skin. One of the ways to achieve this goal is to use a spherical radiator having large aperture angle and comprising a multiplicity of radiating elements. Conventional ways of their manufacture (e.g. composite ceramics) are expensive and time consuming. The authors developed a method of building such an array using a single spherical piece of anisotropic piezoceramics, which is more simple and fast. The goal of this work is to evaluate the array performance, which is characterized by the level of cross-talks between different elements, statistics over resonance frequencies and electric impedances of the elements, etc. Manufactured phased array has aperture diameter and curvature radius of 84 and 54 mm, respectively and comprises 160 elements. Average resonance frequency and electric impedance measured over all elements were 1043 ± 42 kHz and 315 ± 28 Ohm, respectively. To assess the level of cross-talking and surface vibration velocity distribution the approach developed by O. Sapozhnikov et al for quasi-planar sources was used. We validated this approach for the case of strongly focused transducer by examining a single element spherical radiator with the same geometry and a rubber strap, forming a specified figure, bonded to its radiating surface. The reconstructed velocity distribution showed rather low level of inter-element coupling. All these results demonstrated the validity of proposed method for phased array building.

Keywords: Phased Arrays; HIFU
PACS: 43.38.Fx; 43.38.Ja

INTRODUCTION

In recent years we have seen increase of interest in High Intensity Focused Ultrasound (HIFU) applications, including non-invasive surgery [1], cancer treatment [2], histotripsy [3], aesthetics [4, 5], etc. Since for most of applications HIFU frequency range lies in the range 0.8 – 6.0 MHz, respective focal area, where the effect takes place, is very small. Hence, the treatment of a comparatively large target volume using single element focusing transducer requires too much time. Devices that address this problem usually use dynamic focusing and incorporate annular [6, 7] or phased array HIFU transducers [8, 9]. The latter are usually fabricated by mounting separate radiators on a spherical shell [10] or using composite piezoceramics [8]. Both approaches are very expensive, especially if they comprise hundreds of elements. If used intensively and at extreme power, transducer performance can degrade and it should be frequently replaced. It is clear that from the commercial point of view it is very important to find a way for producing low-cost phased array transducers for HIFU applications. Here we present preliminary results of evaluation of a multi-element, low-cost transducer prototype developed in UltraShape®.

CP1113, *8th International Symposium on Therapeutic Ultrasound*, edited by E. S. Ebbini
© 2009 American Institute of Physics 978-0-7354-0650-6/09/$25.00

METHODS

The requirements for the phased array are imposed by its application in a device for improving body appearance [4, 5], and are as follows: operational frequency of 1.0 MHz, depth of focus of 20 ±10 mm, steering within the volume of 15x15x15 mm^3, overall dimensions less than 100 mm and manufacturing cost less than $800. To achieve all these goals we decided to manufacture phased array using a single spherical piezoelement having required geometry and dimensions and to partition the electrode covering its convex surface into a multiplicity of separate segments. The shape, dimensions and amount of segments were determined as a result of transducer modeling.

As a basis for our calculations we considered N circular radiators, each having radius a, which are distributed over the spherical segment with the aperture diameter of 84 mm and radius of curvature of 54 mm. The segment possesses an opening in the center having diameter of 17 mm for inserting an imaging transducer or a cavitation detector. These dimensions ensured that the overall transducer size will not exceed 100 mm and its main focus will be at approximately 20 mm from the transducer-skin interface. We considered a random distribution of the radiators over the segment, since it is known [10, 11] that such distribution allows for reducing of side lobe levels. Our goal was to optimize the design by finding maximal a and minimal N values, which allow for focusing in the specified volume keeping side lobe levels at no more than 30% of the respective focal pressure. The minimal distance between any two radiators was set to 1.0 mm.

It was assumed that the phased array works at 1.0 MHz in tone-burst mode, each burst having 5 periods. The array is loaded by a mineral oil to the depth of 38 mm from its center, and with the water further on. The combined field of the array was calculated by summation of the pressure contribution from every radiator at each point of interest. Phase delays between radiators have been calculated based on distances from points in space to the center of the respective radiator, and sound velocities in the oil and water. For each radiator, acoustic field was calculated by combining Rayleigh integral [12] to obtain a wave field incident on the interface, with angular spectrum expansion method [13] to describe a wave passing through the interface.

The results of the modeling showed that the optimal values of N and a, which comply with our requirements are: $N = 160$, $a = 2.6$ mm. In this case the radiators cover 52% of the spherical segment area. In Table 1 are presented ratios P_F/P_0 and $\gamma=P_L/P_F$ for different points. Here P_F, P_L are the pressure in the focus and the maximum pressure of the side lobes, respectively. $P_0=v_0 \cdot Z_{ac}$; v_0-normal velocity on the radiator surface; Z_{ac} – acoustic impedance of the mineral oil. The point with coordinates (0,0,52) mm corresponds to the calculated focus of the array. Point (0,0,0) is at the center of the spherical shell and Z axis coincides with the axis of the axial symmetry. As one can see, in the most distant points the focal pressure reduces for about 50% and the level of side lobes is about 30% of the respective focal pressure. These are appropriate levels for our application, but if one needs to reduce further the level of side lobes, it is always possible to do by increasing the number of radiators and reducing their dimensions respectively. Analogously, increase of the f-number of the phased array leads to the enlargement of the effectively treated focal volume. Reduction of P_F/P_0 may be compensated by increasing v_0 in corresponding points.

TABLE 1. Field characteristics at different focusing points

Parameter	Coordinate (X,Y,Z), mm								
	(0,0,42)	(5,5,42)	(7,7,42)	(0,0,52)	(5,5,52)	(7,7,52)	(0,0,62)	(5,5,62)	(7,7,62)
P_F/P_0	44.0	32.9	24.4	50.7	38.9	29.5	31.3	25.2	21.36
γ	0.125	0.20	0.29	0.05	0.15	0.24	0.08	0.25	0.32

A prototype multi-element transducer was built from a proprietary piezoceramics developed and manufactured in UltraShape. The ceramics parameters had the following values: acoustic impedance $Z_{ac} \cong 20$ MRayls, mechanical quality factor $Q \cong 25$, piezoelectric constants $d_{33} \cong 280$ pC/N and $d_{31} \cong 75$ pC/N, electric permittivity $\epsilon \cong 850$ and electro-mechanical coupling coefficient $k_t \cong 0.55$. The piezoelement had a shape of a spherical cap with aperture diameter of 84 mm, radius of curvature of 54 mm and thickness of 1.4 mm. In the center of the element there was an opening with diameter of 17 mm. After the element was electroded, polarized and tested, its outer, convex electrode was segmented into 160 circle elements of radius 2.6 mm. This operation was executed using a special laser cutting machine (Smart Solutions Ltd., Tel Aviv, Israel) having accuracy $\pm$ 1μm. The laser energy was adjusted to the level that ensured evaporation of only a thin layer of the silver electrode (30 μm -50 μm). The time required for producing one circle element was about 2 – 3 seconds, and all the operation including installation and calibration took about 25 – 30 min. The cost of array construction was about US \$400. All the elements of the array were wired and it was placed into cylindrical Perspex housing filled with mineral oil. The bottom of the cylinder had an opening covered by a thin 100 μm PVC membrane, which formed acoustically transparent window. Through this window, ultrasound radiated by the array penetrated into acoustic load, which in our case was the water.

MEASUREMENTS AND RESULTS

Complex electrical impedance Z_{el} of each element was measured using Hioki 3532-50 LCR meter (Hioki USA Corp., USA) in the frequency range 600 kHz – 1500 kHz. In the Table 2 are presented the results of measurements, averaged over all 160 elements. Since usually radiators are excited at the frequency f_r corresponding to the minimum of $| Z_{el}|$, we presented the respective values of f_r, $| Z_{el}(f_r)|$, and phase ϕ of $Z_{el}(f_r)$.

Table 2

	f_r, kHz	$| Z_{el}(f_r)|$, Ohm	$\phi(f_r)$, deg
Average	1043	315	-73
STD	42	28	2
STD, %	4.0	8.9	2.8

Our main concern was cross-talking, inevitably existing between neighboring elements in such kind of design, which may significantly deteriorate acoustic field and array performance. To estimate the contribution of cross-talking we examined field distribution in the focal plane and normal velocity distribution over the surface of the phased array. To make things easier for evaluation we excited only 30 of 160 elements according to the scheme shown in Fig. 1a. This way we could analyse the behavior of clusters of neighboring elements as well as separate ones. The elements were excited "in phase" at frequency of 1043 kHz with burst tones having duration of 10 periods. The signal was supplied by Agilent 33220A arbitrary function generator and amplified by AG-1021 power amplifier (T&C Power Conversion, Inc., USA). The total supplied electric power was 60 W. Using Acoustic Intensity Measurement System (AIMS) and hydrophone HNR-0500 (both of Onda Corp., USA) we measured acoustic pressure distribution in the focal plane with the spatial resolution of 0.2 mm. In Fig.1b, 1d are shown calculated and measured field distributions, which look very similar. Since our calculations have been made with the assumption of zero cross-talking, this similarity indicates that the influence of cross-talking on acoustic field is very low. The pressure distribution in the focal plane served as a source for the reconstruction (as described in [14]) of the surface normal velocity distribution over the phased array, which is shown in Fig. 1c. Comparison of Fig. 1a and Fig. 1c shows excellent correspondence between velocity distribution pattern and radiators distribution shown on the scheme. One can easily resolve each radiator in Fig. 1c. This correspondence is an additional confirmation that the level of cross-talking between array elements is rather low.

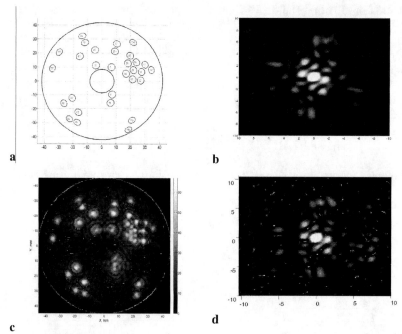

Figure 1. a – element distribution on a spherical shell; **b** – calculated field distribution in the focal plane; **c** – reconstructed surface normal velocity distribution; **d** – measured field distribution in the focal plane.

To validate the method of normal velocity reconstruction [14] for our case of strongly focusing transducer, we tested it on a single focusing piezoelement, having the same geometry as the array, with rubber letters glued to its surface (Fig. 6). The element was excited in the same manner as the phased array and its measured field distribution in the focal plane was used for normal velocity reconstruction over its surface (Fig.7). The result confirms the high accuracy of the method for the case of strongly focusing radiator.

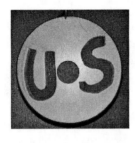 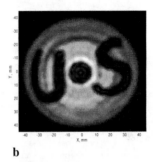

a   b

Figure 2. a – photo of a single piezo-element with glued rubber letters; **b** - reconstructed normal velocity distribution over the surface of a single piezoelement shown in Fig. 2a.

REFERENCES

1. Gail ter Haar, D. Sinnett, I. Rivens, *Phys. Med. Biol.*, **34**, 1743-1750 (1989)
2. Gail ter Haar, *Progr. Bioph. Mol. Biol.*, **93**, 111-129 (2007)
3. Z. Xu, A. Ludomirsky, L.Y. Eun, T.L. Hall, B.C. Tran, J.B. Fowlkes, C.A. Cain, *IEEE Trans. Ultras., Ferroelect., Freq. Contr.*, **51**, 726-736 (2004)
4. S. A. Teitelbaum, J.L. Burns, J. Kubota, M.J. Otto, J. Shirakaba, Y. Suzuki, S.A. Brown, *Plastic and reconstruction surgery*, **120**, 779-789 (2007)
5. J. Moreno, T. Valero-Altes, A.M. Riquelme, M.I. Issaria-Marcosy, J. Royo de la Torre, *Lasers in Surgery and Medicine*, **39**, 315-323 (2007)
6. C.A. Cain, S.A. Umemura, *IEEE Trans. Microwave Theory Tech.*, vol. MTT-34, 542-551 (1986)
7. J.P. Do-Huu, P. Harteman, *Proc. IEEE Ultrason. Symp.*, 705-710 (1981)
8. D.R. Daum, K. Hynynen, *IEEE Trans. Ultras., Ferroelect., Freq. Contr.*,**46**, 1254-1268 (1999)
9. M.Z. Lu, M.X. Wan, F. Xu, X.D. Wang, H. Zhong, *IEEE Trans. Ultras., Ferroelect., Freq. Contr.*, **52**, 1270-1290 (2005)
10. S. Goss, L. Frizzel, J.T. Kouzmanoff, J.M. Barich, J.M. Yang, *IEEE Trans. Ultras., Ferroelect., Freq. Contr.*, 43, 1111-1121 (1996)
11. L.R. Gavrilov, J.W. Hand, *IEEE Trans. Ultras., Ferroelect., Freq. Contr.*, **47**, 125-139 (2000)
12. A.D. Pierce, *Acoustics,* Acoust. Soc. Am., Woodbury, NY, 1989.
13. P.R. Stephanishen, K.C. Benjamin, *JASA*, **71**, 803-812 (1982)
14. O.A. Sapozhnikov, Yu.A. Pishchal'nikov, V. Morozov, *Acoustical Physics*, **49**, 354-360 (2003)

Development of HIFU Therapy System for Lower Extremity Varicose Veins

Ryuhei Ota*, Jun Suzuki[†], Kiyoshi Yoshinaka*,Juno Deguchi[†], Shu Takagi*, Tetsuro Miyata[†], and Yoichiro Matsumoto*

*Department of Mechanical Engineering, The University of Tokyo
7-3-1 Hongo, Bunkyo-ku, Tokyo 113-8656, JAPAN
[†]Vascular Surgery, Department of Surgery, The University of Tokyo,
7-3-1 Hongo, Bunkyo-ku, Tokyo 113-0033, JAPAN

Abstract. High-intensity focused ultrasound (HIFU) treatment utilizing microbubbles was investigated in the present study. It is known that microbubbles have the potential to enhance the heating effects of an ultrasound field. In this study, the heat accompanying microbubble oscillation was used to occlude varicose veins. Alteration of veins was observed after ultrasound irradiation. Veins were resected by stripping. In this study, two vein conditions were adopted during HIFU irradiation; non-compressed and compressed. Compressing the vein was expected to improve occlusion by rubbing the altered intima under compressed conditions. The frequency of the ultrasound was 1.7 MHz, the intensity at the focus was 2800 W/cm^2, and the irradiation time was 20 s. In this study, the contrast agent Levovist® was chosen as a microbubble source, and the void fraction (ratio of total gas volume to liquid) in the vein was fixed at 10^{-5}. Under non-compressed conditions, changes were observed only at the adventitia of the vein anterior wall. In contrast, under compressed conditions, changes were observed from the intima to the adventitia of both the anterior and posterior walls, and they were partly stuck together. In addition, more experiments with hematoxylin-eosin staining suggested that the changes in the vein were more substantial under the latter conditions. From these results, it was confirmed that the vein was occluded more easily with vein compression.

Keywords: high-intensity focused ultrasound, varicose vein, microbubbles, hematoxylin-eosin stain

INTRODUCTION

At present, there are many patients who suffer from varicose veins in the lower extremities. Varicose veins develope as a result of reverse blood flow in the leg veins and are accompanied by pain. Stripping is currently the most reliable therapy for lower varicose veins. Stripping pulls the veins out using a wire and skin incisions. This therapy has a 100-year history and can treat any type of varicose vein. On the other hand, it has two disadvantages. One is the high invasiveness and the other is a two-week hospital stay. To solve these problems, therapeutic research using HIFU has been conducted [1]. As compared with stripping, HIFU is a much less-invasive method and reduces surgical times. It is thought that thermal energy resulting from HIFU to the target vein leads to intima alteration, shrinking of the vein wall, and occlusion of the vein with scarring. As time passes the occluded vein is expected to become fibrotic, resulting in the same effects as treatment by stripping.

CP1113, *8th International Symposium on Therapeutic Ultrasound*, edited by E. S. Ebbini
© 2009 American Institute of Physics 978-0-7354-0650-6/09/$25.00

However, there remain questions over ultrasonic energy absorption by skin and fat, and over the results of insufficient energy to occlude the vein at the focus. To overcome these issues, microbubbles may be used to enhance the heating effects at the focus. In previous studies on HIFU treatment, *in vivo* experiments with microbubbles have been conducted, and found that the heat effects are enhanced by the presence of microbubbles [2-4].

In this study, changes in the veins were observed after HIFU irradiation to a vein resected by stripping. The vein was filled with saline containing microbubbles (the contrast agent Levovist® was used as a microbubble source). Two sets of conditions were used during HIFU irradiation: non-compressed and compressed. It was thought that the vein would be more easily occluded under compressed conditions.

EXPERIMENTAL CONDITIONS

Non-compressed Experiment

Figure 1 shows a schematic representation of the experimental system with the non-compressed vein. In this study, a vein that was resected by stripping was used. The vein was fixed in a column-shaped hole in a polyacrylamide gel, and set at the focus of a piezoelectric transducer. The vein was filled with saline containing Levovist® at a void fraction was 10^{-5}. The PET sheet is far shorter than the ultrasound wavelength. The piezoelectric transducer was 80 mm in diameter and its focal length was 80 mm. The frequency was 1.7 MHz, and the ultrasound intensity at the focus was 2800 W/cm^2, while the irradiation time was 20 s.

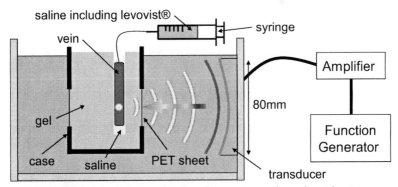

FIGURE 1. Schematic representation of non-compressed experimental system

Compressed Experiment

Figure 2 shows a schematic representation of the experimental system with the compressed vein. The column-shaped hole in the polyacrylamide gel was filled with saline and the column-shaped holder was set up there. The target vein was fixed in the holder, which had a hole so as not to disturb ultrasound propagation. The vein was compressed by placing an acoustic absorbent between the holder and the vein, and the compressed area of the vein was set at the focus of a piezoelectric transducer. The vein was filled with saline containing Levovist®. HIFU irradiation was conducted with the same parameters as for the non-compressed experiment: The void fraction was 10^{-5}, the frequency was 1.7 MHz, and the ultrasound intensity at focus was 2800 W/cm^2.

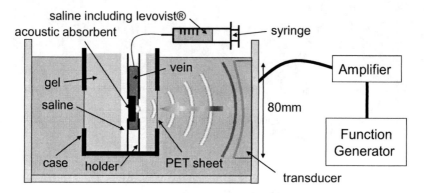

FIGURE 2. Schematic representation of compressed experimental system

RESULTS AND DISCUSSION

Non-compressed Experiment

Figure 3 shows the vein after HIFU irradiation. Neither shrinking of the vein wall nor occlusion of the vein was observed. Changes were observed on the surface of the vein anterior wall, but not in the vein posterior wall. Figure 4 shows the histopathologic examination (hematoxylin and eosin staining) of the vein. HIFU was irradiated from the left side of the figure. Swelling and waxy homogenization of collagen were observed in the adventitia and no changes were seen in the intima. This suggests that the microbubbles, which were present in the anterior of the vein, oscillated and inhibited ultrasound propagation to the posterior wall. In addition, it indicates that the intima of the anterior wall is not changed because of the cooling effects of the saline in the vein.

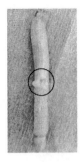 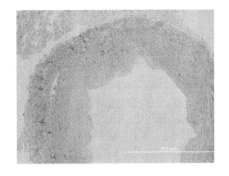

FIGURE 3. Vein after HIFU irradiation   **FIGURE 4.** Hematoxylin-eosin stain

Compressed Experiment

Figures 5 (a), (b) and (c) show the changes in the vein that was compressed during HIFU irradiation. Changes were observed in both the anterior and posterior walls. This is because the heat generated around the anterior wall was easily conducted to the posterior wall. Although water flow through the altered part of the vein was observed, the anterior wall and the posterior wall were partly stuck together. Figure 6 (a) shows hematoxylin and eosin-stained histopathologic examination of a normal varicose vein after stripping. Figure 6 (b) shows the same examination after HIFU irradiation. HIFU was irradiated from the right side of the figure. Denudation of the intima, lift-off of endothelial cells, and loss of cellular contours were observed. In addition, some areas show marked vacuolization of cells or even spongiosis. Thus, the vein is more easily occluded with compression during HIFU irradiation. However, in this experiment, the vein was not completely occluded. In order to effectively conduct HIFU treatment, the target vein must be occluded completely and controlling the alteration range is essential.

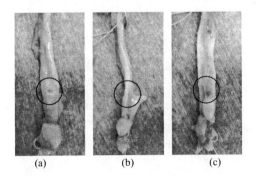

(a)   (b)   (c)

FIGURE 5. Vein after HIFU irradiation; (a) front view, (b) side view, (c) back view

365

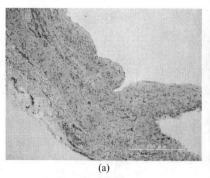 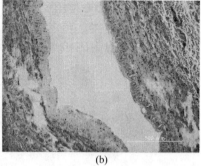

(a)   (b)

FIGURE 6. Hematoxylin-eosin stain; (a) control, (b) after HIFU irradiation

CONCLUSION

In this study, HIFU was applied to non-compressed and compressed veins, and the contrast agent Levovist® was used as a microbubble source in order to enhance the heating effects at the focus. Changes in each vein were observed with hematoxylin-eosin staining. Under non-compressed conditions, changes were only seen in the anterior wall. Under compressed conditions, changes were observed from the intima to the adventitia in both the anterior and posterior walls, and the walls were partly stuck together. These results suggest that compressing the target vein during HIFU irradiation is very effective in occluding varicose veins.

ACKNOWLEDGEMENTS

This work was partially supported by a grant for Center for Translational Systems Biology and Medicine Initiative (TSBMI) and Scientific Research (A)18206020, from the Ministry of Education, Culture, Sports, Science and Technology of Japan.

REFERENCES

1. Samuel P. Rene M. et al., in Vitro Experimental Study on The Treatment of Superficial Venous Insufficiency with High-Intensity Focused Ultrasound, 2006, Ultrason. in Med. & Biol., vol. 32, pp. 883-891.
2. Kaneko Y., D. thesis, The University of Tokyo, 2006.
3. Holt R. G. and Roy R. A., Measurements of bubble-enhanced heating from focused, MHz-frequency ultrasound in a tissue-mimicking material, 2001, Ultrason. in Med. & Biol., vol. 27, pp. 1399-1412.
4. Kaneko Y., Iida N., et al., Effective Heat therapy Controlling Heat Deposition of Microbubbles in the Ultrasound Field, 2006, Proc. 6th ISTU, pp. 157-163.

Thermal ablation system using high intensity focused ultrasound (HIFU) and guided by MRI

C.Damianou [a,b], K. Ioannides [c], V. HadjiSavas [a], N. Milonas [a], A. Couppis [a], D. Iosif [a], M. Komodromos [a], F. Vrionides [a],

[a] Frederick University Cyprus,
Mariou Agathangelou, 308,Limassol, Cyprus,
[b] MEDSONIC LTD, Ponidos 6, 4103 Ayios Athanasios, Cyprus,
[c] Polikliniki Ygia, Limassol, Cyprus.

Abstract. In this paper magnetic resonance imaging (MRI) is investigated for monitoring lesions created by high intensity focused ultrasound (HIFU) in kidney, liver and brain in vitro and in vivo.

Spherically focused transducers of 4 cm diameter, focusing at 10 cm and operating at 1 and 4 MHz were used. An MRI compatible positioning device was developed in order to scan the HIFU transducer.

The MRI compatibility of the system was successfully demonstrated in a clinical high-field MRI scanner. The ability of the positioning device to accurately move the transducer thus creating discrete and overlapping lesions in biological tissue was tested successfully.

A simple, cost effective, portable positioning device has been developed which can be used in virtually any clinical MRI scanner since it can be sited on the scanner's table. The propagation of HIFU can use either a lateral or superior-inferior approach. Both T1-w FSE and T2-w FSE imaged successfully lesions in kidney and liver. T1-w FSE and T2-w FSE and FLAIR shows better anatomical details in brain than T1-w FSE, but with T1-w FSE the contrast between lesion and brain is higher for both thermal and bubbly lesion. With this system we were able to create large lesions (by producing overlapping lesions). The length of the lesions in vivo brain was much higher than the length in vitro, proving that the penetration in the in vitro brain is limited by reflection due to trapped bubbles in the blood vessels.

Keywords. ultrasound.MRI.positioning.robot.
PACS: 87.50.Y, 43.80.+p

INTRODUCTION

In this paper a positioning device for scanning a High Intensity Focused Ultrasound (HIFU) transducer is described which is simple, cost effective, portable and universal. The transducer is scanned inside a Magnetic Resonance Imaging (MRI) scanner. The positioning device is universal because it can be placed on the table of a MRI

CP1113, 8th International Symposium on Therapeutic Ultrasound, edited by E. S. Ebbini
© 2009 American Institute of Physics 978-0-7354-0650-6/09/$25.00

scanner and therefore it can be integrated with all MRI scanners available. The system of patent [1] is placed inside the table of a GE MRI scanner and therefore it can not be integrated with the other commercial MRI scanners. Also the current device includes a flexible coupling system, and thus it can be used in all the anatomies accessible by HIFU (liver, kidney, breast, brain and pancreas).

Several examples of MRI compatible positioning devices (robot) have been developed for other applications. Systems have been developed to perform breast interventions [2–5], to perform brain biopsies [6], to perform prostate procedures [7–8], and one to perform general purpose procedures with the "doubledonut" scanner [9]. Although these studies have demonstrated the technical feasibility of MR compatible manipulators, these devices are highly specialized for a certain anatomy or MR scanner design.

In this paper the goal was to investigate the effectiveness of MRI to monitor therapeutic protocols of HIFU in the kidney, liver and brain. Thus, we have used the basic pulse sequences T1-w and T2-w fast spin echo (FSE). These MRI pulse sequences have been successful in other organs regarding their ability to identify thermal lesions.

MATERIAL AND METHODS

HIFU/ MRI system

Fig. 1 shows the block diagram of the HIFU/MRI system which includes the following subsystems:
a) HIFU system, b) MR imaging, c). Positioning device (robot) and associate drivers, d). temperature measurement, e). Cavitation detection, f). MRI compatible camera, g). Software.

The HIFU system consists of a signal generator (HP 33120A Agilent technologies, Englewood, CO, USA), a RF amplifier (250 W, AR, Souderton, PA, USA), and a spherically shaped bowl transducer (Etalon, Lebanon, IN, USA) made from piezoelectric ceramic which is non-magnetic. Two transducers were used operating at 4 MHz (kidney and liver ablation) and 1 MHz (brain). The focal length of both transducers is 10 cm and the diameter is 4 cm. The transducer is rigidly mounted on the MR compatible positioning system (MEDSONIC LTD, Limassol, Cyprus). The 3-d positioning device and the transducer were tested inside a MRI scanner (Signa 1.5 T, by General Electric). A spinal or a brain coil was used to acquire the MRI signal.

Positioning device

The robot has been developed initially for three degrees-of-freedom, but it can be easily developed for 5 degrees of motion. Since the positioning device is placed on the table of the MRI scanner its height should be around 55 cm (bore diameter of the MRI scanner). The length of the positioning device is 45 cm and its width 30 cm. The weight of the positioning device is only 6 kg and therefore it is considered portable. Fig. 2 shows a photograph of the top view of the robot

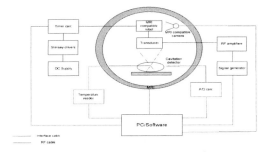

FIGURE 1. HIFU system under MRI guidance showing the various functionalities of the HIFU/MRI system.

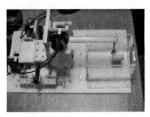

Fig. 2 Picture of the robot (top view).

RESULTS

Figure 3 shows the MRI image in a plane perpendicular to the beam by using T2-weighted FSE. Note that spatially the necrosis is continuous, thus resulting to absolutely no untreated spaces. The continuous necrosis coverage was visually confirmed after gross examination of the kidney. On the same tissue, a single lesion (reference) was created using the same exposure (1500 W/cm^2 for 5 s) in order to show the size of a discrete lesion for this specific exposure.

Figure 4 shows the MRI image using T2-weighted FSE of a large lesion in the kidney in a plane perpendicular to the beam. This lesion was created by using a 4x5 grid of lesions. The intensity used was 2000 W/cm^2 at 5 s and the spacing between the lesions was 3 mm. Note that the necrosis coverage is incomplete, resulting to some untreated spots.

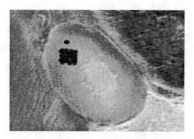

Fig. 3. MR images (in a plane perpendicular to the transducer beam) of large lesion (full coverage of the intended target) using T2-weigthed FSE with TE=32 ms. The spatial average intensity was 1500 W/cm^2 for 5 s.

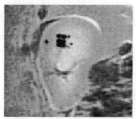

Fig. 4. MR images (in a plane perpendicular to the transducer beam) of large lesion (partial coverage of the intended target) using T2-weigthed FSE with TE=32 ms. The spatial average intensity was 2000 W/cm^2 for 5 s.

Fig. 5 shows ablation in rabbit *in vivo* using a 4x4 grid with intensity of 2000 W/cm^2 for 20 s. This large lesion was created using thermal mechanisms and therefore the lesion appears bright. The contrast of thermal lesions is definitely much better than the case of bubbly lesions.

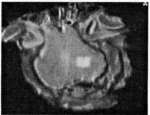

Fig. 5 MRI image using T1-w FSE of large thermal lesion created *in vivo* using 2000 W/cm^2 for 20 s.

DISCUSSION

The robot presented in this paper is utilized in the research setting for performing experiments either in vitro tissue or in vivo animals. The positioning device is placed on

370

the table of the MRI scanner and access of ultrasound to the brain is achieved either from superior to inferior or laterally. Since the positioning device is placed on the table of the MRI scanner, this device can be used in all the available MRI scanners (ie it is a universal positioning device).

Another advantage of this device is that it is much simpler and inexpensive than the existing system, while maintaining high standards of repeatability and readability. Another advantage of this positioning device is that it is lightweight (approximately 6 Kg) and therefore it can be transported from one MRI scanner to another (ie it is portable).

Previous literature [10]demonstrated that lesions can be monitored with excellent contrast in rabbit brain (in vivo) using T1-w FSE with TR=500 ms. The lesions imaged in the previous studies and also in this study appeared bright with T1-w FSE, whereas brain tissue appeared gray. However in the previous studies only thermal lesions were shown. In this paper we have explored extensively the use of MRI to image both lesions created under thermal mechanisms and mechanisms that create bubbly lesions (cavitation or boiling).

The contrast between lesion and brain tissue out of the 3 pulse sequences used is best with T1-w FSE. The signal intensity of the brain tissue is homogeneous using this method, and therefore the contrast with thermal lesions or with bubbly lesions is excellent. Best contrast is observed for TR above 500 ms.

ACKNOWLEDGEMENTS

The work was supported by the Research Promotion Foundation (RPF) of Cyprus under the projects SONOTHERM and SONOCARDIO and by the ministry of industry of Cyprus under the project SONOMRI.

REFERENCES

[1]. Yehezkeli O., Freundlich D., Magen N., Marantz C., Medan Y., Vitek S., Weinreb A., WO0209812 (2002)

[2]. Kaiser, W. A., Fischer, H., Vagner, J., and Selig, M., Invest. Radiol. **35**, 513–519 (200)

[3]. Felden, A., Vagner, J., Hinz, A., Fischer, H., Pfleiderer, S. O., Reichenbach, J. R., and Kaiser, W.. *Biomed. Tech.* **47**, 2–5. (2002)

[4]. Tsekos, N. V., Shudy, J., Yacoub, E., Tsekos, P. V., and Koutlas, I. G. *2nd IEEE International Symposium on Bioinformatics and Bioengineering*, Washinghton, DC. (2001)

[5]. Larson, B. T., Erdman, A. G., Tsekos, N. V., Yacoub, E., Tsekos, P. V., and Koutlas, I. G. ASME J. *Biomech. Eng.* **126**, 458–465. (2004)

[6]. Masamune, K., Kobayashi, E., Masutani, Y., et.al. *J Image Guided Surgery* **1**:242–8. (1995)

[7]. Chinzei, K., and Miller, K. *Med Sci Monit* **7**, 153–163. (2001)

[8]. Susil, R. C., Krieger, A., Derbyshire, J. A., Tanacs, A., Whitcomb, L. L., Fichtinger, G., and Atalar, E.. *Radiology* **228**, 886–894. (2003)

[9]. Jolesz, F. A., Morrison, P. R., Koran, S. J., Kelley, R. J., Hushek, S. G., Newman, R. W., Fried, M. P., Melzer, A., Seibel, R. M., and Jalahej, H.. J. *Magn. Reson. Imag.* **8**, 8–11. (1998)

[10]. Hynynen K. McDannold N. Vykhodtseva N. Jolesz F. Noninvasive, *Radiology* **230**:640-646. (2001).

371

MR guided FUS therapy with a Robotic Assistance System

Jürgen W. Jenne, Axel J. Krafft, Florian Maier, Jaane Rauschenberg, Wolfhard Semmler, Peter E. Huber and Michael Bock

German Cancer Research Center, INF 280, 69120 Heidelberg, Germany

Abstract. Magnetic Resonance imaging guided Focus Ultrasound Surgery (MRgFUS) is a highly precise method to ablate tissue non-invasively. To date, there is only one commercial MRgFUS system available and only a few are in a prototype stage. The objective of this ongoing project is to establish an MRgFUS therapy unit as add-on for a commercially available robotic assistance system originally designed for percutaneous needle interventions in whole-body MR scanners.

A FUS treatment head was designed and built as add-on to the fully MR compatible robotic assistance system Innomotion™ (Innomedic, Herxheim, Germany), which features six degrees of freedom. The treatment head consists of a water filled flexible bellow with an integrated ultrasound transducer ($f = 1.7$ MHz; $f' = 68$ mm, NA = 0.44), a thin Mylar window for ultrasound coupling and a dedicated MR receive coil. The transducer itself is directly connected to the head of the robotic system. For FUS application, the therapy head will be coupled from above to the targeted region. The system was tested in a clinical 1.5 T whole body MR scanner on transparent PAA-gel phantoms and in animal trials with pigs.

In vivo and in vitro trials proved the new add-on MRgFUS system as highly MR compatible. Additionally, the positioning accuracy of the US focus was better than 0.7mm. Hence, a well-defined confluent tissue ablation under MR guidance and online thermometry in animal experiments were possible. In practice, the coupling of the FUS head from above clearly facilitates the ultrasound coupling process.

The next steps will include the integration of dedicated MRgFUS planning and treatment software as well as real time motion correction for MR thermometry.

Keywords: High intensity focused ultrasound, Focused Ultrasound Surgery, Magnetic Resonance Imaging, MR guided FUS, MR thermometry.
PACS: 87.61.Ff

INTRODUCTION

Magnetic Resonance imaging guided Focus Ultrasound Surgery (MRgFUS) realizes an ideal non-invasive method to thermally ablate, even deep-seated tissue target volumes under the accurate control and guidance of magnetic resonance imaging (MRI).

Within the last decade the feasibility and the safety of FUS has been tested in a growing number of clinical studies on several benign and malign diseases. Actually the clinical studies focus on solid tumors, e.g. liver or kidney tumors, prostate cancer and uterine fibroids. A necessary prerequisite for a safe and effective FUS therapy is a

CP1113, *8th International Symposium on Therapeutic Ultrasound*, edited by E. S. Ebbini
© 2009 American Institute of Physics 978-0-7354-0650-6/09/$25.00

reliable imaging method for therapy guidance and monitoring in order to provide the opportunity for a complete ablation of the targeted volume.

The imaging modality best suited for FUS therapy guidance is MRI with its excellent soft tissue contrast and the ability to monitor the FUS induced temperature changes online. However, the high initial costs for the MR compatible therapy unit and the MR scanner itself are major disadvantages of MRgFUS. Furthermore, the limited space, the strong magnetic and the presence of radiofrequency fields demand a complex and an expensive technology. To date, only a few MRgFUS treatment units are commercially available and are mostly arranged in a prototype stadium [1].

An important component of an MRgFUS therapy unit is an actuator, which allows the focal spot or continuous scanning of the target volume. The related need for any mechanical movements of the ultrasound source can be reduced by using phased array ultrasound transducers. However, due to limited beam steering abilities of these transducers, mechanical source motion remains necessary.

Today, commercial and experimental MRgFUS systems are typically integrated into the patient table of the MR scanner. These transducers can only be moved over a very limited spatial range. In addition, these systems use a specially designed patient table and thus, are dependent on the MR type and manufacturer.

The objective of this ongoing project is to establish an MRgFUS therapy unit as add-on for a commercially available robotic assistance system (Fig. 1), which was designed for percutaneous needle interventions in whole-body MR scanners.

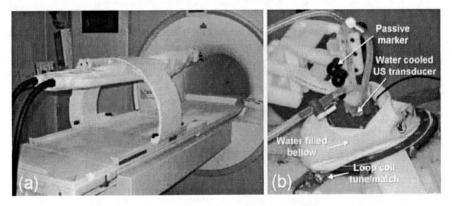

FIGURE 1: (a) Robotic assistance system normally used for needle interventions. (b) Newly developed add-on ultrasound treatment unit connected to the head of the robotic system.

MATERIAL AND METHODS

A FUS treatment head was designed and built as add-on to the fully MR compatible robotic assistance system Innomotion^{TM} (Innomedic, Herxheim, Germany), which features six degrees of freedom. Five of them are controlled by fully MR compatible pneumatic actuators. Designed for MR guided interventions with needles the system features a distal instrument holder with four passive MR markers for localization (Fig. 1).

The constructed treatment head (Fig. 1b) consists of a water filled flexible bellow with an integrated ultrasound transducer (prototype, Siemens Medical Solutions, Erlangen, Germany, focal length: 68 mm, NA = 0.44; elliptical focus: 8.1 mm length; 1.1 mm diameter), a thin Mylar window for ultrasound coupling and a dedicated, in-house developed MR receive coil (single loop coil, coil diameter: 17 cm) [2]. The transducer itself is directly linked to the head of the robotic system, so that the sonication axis coincided with the original needle axis. Consequently, the system's intervention planning software could be used. The transducer was connected to a RF power amplifier located outside the RF cabin using a specially designed transmission line with integrated filters (< 100dB @ 63MHz) to suppress unwanted coupling with the MR signal at 63 MHz. For FUS application, the therapy head will be coupled from above to the targeted region.

The system was tested in a clinical 1.5 T whole body MR scanner (Magnetom Symphony, Siemens Medical Solutions, Erlangen, Germany) equipped with a 30 mT/m gradient system.

The positioning accuracy of the setup was assessed by defined sonications of a tissue mimicking transparent polyacrylamide (PAA) gel phantom. The PAA-phantom was enriched with egg white as temperature sensitive indicator and guaranteed well-defined acoustic parameters [3]. The relative positions of the FUS induced lesions (Fig. 2) were measured by calipers and on T2w MR images (spin echo, TR = 4000 ms, TE = 143 ms, SL = 3 mm, FOV = 250×250 mm^2, matrix: 384×384).

The performance of the combined robotic assisted FUS treatment system was investigated in an in vivo experiment with a fully anesthetized, 3 month old domestic pig. A defined area at the pig's right hind leg muscle was treated (several sonications of about 60 s) under MR guidance. Initially, planning images were acquired, a target was defined with the assistance system's planning software and the FUS transducer was positioned and oriented by the robot. Based on the proton resonance frequency (PRF) shift, local online temperature mapping (FLASH, TR = 20 ms, TE = 15 ms, SL = 5 mm, FOV = 300×300 mm^2, matrix: 256×256) was performed. The thermally induced tissue lesions were afterwards evaluated on T2w MR images (turbo spin echo, TR = 4000 ms; TE = 118 ms; SL = 3 mm; FOV = 350×350 mm^2; matrix: 256×256).

RESULTS

An MR image (coronal slice orientation) of several thermally induced lesions at pre-defined positions in the PAA-phantom is shown in Fig. 2 to asses the accuracy of the robotic assisted US focus positioning. Both caliper and MR image based measurements showed a maximal spatial deviation of 0.7 mm at a positioning distance of 30.0 mm. A confluent lesion could be successfully created by using 1 mm re-positioning steps between five individual sonications.

In Fig. 3a five individual PRF-based temperature images are overlaid to one of the corresponding magnitude images (sagittal slice orientation) of the corresponding sonication series of porcine muscle tissue. A maximal temperature increase of about 30 K was measured for each sonication. The continuous temperature measurements allowed to calculate a thermal dose distribution (Fig. 3b) using the approach of cumulative equivalent minutes (*CEM*) [4] and hence, to quantify the volume of the destroyed tissue areas (a threshold value of the lethal thermal dose of *CEM* = 240 min was assumed). Fig. 3c shows the corresponding T2w post-sonication MR image (sagittal slice orientation). All three images delineate a well-defined confluent lesion of about 3 cm in diameter.

In all the performed experiments the MRgFUS setup consisting of the robot and the add-on FUS head proved fully MR compatible. Especially positioning and subsequent sonication were possible without imaging artifacts.

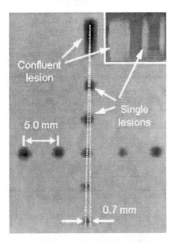

FIGURE 2: Enlarged MR image and photograph (insert) of the thermally induced lesions in the PAA-phantom. Five individual sonications at a distance of 1.0 mm were used to create a confluent lesion

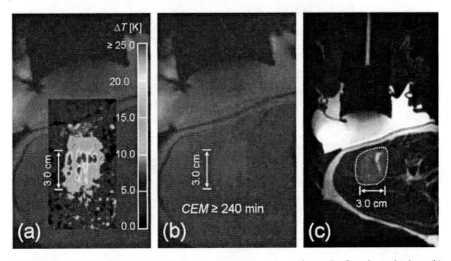

FIGURE 3: (a) Overlay of 5 individual temperature maps at the end of each sonication. (b) Corresponding map of lethal thermal dose (according to [4]). (c) Section of post-sonication MR image to analyze the created lesion.

DISCUSSION

We were able to demonstrate that the combination of a commercially available robotic assistance system intrinsically dedicated for MR guided needle interventions with a specially designed add-on ultrasound treatment applicator proved as a complete MRgFUS therapy unit. The system showed a high positioning accuracy and was fully MR compatible. As the robotic system provides a wide range of flexibility in positioning of the treatment head and as it offers an access to the patient from above, a more flexible positioning of the FUS transducer becomes possible. Additionally, the critical process of coupling the US treatment unit to the patient's skin can be performed under visible control of the user. However, specifically designed treatment heads might be necessary to enable the treatment of different organs.

Beside technical improvements, e.g. the MR receive coil, the next steps will include the integration of dedicated MRgFUS planning and treatment software as well as motion correction for MR thermometry techniques.

REFERENCES

1. McDannold N, Tempany CM, Fennessy FM, So MJ, Rybicki FJ, Stewart EA, Jolesz FA, and Hynynen K. Radiology **240**, 263-272 (2006).
2. Krafft AJ, Jenne JW, Rauschenberg J, Semmler W, Stafford RJ, Bock M. MR-guided HIFU Thermotherapy with a Robotic Assistance System. Proc. Intl. Soc. Mag. Reson. Med. **16,** #65 (2008)
3. Wilzbach Divkovic G, Liebler M, Braun K, Dryer T, Huber PE, Jenne JW. Thermal Properties and Changes of Acoustic Parameters in an Egg White Phantom During Heating and Coagulation by High Intensity Focused Ultrasound. Ultrasound Med. Biol. **33**, 981-986 (2007).
4. Sapareto SA, Dewey WC. Thermal Dose Determination in Cancer Therapy. Int. J. Radiation Oncology Biol. Phys. **10**, 787-800 (1984).

A 1372-element Large Scale Hemispherical Ultrasound Phased Array Transducer for Noninvasive Transcranial Therapy

Junho Song[a,b] and Kullervo Hynynen[a,b]

[a] Sunnybrook Health Science Centre, 2075 Bayview Ave, Toronto, ON, Canada, M4N 3M5
[b] Medical Biophysics, University of Toronto, ON, Canada, M4N 3M5

Abstract. Noninvasive transcranial therapy using high intensity focused ultrasound transducers has attracted high interest as a promising new modality for the treatments of brain related diseases. We describe the development of a 1372 element large scale hemispherical ultrasound phased array transducer operating at a resonant frequency of 306 kHz. The hemispherical array has a diameter of 31 cm and a 15.5 cm radius of curvature. It is constructed with piezoelectric (PZT-4) tube elements of a 10 mm in diameter, 6 mm in length and 1.4 mm wall thickness. Each element is quasi-air backed by attaching a cork-rubber membrane on the back of the element. The acoustic efficiency of the element is determined to be approximately 50 %. The large number of the elements delivers high power ultrasound and offers better beam steering and focusing capability. Comparisons of sound pressure-squared field measurements with theoretical calculations in water show that the array provides good beam steering and tight focusing capability over an efficient volume of approximately 100 x 100 x 80 mm³ with nominal focal spot size of approximately 2.3 mm in diameter at -6 dB. We also present its beam steering and focusing capability through an ex vivo human skull by measuring pressure-squared amplitude after phase corrections. These measurements show the same efficient volume range and focal spot sizes at -6dB as the ones in water without the skull present. These results indicate that the array is sufficient for use in noninvasive transcranial ultrasound therapy.

Keywords: HIFU; therapeutic ultrasound; hemispherical transducer.
PACS: 43.38.-p, 43.38.Hz

INTRODUCTION

Previous studies have shown that ultrasound energy can be delivered through a human skull to induce tumor tissue destruction [1-3]. However, the skull severely distorts the propagating ultrasound beam and degrades the focusing quality of an ultrasound transducer. To maximize the transmission of ultrasound energy through the skull and achieve reliable focusing, various techniques have been proposed, such as optimization of a driving frequency [4-5], use of a large scale phased array along with other imaging modalities, and implementation of phase and amplitude correction algorithm [6-8].

The objective of the study is to design, fabrication and characterization of a large-scale hemispherical ultrasound phased-array for low frequency transcranial ultrasound therapy. The functionality of the array, including its beam steering and focusing capabilities, is evaluated with an ex vivo human skull.

CP1113, 8th International Symposium on Therapeutic Ultrasound, edited by E. S. Ebbini
© 2009 American Institute of Physics 978-0-7354-0650-6/09/$25.00

MATERIALS AND METHODS

The prototype of a 31 cm in diameter hemispherical ultrasound phased array was constructed with 1372 custom-made lead zirconate titanate (PZT-4) elements as shown in Figure 1. The array was constructed using recently developed transducer fabrication method [9] to reduce the electrical impedance of the elements such that it can be driven with the standard driving amplifiers without employing a matching circuit. The array was made of cylindrical, tube-shaped PZT elements, which had the same dimension of a 10 mm outer diameter, 6 mm height, and 1.4 mm wall thickness. The fundamental and 3rd harmonic frequencies of the array elements were 306 kHz and 840 kHz, respectively.

A concentric array pattern was designed to fully utilize the entire inner surface area of the hemispherical dome. The pattern consisted of one center element and 23 rings of elements. The center of the elements in the 23rd ring was located at a 4 mm below the geometric focal plane which was normal to an acoustic axis. The gaps between the neighboring elements in any directions were less than 0.5 mm. A RF driving system developed in-house with 2000 independent channels was used to drive the array.

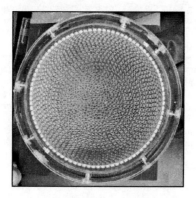

FIGURE 1. A picture of a fully assembled 1372 element hemispherical phased array.

Figure 2 showed the overall experimental setup. A 45 x 50 x 120 cm^3 water tank was covered with anechoic rubber to minimize any acoustic reflections from the tank walls. The tank was filled with degassed deionized (DI) water whose dissolved oxygen level was approximately 0.8 ppm. The array was rigidly placed on the bottom of the tank facing up to the water surface. The ultrasound pressure field radiated from the array was measured with a 0.2 mm in diameter polyvinylidene fluoride (PVDF) needle hydrophone (Precision Acoustics, Dorchester, UK). The hydrophone was affixed to a Parker/Velmax 3-D scanning system (Parker, Hannifi, PA, USA; Velmax Inc, Broomfield, NY, USA) and parallel with the acoustic axis of the array. The phase correction was performed for all the experiments in the study to eliminate any system induced phase delay and to assure the best possible focusing.

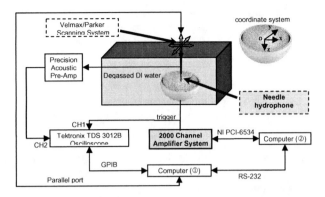

Figure 2. Experimental setup for the hemispherical ultrasound phased array

RESULTS AND DISCUSSION

The amplitude of the electrical impedance and phase angle of a single cylindrical PZT array element were measured in degassed DI water by using a network/spectrum analyzer (HP 4195A, Agilent Technology, Santa Clara, CA, USA). The fundamental and third harmonic frequencies were measured at 306 kHz and 840 kHz, respectively. These frequencies corresponded to the length mode resonance frequencies of the cylindrical PZT transducer. The electrical impedance at the fundamental frequency (f = 306 kHz) was 142.6 ± 4.4 Ω with a zero phase angle. Similarly, its electric impedance at the third harmonic frequency (f = 840 kHz) was 182.82 ± 5.4 Ω with a phase angle of -63.17° ± 2.74°. These measurements clearly showed that the introduction of the cylindrical PZT transducer in the phased array fabrication and driving them at length mode provided at least an order of magnitude reduction in the electrical impedance, compared with standard PZT plate transducers driven at thickness mode. The overall electrical-to-acoustic power conversion efficiency of the element were measured to be 52.5 ± 1.1% at 306 kHz and 35.0 ± 1.3 % at 840 kHz, respectively.

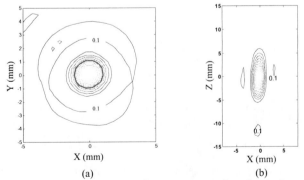

(a)   (b)

FIGURE 3. Normalized sound pressure-squared measurement surface plots in the xy and xz plane at the geometric focus when the array is driven at the fundamental frequency (f = 306 kHz).

Figure 3 showed the normalized sound pressure-squared (PS) measurement surface plots in the *xy* and *xz* plane at the geometric focus when the array is driven at the fundamental frequency (f = 306 kHz). The focal beam spot size, measured at a 50 % value of its peak amplitude, was approximately 2.3 mm and 6.5 mm in the *xy* and *xz* planes, respectively. Figure 4 showed the pressure squared field measurements at different foci along the lateral (*x*) and axial (*z*) axes in water when the array was driven at 306 kHz. Inferring from these measurements, the range of the 50% of the PS peak, or the effective beam steering range, was predicted to be 100 mm (-50 ~ 50 mm) x 100 mm (-50 ~ 50 mm) in the *xy* plane and 80 mm (-40 ~ 40 mm) in the axial direction, respectively. Such wide effective range would require only a rough placement of the patient's head with electronic aiming of the beam to the exact target locations. In addition, it allows fast electronic beam steering for advanced multi-location sonication patterns.

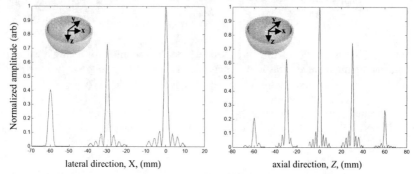

FIGURE 4. Normalized pressure squared field measurement in the *x-y* (a) and *x-z* (b) planes at the geometric focus when the array is driven at 306 kHz.

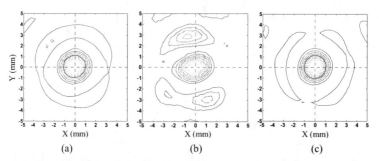

FIGURE 5. Normalized sound pressure-squared measurement contour plots in the *xy* plane at the geometric focus, (0,0,0). The driving frequency of the transducer is 306 kHz. The plots are shown the measurements in water: (a) without a skull, (b) with a skull but no phase correction is used, and (c) with a skull when phase correction is used. The contour interval is 10% of the peak value.

Figure 5 showed the normalized PS field measurements at 306 kHz obtained without (a) or with (c) an *ex vivo* skull present. When phase correction was performed, the beam profile and spot size were almost identical. As shown in Figure 5 (b), a significant focus distortion through the human skull was observed when the skull specific phase correction was not performed. The skull measurement showed that the 306 kHz beam could be focused without skull specific phase correction but with increased beam diameter and side lobes. The skull specific corrections restored a sharp focus.

CONCLUSION

This study demonstrated the feasibility of constructing electronically focused and steered ultrasound phased array using cylindrical piezoelectric transducer elements. The elements allow the electrical impedance to be reduced at least an order of magnitude such that effective operation can be achieved without electronic matching circuits. The 1372 element array was shown to be sufficient to produce excellent focusing through the *ex vivo* human skull and an adequate beam steering range for clinical brain treatments. The lower frequency would be suitable for cavitation enhanced treatments such as focal drug delivery and the higher frequency for thermal and thrombolytic therapies.

ACKNOWLEDGMENTS

This research was supported by NIH Grants (EB 00705 and EB003268). The author thanks Ping Wu for her great amount of time and support on the array fabrication, and Samuel Gunaseelan for his technical assistant and support on the electronics.

REFERENCES

1. F.J. Fry. Transskull transmission of an intense focused ultrasonic beam. Ultrasound Med. Biol. 1977; 3: pp.179-184.
2. K. Hynynen, F.A. Jolesz. Demonstration of potential noninvasive ultrasound brain therapy through an intact skull. Ultrasound Med. Biol. 1998; 24(2): pp.275-283
3. F. Marquet F, M. Pernot, J.F. Aubry, M. Tanter, A.L. Boch, M. Kujas, D. Seihean, and M. Fink. Noninvasive Transcranial Brain Therapy Guided by CT Scans: an In Vivo Monkey Study. AIP Conf. Proc. The 6th Interational Symposium on Therapeutic Ultrasound, 2007; 911: pp.554-560.
4. F.J. Fry, J.E. Barger. Acoustical properties of the human skull. J Acoust Soc Am 1978; 63: pp. 1576-1590
5. X. Yin, K. Hynynen. A numerical study of Transcranial focused ultrasound beam propagation at low frequency. Phys. Med. Biol. 2005; 50: pp.1821-1836.
6. G.T. Clement, J. Sun, T. Giesecke and K. Hynynen. A hemisphere array for non-invasive ultrasound brain therapy and surgery. Phys. Med. Biol. 2000; 45: pp.3707-3719.
7. G.T. Clement, K. Hynynen. A non-invasive method for focusing ultrasound through the human skull. Phys. Med. Biol 2002; 47: pp.1219-1236.
8. K. Hynynen, G.T. Clement, N. McDoannold, N. Vykhodtseva, R. King, P.J. White, S. Vitek, and F.A. Jolesz. 500-Element Ultrasound Phased Array System for Noninvasive Focal surgery of the brain: A preliminary Rabbit study with ex vivo Human skulls. Magnetic Resonance in Medicine 2004; 52: pp.100-107.
9. K. Hynynen. A method to control the electrical impedance of phased array elements. IEEE Ultras. Symp. 2006, pp.1052-1055.

Multi-Channel RF System for MRI-Guided Transurethral Ultrasound Thermal Therapy

Nicolas Yak[a], Matthew Asselin[a], Rajiv Chopra[a,b], Michael Bronskill[a,b]

[a]Sunnybrook Health Sciences Centre, 2075 Bayview Ave., Toronto, ON, Canada, M4N 3M5.
[b]Department of Medical Biophysics, University of Toronto

Abstract. MRI-guided transurethral ultrasound thermal therapy is an approach to treating localized prostate cancer which targets precise deposition of thermal energy within a confined region of the gland. This treatment requires a system incorporating a heating applicator with multiple planar ultrasound transducers and associated RF electronics to control individual elements independently in order to achieve accurate 3D treatment. We report the design, construction, and characterization of a prototype multi-channel system capable of controlling 16 independent RF signals for a 16-element heating applicator. The main components are a control computer, microcontroller, and a 16-channel signal generator with 16 amplifiers, each incorporating a low-pass filter and transmitted/reflected power detection circuit. Each channel can deliver from 0.5 to 10W of electrical power and good linearity from 3 to 12MHz. Harmonic RF signals near the Larmor frequency of a 1.5T MRI were measured to be below -30dBm and heating experiments within the 1.5T MR system showed no significant decrease in SNR of the temperature images. The frequency and power for all 16 channels could be changed in less than 250ms, which was sufficiently rapid for proper performance of the control algorithms. A common backplane design was chosen which enabled an inexpensive, modular approach for each channel resulting in an overall system with minimal footprint.

Keywords: MRI-guided; Transurethral; Ultrasound Thermal Therapy; Prostate; RF; Signal Generator; Amplifier; Multi-Channel
PACS: 84.30.-r, 84.30.Jc, 84.30.Ng, 84.30.Vn, 84.61.-c

INTRODUCTION

Prostate cancer is a leading cause of death for men in North America [1]. Although existing treatments for localized prostate cancer are able to achieve effective disease control, they are often associated with significant long-term complications to urinary, rectal and sexual function [2]. One promising technique that aims to reduce these complication rates is MRI-guided transurethral ultrasound therapy [3,4].

Thermal coagulation of prostate tissue is achieved using ultrasound transducers introduced within the gland through the patient's urethra. Modulation of transducer power and frequency enables control over depth of heating, while simultaneous rotation of the device enables coagulation of prostate tissue volumes.

A transurethral device consisting of a single ultrasound transducer is unable to shape a heating pattern to the 3 dimensional volume of the prostate gland. As shown in Figure 1, multiple transducers can be incorporated to increase control over the 3D

CP1113, *8th International Symposium on Therapeutic Ultrasound*, edited by E. S. Ebbini
© 2009 American Institute of Physics 978-0-7354-0650-6/09/$25.00

heating pattern to compensate for various sizes and shapes of glands. Preliminary experiments within our group suggest that individual elements with a length of 3mm are capable of producing adequate output acoustic power for this application. Analysis of a patient database of MRI-segmented prostate suggests that human prostate lengths range from 27-50mm; thus 16 3mm ultrasound transducers are required to cover the entire prostate. Consequently, 16 independent channels of RF electronics are necessary to control their output power.

We present a description of the requirements, design, and performance of a prototype, 16-channel RF system capable of driving each ultrasound transducer independently to conform to the varying shapes and sizes of prostate glands.

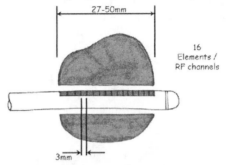

FIGURE 1. Simplified prostate in the sagittal view demonstrating the need for a 16-element transducer to cover a 50mm prostate

REQUIREMENTS

A block diagram of the system signal flow is shown in Figure 2. At the heart of the transurethral ultrasound therapy system is a control computer which receives MR images in the form of temperature maps, typically every 5 seconds. Based on the acquired temperature information, a control algorithm updates the parameters necessary to continue a safe and effective treatment [4]. In particular, by modulating power and frequency for the ultrasound transducers, it ensures accurate shaping of the heating pattern to the targeted volume [5].

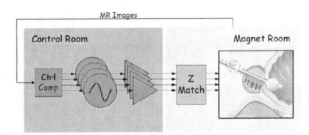

FIGURE 2. Block diagram demonstrating RF signal flow through the system and the importance of an MRI-compatible multi-channel RF system

The specifications derived for the 16-channel prototype unit were:

1) Output up to 10W of electrical power per channel, between 3-12MHz
2) Electrical noise/harmonics below -30dBm within the MRI bandwidth
3) Time for updating power and frequency of 16 channels to be less than 250msec
4) Small footprint/mobile

As illustrated in Figure 2, the electronics are not located within the magnet room and, thus, material selection is not required to be MRI compatible. However, the RF signals propagating into the magnet room to the ultrasound transducers must not contain any high frequency harmonics that might interfere with image acquisition (requirement 2 in the above listing). In addition to these requirements, a mobile system with small footprint to reduce the size of equipment in the control room was desired.

DESIGN

The multi-channel RF system prototype is composed of 16 signal generator modules and 16 associated amplifier modules. The control computer interfaces with the RF system via an 8-bit microcontroller enabling independent communication with each channel.

The microcontroller communicates with the signal generator modules, direct digital synthesizers (DDS), to create a waveform of the desired frequency. Subsequently, these synthesized waveforms are passed to digital potentiometers (DigiPOTs) for modulating the signal amplitudes. Finally, a low-pass filter (f_c = 15MHz) suppresses higher-order harmonics introduced by the digital reconstruction of the RF signal by the DDS.

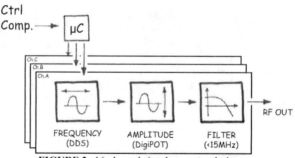

FIGURE 3. 16-channel signal generator design

The RF signal from the signal generator module is amplified (Figure 4) through a Class AB amplifier providing a good compromise between linearity and power efficiency. To suppress further any high-order harmonics introduced by the amplifier, an additional low-pass filter with a cut-off frequency of 40MHz is introduced. To ensure patient safety, the amplified RF-signal passes through a bi-directional coupler to enable real-time monitoring of forward and reflected power levels to ensure accurate power levels are being delivered to the transducers.

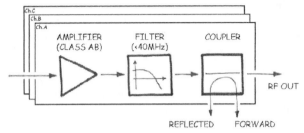

FIGURE 4. 16-channel wideband high-power amplifier design

PERFORMANCE

Figure 5(a) illustrates the electrical output power for one prototype channel with respect to the input to the channel via the DigiPOT. This measurement was repeated for the range of frequencies required. Figure 5(a) demonstrates smooth, continuous control over the output power from 0.5-10W. There are small differences in performance at different frequencies and the output power is not linear with the digital input value. In practice, however, this is not a limitation because the treatment is operated at 2 discrete frequencies, therefore a flat frequency response is not critical, and look-up tables can easily be implemented to ensure accurate power delivery.

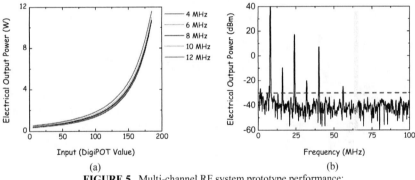

(a)   (b)

FIGURE 5. Multi-channel RF system prototype performance:
(a) system RF output power, (b) system output frequency spectrum

Figure 5(b) illustrates the output frequency spectrum measured for a 10W 8MHz signal from one channel of the prototype system. Harmonic levels in the bandwidth of a 1.5T MRI system (around 64MHz) are well below the -30dBm level which meets our specification for avoiding interference with the MRI system which could degrade temperature measurement during treatment delivery. On a 3T MRI system (at 128MHz), the harmonic level is expected to be even lower. We measure a dynamic range of at least 80dB between the fundamental frequency and harmonic level at 64MHz.

The timing performance of the 16-channel prototype system was also measured. The time required to update the frequency and amplitude parameters for one channel was measured to be 11.5ms, and this scaled linearly for all 16 channels to 184ms. The system required 5.9ms to shut down a single channel; however, this did not scale linearly with channel number and only 8.4ms was required to stop all 16-channels. This was attributed to the structure of the messaging between the control computer and the microcontroller, whereby a single command is sent to shut down all channels while two commands per channel are necessary to update both frequency and amplitude.

TABLE 1. Signal update time for 1-channel and 16-channels

Parameter	1 Channel (ms)	16 Channels (ms)
Time to Update (Freq+Ampl)	11.5	184
Time to turn OFF	5.9	8.4

DISCUSSION & CONCLUSIONS

A 16-channel RF system for MRI-guided transurethral ultrasound therapy has been designed and fabricated. The measured system performance met all our requirements for output power and frequency, harmonic/noise levels in the bandwidth of a 1.5T MRI system, quick and efficient update times, and flexibility for expansion of the channel count.

The system will undergo additional testing with tissue-mimicking gel phantoms and pre-clinical studies to evaluate its performance further under full experimental conditions.

ACKNOWLEDGMENTS

Financial support for this project was received from the Terry Fox Foundation, the Ontario Research and Development Challenge Fund, the Ontario Institute of Cancer Research, and the Canadian Institutes of Health Research.

REFERENCES

1. Canadian Cancer Statistics 2006, 2006.
2. L. Potosky, W. W. Davis, R. M. Hoffman, J. L. Stanford, R. A. Stephenson, D. F. Penson, and L. C. Harlan. (2004) "Five-year outcomes after prostatectomy or radiotherapy for prostate cancer: the prostate cancer outcomes study." J Nat Cancer Inst, 96 (18): 1358-1367.
3. C. Mougenot, R. Salomir, J. Palussiere, N. Grenier, C. T. Moonen. (2004) "Automatic spatial and temporal temperature control for MR-guided focused ultrasound using fast 3D MR thermometry and multispiral trajectory of the focal point." Magn Reson Med, 52 (5): 1005-15.
4. R. Chopra, N. Baker, V. Choy, A. Boyes, K. Tang, D. Bradwell, and M.J. Bronskill. (2008) "MRI-compatible transurethral ultrasound system for the treatment of localized prostate cancer using rotational control." Med Phys, 35 (4): 1346-1357.
5. R. Chopra, M. Burtnyk, M.A. Haider, and M.J. Bronskill. (2005) "Method for MRI-guided conformal thermal therapy of prostate with planar transurethral ultrasound heating applicators." Phys Med Biol, 50: 4957–4975.

Multi-Angle Switched HIFU: A New Ultrasound Device for Controlled Non-Invasive Induction of Small Spherical Ablation Zones – Simulation and Ex-Vivo Results

Petr Novák[a], Azemat Jamshidi-Parsian[a], Donny G. Benson[a], Jessica S. Webber[a], Eduardo G. Moros[a], Gal Shafirstein[b], and Robert J. Griffin[a]

Departments of [a]Radiation Oncology and [b]Otolaryngology, University of Arkansas for Medical Sciences, Little Rock, AR 72205, USA

Abstract. Current HIFU devices produce elongated elliptical lesions (cigar shaped) in a single energy deposition. This prohibits the effective use of HIFU in small animal research as well as in clinical treatment where small volumes of tissue surrounded by critical structures need to be destroyed. We developed an ultrasound ablation device that non-invasively creates spheroidal lesions of an arbitrary diameter of up to 1 cm in a depth of up to 5 cm. The device consists of two focused ultrasound transducers aimed to the ablation target volume from two directions at a 90 degree angle. The operation of the transducers is switched back and forth so that only one transducer is energized at a time. A transient analysis of this ablation approach was performed using coupled simulations of acoustical pressure distributions, resulting temperature distributions, and thermal dose deposited to soft tissue. A prototype of the device was developed and tested in-vitro in a phantom and later in ex-vivo experiments in pig liver. The experimental results agreed with the numerical simulations and confirmed the ability of the multi-angle switched HIFU (MASH) device to create small spheroidal lesions in soft tissue within 2 minutes without significantly affecting the surrounding tissues.

Keywords: high intensity focused ultrasound; thermal ablation; tumors; new device

PACS: 43.64.+r, 44.10.+i

INTRODUCTION

Thermal ablation with high-intensity focused ultrasound (HIFU) has become an important approach complementing traditional surgical techniques in a range of clinical applications [1-4]. HIFU permits non-invasive interventions delivered to a well defined tissue volume while sparing the surrounding tissues [5]. It heats isolated tissue volumes to 55 °C or more and maintains this temperature for a few seconds. Such temperature elevation has been shown to lead to coagulative necrosis and immediate cell death in the affected area [6, 7].

Here we present a simple yet effective strategy for HIFU ablation in order to create spheroidal lesions of approximately 1 cm or smaller in diameter. The goal was to design a system that can spare the skin and overlying tissue in experimental models of cancer while ablating a precise and predictable volume within an implanted tumor. A system able to achieve this type of heating will allow combination treatments with chemotherapy or radiation therapy to be studied in a reproducible fashion and improve

CP1113, *8th International Symposium on Therapeutic Ultrasound*, edited by E. S. Ebbini
© 2009 American Institute of Physics 978-0-7354-0650-6/09/$25.00

our ability to document the biological and physiological effects of HIFU heating on solid tumor tissue.

MATERIALS AND METHODS

Two HIFU transducers were aligned at a 90° angle so that their focal zones overlap at the point of maximum acoustical pressure [8]. Additionally, software was written to operate the transducers in alternating fashion so that no more than one of them is energized at a time. First, a range of transducer parameters was selected for simulation. Transducers of 25.4 mm and 38.1 mm in diameter, radius of curvature 50.8 mm and 63.5 mm, and resonant frequencies of 2.25MHz and 3.5 MHz were picked as appropriate for possible MASH designs (8 unique configurations in total). These transducer parameters were chosen based on the selection of transducers available from our supplier. The diameter of the transducer needed to be large enough to generate enough acoustical power assuming $10W/cm^2$ as a reasonable intensity maximum. The radius of curvature and the frequency were selected with respect to the required penetration depth and to the 6dB beam-width calculated as [9]:

$$BW_{6dB} = 1.028 * FL * \lambda / D,$$

(1)

where BW_{6dB} is the 6dB beam-width, FL is the focal length (same as radius of curvature for a spherically focused transducer used), λ is the acoustical wavelength in the media, and D is the diameter of the transducer.

Second, the acoustical free-field intensity of an air-backed ultrasound transducer was calculated by evaluating the Rayleigh-Sommerfeld integral over the surface of a transducer [10]:

$$I(x,y,z) = \frac{1}{2\rho c}\left[\frac{i\rho ck}{2\pi}\int_S \frac{ue^{-ik(r-r')}}{r-r'}dS\right]^2,$$

(2)

where $\rho = 1050$ kg m^{-3} is tissue density, $c = 1500$ m s^{-1} is the speed of sound, $k = 2\pi/\lambda$ is the wave number (λ is the wavelength), u is the complex surface velocity of the source, and S is the area of the ultrasound source. The calculation was implemented in Matlab.

Third, temperature elevation caused by acoustical field was simulated by solving the bioheat transfer equation (not shown) [11]. Since the attenuation coefficient depends on thermal dose, solving the bioheat transfer equation needed to be coupled to the calculation of attenuation coefficient. This meant the attenuation coefficient had to be interactively updated during the bioheat transfer equation calculation in respect to temperature simulated for a particular point in space. The simulation was performed using COMSOL Multiphysics (v.3.3, Comsol AB, Stockholm, Sweden) with transient

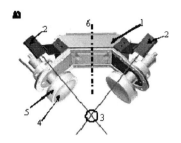 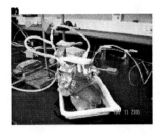

FIGURE 1. A) CAD of the MASH prototype with removed water bolus: 1 – holder, 2 – laser pointers used for optical demarcation of the center of the overlapped ultrasound focal zones, 3 – overlapped focal zone, 4 – ultrasound transducer, 5 – transducer enclosure, 6 – main axis of the device. B) Photograph of the MASH during in-vitro ablation of pig liver.

analysis using finite element method and Matlab (R2007b, Mathworks, Natick, MA) working in a loop.

The body of the MASH applicator was designed as a holder that kept the transducers in preset positions to each other at all times and allowed easy manipulation of both transducers as one unit (Figure 1A). A removable frame was designed on the front face of the holder where an ultrasound compatible material (Probe Cover #E1000SK, GE Healthcare) could be attached so that the entire volume around the transducers can be filled with degassed water and serve as a coupling bolus between the ultrasound transducers and tissue (Figure 1B). The ultrasound transducers were driven with a multi-channel RF generator (500-008, Advanced Surgical Systems, Tucson, AZ) providing up to 100W per channel. The RF generator was connected to a PC via RS-232 and controlled with custom software designed for this purpose.

RESULTS

An example of temperature buildup during MASH simulated ablation is shown in Figure 2A. The temperature was always maximal at the intersection of the two focal zones. Figure 2B shows thermal dose plot corresponding to temperature distributions shown in Figure 2A. A contour demarking points with a thermal dose (TD) > 250 CEM43 is shown that predicts the immediate extent of ablation with MASH. The effect of blood perfusion on the MASH ablation outcome was studied for perfusion rates 0, 5, and 9 kg m^{-3} s^{-1}. Tissue was considered ablated at points where the thermal damage reached at least 240 t43-equivalent minutes [12]. The ultimate criteria for ablation assessment were the size and shape of created lesion and the total ablation time. Figure 2C shows the dependence of the lesion diameter on the overall ablation time, the on-off sequence and kinetics of power-switching, and the perfusion rate.

Figure 3 shows examples of lesions thermally induced with the MASH in actual tissue (fresh porcine liver). A typical cigar-shaped lesion (Figure 3A) was achieved within 50 seconds using 75W electrical power at 50% duty cycle (200ms power on and 200ms off). Figure 3B is a photograph of an axial-lateral cut (considering the coordinates of the ultrasound transducers) of liver ablated for 140s at 40W with a 200ms/200ms/200ms (t1_on/t2_on/t_delay) power-switching scheme. The resulting lesion had a 6 mm diameter rounded shape very different from the cigar-shaped lesion. No ablation of tissue between the lesion and the surface of the tissue sample along the

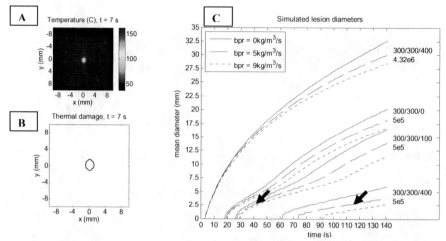

FIGURE 2. Simulation results of thermal ablation with MASH. A) Calculated temperature distribution for time, power-switching scenario, power, and perfusion rate (bpr). B) Simulated lesion size and shape corresponding to case (A). C) Simulated lesion diameters and dependence on blood perfusion. The same lesion size and shape was found to be achievable with several power-switching scenarios (see arrows).

path of either ultrasound beam was visible. Figure 3C is a lesion resulting from a 110 s ablation at 40W and 300ms/300ms/400ms power switching scheme. Figure 3D is after an axial-lateral bisection through the liver (same as Figure 3C), and 129s total ablation time.

DISCUSSION

In this study, we investigated the feasibility of combining spherically focused ultrasound transducers for thermal induction of small spheroidal lesions in soft tissues. The concept of two ultrasound transducers aligned at a 90-degree angle with overlapping focal zones was employed in a numerical simulation and by using a gel phantom (not shown) and pig liver. The transducers were operated in an alternating manner, so that there was no more than one transducer energized at a time allowing for possible power-off intervals during the course of ablation. The device was envisioned to facilitate and simplify HIFU induction of small spherical lesions at a variety of thermal doses and dose rates, which may be of great value for animal research, veterinary medicine, and potentially human clinical medicine as well.

The finite element simulation of acoustical pressure and heat transfer in soft tissue indicated power switching scenarios which take advantage of heat transfer properties

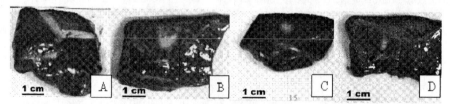

FIGURE 3. Photographs of axial-lateral sectioned lesions induced with MASH in pig liver.

390

(mainly thermal conduction) result in a spherical shape of the induced lesion. As expected, the shape of the lesion approximated a sphere when the thermal properties were allowed to impact the overall temperature distribution during the ablation (i.e., the temperature rise was relatively slow). The current acoustical model is limited to acoustical powers where nonlinear propagation of ultrasound has a negligible influence on the location of generated temperature increase maximum and where no cavitations are anticipated as these phenomena are not accounted for. The error of using such model was shown to be insignificant for acoustical powers employed in this study (Figure 3) however application of the device in clinical settings will require more rigorous investigation.

Our results indicated that several power-switching scenarios of the MASH can lead to the same size and shape of lesion yet with significantly different impact of the blood perfusion on obtaining these lesions (Figure 3C). The shape and size of the lesions we were able to induce in pig liver confirmed the feasibility of the MASH concept for thermal induction of small spherical ablation zones (Figure 3). This study has shown the potential of using the MASH concept for non-invasive thermal induction of small spherical lesions in experimental models of cancer. Further characterization of MASH alone and in combination with other therapy in small animal models is warranted.

ACKNOWLEDGEMENTS

Supported by NCI CA44114 and Central Arkansas Radiotherapy Institute (CARTI)

REFERENCES

1. Wu, F., et al., *Pathological changes in human malignant carcinoma treated with high-intensity focused ultrasound.* Ultrasound in Medicine and Biology, 2001. **27**(8): p. 1099-1106.
2. Beerlage, H.P., et al., *Transrectal high-intensity focused ultrasound using the ablatherm device in the treatment of localized prostate carcinoma.* Urology, 1999. **54**(2): p. 273-277.
3. Hynynen, K., et al., *MR imaging-guided focused ultrasound surgery of fibroadenomas in the breast: A feasibility study.* Radiology, 2001. **219**(1): p. 176-185.
4. Stewart, E.A., et al., *Clinical outcomes of focused ultrasound surgery for the treatment of uterine fibroids.* Fertility and Sterility, 2006. **85**(1): p. 22-29.
5. ter Haar, G., *Acoustic surgery.* Physics Today, 2001. **54**(12): p. 29-34.
6. Sapareto, S.A. and W.C. Dewey, *Thermal Dose Determination in Cancer-Therapy.* International Journal of Radiation Oncology Biology Physics, 1984. **10**(6): p. 787-800.
7. Dewhirst, M.W., et al., *Basic principles of thermal dosimetry and thermal thresholds for tissue damage from hyperthermia.* International Journal of Hyperthermia, 2003. **19**(3): p. 267-294.
8. Chauhan, S., M.J.S. Lowe, and B.L. Davies, *A multiple focused probe approach for high intensity focused ultrasound based surgery.* Ultrasonics, 2001. **39**(1): p. 33-44.
9. *The Ultrasonic Transducer.* 2008 [cited 2008 March]; Available from: Company website [http://www.bostonpiezooptics.com/].
10. Oneil, H.T., *Theory of Focusing Radiators.* Journal of the Acoustical Society of America, 1949. **21**(5): p. 516-526.
11. Pennes, H.H., *Analysis of Tissue and Arterial Blood Temperatures in the Resting Human Forearm.* Journal of Applied Physiology, 1948. **1**(2): p. 93-122.
12. Liu, H.L., et al., *A novel strategy to increase heating efficiency in a split-focus ultrasound phased array.* Medical Physics, 2007. **34**(7): p. 2957-2967.

Endocavitary Ultrasound Applicator for Hyperthermia Treatment of Cervical Cancer

Jeffery Wootton[a,b], Xin Chen[b], Titania Juang[b], Viola Rieke[c], I-Chow Joe Hsu[b], and Chris Diederich[a,b]

[a]Joint Graduate Group in Bioengineering, Univ. of California, Berkeley and San Francisco
[b]Thermal Therapy Research Group, Dept. of Radiation Oncology, Univ. of California, San Francisco
[c]Dept. of Radiology, Stanford University Medical Center

Abstract. An endocavitary ultrasound applicator has been developed for targeted heat delivery to the cervix. The device has multiple sectored tubular transducers for truly 3-D heating control (angular and along the length) and is integrated with an intracavitary HDR brachytherapy applicator for sequential administration of conformal heat and radiation. Brachytherapy treatment planning data are inspected to determine target thermal treatment volumes. Heat treatments are simulated with an acoustic and biothermal model of cervical tissue. Power control to individual elements and sectors is implemented for global maximum and pilot point control to limit rectum and bladder temperature. A parametric analysis of device parameters, tissue properties, and catheter materials is conducted to assess their effects on heating patterns and inform device development. Acoustic output of all devices was characterized. MR thermal imaging is used to analyze 3-D conformal heating capabilities in *ex vivo* tissue and compare to theoretical predictions. Devices were fabricated with 1-3 transducers at 6.5-8 MHz with sectors from 90-180° and heating length from 15-35 mm housed within a 6 mm diameter water-cooled PET catheter. Directional heating from sectored transducers can extend lateral penetration of therapeutic heating (41°C) > 2 cm while maintaining rectum and bladder temperatures within 12 mm below thermal damage thresholds. MR artifacts extended <2 mm beyond the device and real time thermal imaging was used to guide power selection to shape heating profiles in axial and coronal slices. Endocavitary delivery of ultrasound thermal therapy is feasible and 3-D conformal capabilities will benefit targeted cervical hyperthermia.

Keywords: hyperthermia; thermal therapy; cervical cancer; minimally-invasive therapy; intracavitary; multi-sectored transducers; magnetic resonance thermal imaging
PACS: 43.80.Gx, 43.80.Sh, 87.50.yt

INTRODUCTION

Cervical cancer causes more than 250,000 deaths per year worldwide [1]. Although stage I (FIGO) disease can generally be well managed, treatment of more advanced tumors is often unsuccessful; 5-year survival for stage II disease is 70%, dropping to 40% for stage III and 15% for stage IV [2]. The current standard of care calls for cisplatin-based chemotherapy (ChT) combined with radiation therapy (RT) consisting of external beam radiation and high-dose-rate (HDR) brachytherapy. Hyperthermia (HT), or temperature elevation to 41-43°C, improves tumor control by enhancing damage from RT and ChT. Recent data from the Dutch Deep Hyperthermia Trial show improvements in survival of nearly 100% after 12 years of follow-up when HT

CP1113, *8th International Symposium on Therapeutic Ultrasound*, edited by E. S. Ebbini
© 2009 American Institute of Physics 978-0-7354-0650-6/09/$25.00

is combined with RT [3]. Although these are highly positive results, deep regional heating equipment used in these treatments elevates temperature throughout the pelvis, limiting attainable thermal dose within the target and potentially resulting in overheating of non-targeted tissue [4, 5]. More localized therapy should further improve hyperthermia efficacy while minimizing toxicity.

An endocavitary ultrasound applicator has been developed for locally targeted heating to the uterine cervix. A linear array of sectored tubular transducers provides control of power output angularly and along the length of the device for truly 3-D conformal heating. Compared to deep regional heating equipment, the device has much improved thermal dose localization to the cervix, is far less costly, easier to use and disseminate, and does not require electromagnetically shielded treatment rooms. The device is integrated with a tandem and ring brachytherapy applicator to allow for sequential or simultaneous delivery of heat and radiation and to align heating with conformal radiation dose.

METHODS

Anatomical data from 25 HDR brachytherapy treatment plans using tandem and ring applicators were inspected. The dimensions of gross tumor volumes and target radiation treatment volumes defined by the physician were recorded. The location of sensitive tissues that must be protected during thermal therapy was noted.

The effects of ultrasound transducer parameters on heating profiles in uterine tissue were assessed with acoustic and biothermal simulation. The extension of therapeutic heating (as measured by the 41°C contour) after achieving steady-state temperature elevation was evaluated along with the ability to tailor heating to target volumes while avoiding sensitive tissue. Parameters that were varied include number of transducers, transducer length, diameter, axial sectoring, frequency, and blood perfusion. The influence of the catheter on thermal penetration was evaluated by varying thickness (0.125 – 0.5 mm), attenuation (20 – 80 Np m^{-1} MHz^{-1}), and cooling flow (convective heat transfer coefficient h = 500 – 1000 W m^{-2} °C^{-1}) at low (1 kg m^{-3} s^{-1}) or high (3 kg m^{-3} s^{-1}) blood perfusion. PID control limited maximum temperature to 45°C.

Devices constructed with input from simulations were acoustically characterized and their heating performance evaluated in *ex vivo* tissue with benchtop thermometry or MR thermal monitoring. Acoustic intensity plots were obtained by scanning a hydrophone at 8 mm distance along the length of the device while the device was rotated. Thermocouples were placed 1 cm from the applicator during benchtop trials and temperature was recorded during 10 minutes of heating. MR susceptibility artifacts were measured and MR temperature monitoring was used to guide power control in simple heating tests.

RESULTS AND DISCUSSION

Figure 1 provides an overview of the anatomy of the treatment region and demonstrates the proximity of the rectum and bladder to the cervix. The gross tumor volume to target during hyperthermia in the cervix is typically 2-4 cm in diameter and 2-4 cm along the length of the tandem. The bladder can lie within 12 mm of the uterine cavity anteriorly and the rectum within 15 mm of the uterine cavity posteriorly. Dominant heating should be targeted laterally into the parametrium to avoid thermal damage to the bladder and rectum. Interstitial catheters implanted during brachytherapy can act as conduits for thermocouples to monitor thermal treatments.

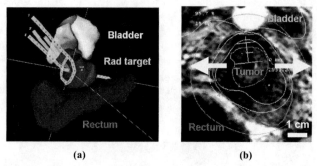

(a) (b)

FIGURE 1. (a) A 3-D reconstruction of a HDR brachytherapy treatment plan with tandem and ring applicator, interstitial catheters, and organs at risk. (b) An MR image of a treatment plan shows the bladder (anterior) and rectum (posterior) in close proximity to the gross tumor volume.

Biothermal simulations demonstrated the capability of the applicator to extend the 41°C contour greater than 4 cm diameter and tailor heating in the axial and sagittal planes. Dead zones (~30 degrees) in heating near sector notches can be aimed towards the bladder and rectum to prevent overheating of these structures. Cooling flow in the device can prevent transducer overheating and protect the uterine endometrium. Catheter material properties had a moderate influence on thermal penetration but not so great an effect as uterine blood perfusion. Figure 2 illustrates the influence of catheter material and uterine blood perfusion on heating performance (7 MHz transducer). Increasing the maximum temperature from 45°C to 47°C would extend thermal penetration even further than demonstrated.

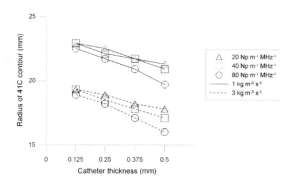

FIGURE 2. The effects of catheter thickness, attenuation, and uterine blood perfusion on thermal penetration as assessed by the radial extension of the 41°C contour (h = 1000 W m^{-2} °C^{-1})

Applicators were constructed according to input from biothermal simulations. The devices have 1 – 3 tubular radiators of 10 – 15 mm for a heating length of 15 to 35 mm. The 3.5 mm diameter transducers operate at 6.5 – 8 MHz and are unsectored, bisectored, or trisectored with sector angles of 135°-135°-90°. PET catheters with 0.20 mm wall were tipped and bent to 30° to mimic the intrauterine brachytherapy tandem. Annular cooling flow protects the transducers and catheter from overheating.

Rotational acoustic intensity plots were used to assess acoustic dead zones and variations in output radially and along the device length. Dead zones were 20 - 30° at the sector cuts and several mm between transducers. Higher intensity regions were typically seen at the ends of the transducers and slightly removed from the center of the sectors. The 90° sector had more uniform output than the larger sectors.

Heating trials with benchtop thermometry demonstrated thermal patterns that closely follow the rotational acoustic intensity plots. Figure 3 shows an acoustic intensity plot next to a temperature map during *ex vivo* heating with the same device. Temperature drops at the sector breaks that could be utilized for thermal protection of sensitive structures were prominent. Temperature elevation within sectors was fairly uniform with some slight dips at low intensity zones. Thermal smearing will likely mitigate these dips in longer treatments.

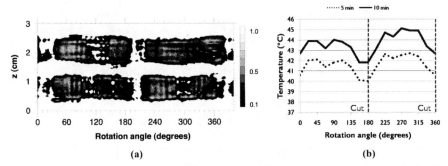

FIGURE 3. The rotational acoustic intensity plot (a) of a bisectored applicator shows acoustic dead zones between sectors and between transducers as well as low intensity zones within the transducers. The thermal map (b) after 10 minutes of heating in *ex vivo* porcine tissue (~3W/sector) correlates with the acoustic output from the device.

MR thermal imaging was feasible and produced more detailed maps of heating. Most devices produce artifacts <1 mm at 3T. Real-time MR temperature monitoring was used to control power to individual sectors and transducers. Figure 4 shows a thermal map taken during heating of *ex vivo* tissue demonstrating control over the temperature profile in the coronal plane.

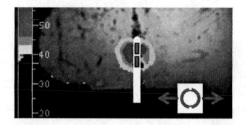

FIGURE 4. MR thermal image from a coronal slice during *ex vivo* heating demonstrates power control along the device length and to individual sectors. Transducers are oriented in the axial plane as shown.

SUMMARY

An endocavitary ultrasound hyperthermia applicator was developed using theory and experiment. Devices were built with non-sectored, bi-sectored, or tri-sectored tubular radiators housed in a water-cooled catheter. The applicator demonstrated feasibility to heat clinical tumor volumes with >2 cm lateral penetration of 41°C at low maximum temperature. Dead zones in acoustic output at sector cuts correspond to reduced heating, which can be used for thermal protection of the rectum and bladder. The applicator produces little MR artifact and real-time MR thermal monitoring was used to demonstrate power control radially and along the length of the device. The ultimate heating performance of the ultrasound applicator will depend on cooling flow, catheter material and, more importantly, the tissue perfusion.

ACKNOWLEDGEMENTS

The authors would like to acknowledge the support of NIH R01CA122276.

REFERENCES

1. D. M. Parkin, F. Bray, J. Ferlay, P. Pisani, Global Cancer Statistics, 2002, *CA. Cancer J. Clin.* **55(2)**, 74-108 (2005).
2. M. Quinn, J. Benedet, F. Odicino, P. Maisonneuve, U. Beller, W. Creasman, et al., Carcinoma of the Cervix Uteri. FIGO 6th Annual Report on the Results of Treatment in Gynecological Cancer., *Int. J. Gynecol. Obstet.* **95(Supplement 1)**, S43-S103 (2006).
3. M. Franckena, L. J. A. Stalpers, P. C. M. Koper, R. G. J. Wiggenraad, W. J. Hoogenraad, J. D. P. van Dijk, et al., Long-Term Improvement in Treatment Outcome After Radiotherapy and Hyperthermia in Locoregionally Advanced Cervix Cancer: An Update of the Dutch Deep Hyperthermia Trial, *Int. J. Radiat. Oncol. Biol. Phys.* **70(4)**, 1176-1182 (2008).
4. P. Wust, B. Hildebrandt, G. Sreenivasa, H. Riess, et al., Hyperthermia in combined treatment of cancer, *Lancet Oncol.* **3(8)**, 487-97 (2002).
5. G. Sreenivasa, J. Gellermann, B. Rau, J. Nadobny, P. Schlag, P. Deuflhard, et al., Clinical use of the hyperthermia treatment planning system HyperPlan to predict effectiveness and toxicity, *Int. J. Radiat. Oncol. Biol. Phys.* **55(2)**, 407-19 (2003).

Functional Neurosurgery in the Human Thalamus by Transcranial Magnetic Resonance Guided Focused Ultrasound

Beat Werner[a], Anne Morel[b], Daniel Jeanmonod[b] and Ernst Martin[a]

[a] *MR-Center, University Children's Hospital Zurich, Switzerland*
[b] *Laboratory for Functional Neurosurgery, Neurosurgical Department, University Hospital Zurich, Switzerland*

Abstract. Potential applications of Transcranial Magnetic Resonance guided Focused Ultrasound (TcMRgFUS) include treatment of functional brain disorders, such as Parkinson's disease, dystonia and tremor, neurogenic pain and tinnitus, neuropsychiatric disorders and epilepsy. In this study we demonstrate the feasibility of non-invasive TcMRgFUS ablation of clinically well established targets in the human thalamus that are currently accessed stereotactically by interventional strategies based on the concept of the thalamocortical dysrhythmia (TCD). Thermal hotspots suitable for clinical intervention were created successfully in anatomical preparations of human ex-vivo heads under pseudo clinical conditions. The hotspots could be positioned at the target locations as needed and local energy deposition was sufficient to create tissue ablation. Numerical simulations based on these experimental data predict that the acoustic energy needed to create ablative lesions in-vivo will be within limits that can safely applied.

Keywords: HIFU, Brain, Functional Neurosurgery, Non-invasive, Transcranial.
PACS: 43.35.Wa.

INTRODUCTION

Non-invasive brain surgery by Transcranial Magnetic Resonance guided Focused Ultrasound (TcMRgFUS) could not be realized until recently due to inherent physical constrains and technical complexities [1]. TcMRgFUS surgery offers precise treatment of deep seated brain tumors and functional brain disorders without the risks and side effects of classical operation techniques such as collateral damage to brain structures, e.g. the risk of bleeding or post surgical infections while accessing the operation field. In our research project we are developing non-invasive TcMRgFUS surgical processes on the basis of a set of well established minimally-invasive stereotactic neurosurgical procedures for the treatment of chronic and therapy-resistant functional brain disorders that share the thalamocortical dysrhythmia (TCD) as an underlying basic physiologic mechanism. These selective and regulatory procedures are the medial thalamotomy,

CP1113, *8th International Symposium on Therapeutic Ultrasound*, edited by E. S. Ebbini
© 2009 American Institute of Physics 978-0-7354-0650-6/09/$25.00

the pallidothalamic and cerebellothalamic tractotomies and the anteromedial pallidotomy [2].

The clinical feasibility of non-invasive tumor surgery in the brain by transcranial focused ultrasound has been demonstrated previously [1, 3]. The aim of this study was to demonstrate the feasibility of creating thermal hotspots in the human thalamus suitable for functional neurosurgery by applying high intensity focused ultrasound to anatomical preparations of human ex-vivo heads. Specifically, based on the geometric properties of the stereotactic targets for our envisioned application, we demonstrated under pseudo-clinical conditions the ability to efficiently and precisely create tissue ablating hotspots of ca. 5mm in diameter at the location of the thalamic nuclei to be targeted later in-vivo.

Material & Methods

Fresh human ex-vivo heads were fixated in 20% alcohol for 3-4 months. In order to avoid experimental artifacts from trapped air in brain tissue and intracranial cavities [4] the skull calvaria was temporarily removed to allow for opening the ventricles towards the cortex and cleaning the subarachnoidal spaces from all tissue, vessels and membranes. Skull calvaria and skin were then put back in place to give a specimen that, for the purpose of these experiments, represented an intact human head.

The anatomically prepared heads were mounted on a frame similar to the stereotactic frame to be used in the clinical application and positioned appropriately in the hemispheric ultrasound transducer.

All sonications were done with the InSightec (InSightec Ltd, Haifa, Israel) ExAblate 4000 system (hemispheric 1024-element phased-array transducer, 660kHz, 2000W,) integrated with a 3.0T GE Signa HDx MR-scanner (GE Healthcare, Milwaukee, USA). The head preparations were sonicated repeatedly at various intensities in the three stereotactic targets to be applied in the envisioned clinical intervention: centro-lateral nucleus, pallido-thalamic tract and antero-medial pallidum.

The stereotactic targets were localized on T1-weighted MR-images using the multi-architectonic Morel atlas of the human thalamus and basal ganglia [5] and graphically prescribed for sonication in the planning software of the FUS system.

Precision and biological effects of the sonications were assessed by proton resonance frequency (PRF) shift MR-thermometry, the Dewey-Sapareto thermal dose model (both implemented in the FUS system) and numerical simulations using a commercial FDTD thermal solver (SEMCAD X, ITIS foundation / speag, Zurich, Switzerland).

Results

All stereotactic targets could be reached without repositioning the stereotactic frame. The hot-spots were reproducibly located precisely (1mm) at the targeted position. They were sharply delineated with a steep temperature gradient towards the border and their size matched the size of the targets (5mm).

The FUS system was able to drive peak temperature elevations at the target of more than 45°C, which exceeds clinical requirements by far.

Numerical simulations based on the driving power/temperature gain measurements yielded a power estimate of 450W for the clinical ablation protocol to be used in-vivo. This complies well with experimentally established safety margins [6].

No histological verification of the ablations in the thalamic brain tissue of the ex-vivo human preparations could be achieved. This was attributed to the fact that the tissue was already thoroughly fixated when heated by the focused ultrasound sonications.

Conclusions

This study successfully demonstrated the feasibility and high precision of non-invasive functional neurosurgery in the human thalamus and subthalamic area by TcMRgFUS under pseudo-clinical conditions. Based on the results of this study, a clinical phase I trial for central lateral thalamotomy in patients with chronic, therapy-resistant neurogenic pain has been initiated.

ACKNOWLEDGMENTS

This work was supported by Swiss National Science Foundation, National Centre of Competence in Research Co-Me, University Children's Hospital Zurich, University Zurich and Swiss Federal Institute of Technology Zurich.

REFERENCES

1. F. A. Jolesz, N. McDannold, *J. Magn. Reson. Imaging* **27**, 391-399 (2008).
2. D. Jeanmonod, M. Magnin, A. Morel, M. Siegemund, A. Cancro, M. Lanz, R. Llinás, U. Ribary, E. Kronberg, J. Schulman and M. Zonenshayn, *Thalamus & Related Systems* **1**, 245–254 (2001).
3. K. Hynynen, GT. Clement, N. McDannold, *Magn. Reson. Med.* **52**, 100-107 (2004).
4. B. Werner, T. Loenneker, D. Jeanmonod, E. Martin, *Proceedings ISTU 2007*.
5. A. Morel, "Stereotactic Atlas of the Human Thalamus and Basal Ganglia", ISBN 978-0824728946, Informa Healthcare (2007).
6. InSightec Ltd. (private communication).

ULTRASOUND-ENHANCED GENE AND DRUG DELIVERY

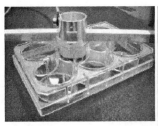
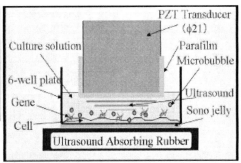

Ultrasound	Frequency	2.1 MHz
	Wave profile	Burst 40/360 (on/off)
	Exposure time (s)	10, 20, 30, 50, 100, 200
	Intensity (W/cm^2)	1.3, 5.4, 12.0, 16.3, 20.8, 26.3
Microbubbles	Levovist$^®$	10% (v/v) (void fraction, 8×10^{-5})
	Sonazoid$^®$	0–30% (v/v) (void fraction, 0-24×10^{-4})
Cell	Fibroblast cells	NIH3T3
Gene	GFP plasmid	15 µg/ml

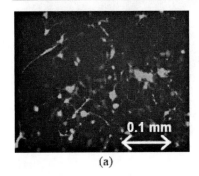
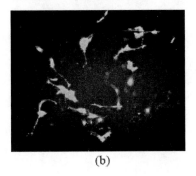

(a)   (b)

Therapeutic Ultrasound Enhancement of Drug Delivery to Soft Tissues

George Lewis Jr[a], Peng Wang[b], George Lewis Sr.[c], William Olbricht[a,b]

[a]Department of Biomedical Engineering, and [b]School of Chemical and Biomolecular Engineering
Cornel University, Ithaca, NY 14850
[c]Transducer Engineering, Inc. P.O. Box 4034, Andover, MA 01810

Abstract. *Effects of exposure to 1.58MHz focused ultrasound on transport of Evans Blue Dye (EBD) in soft tissues are investigated when an external pressure gradient is applied to induce convective flow through the tissue. The magnitude of the external pressure gradient is chosen to simulate conditions in brain parenchyma during convection-enhanced drug delivery (CED) to the brain. EBD uptake and transport are measured in equine brain, avian muscle and agarose brain-mimicking phantoms. Results show that ultrasound enhances EBD uptake and transport, and the greatest enhancement occurs when the external pressure gradient is applied. The results suggest that exposure of the brain parenchyma to ultrasound could enhance penetration of material infused into the brain during CED therapy.*

Keywords: Therapeutic ultrasound, Drug delivery, Acoustic targeted drug delivery, Convection enhanced delivery
PACS: 43.80.Gx, 43.80.Sh, 43.80.Vj

INTRODUCTION

Over the last decade, a driving factor in pharmaceutical development and drug delivery has been the ability to target disease at the cellular and tissue levels. Local delivery of therapeutics often allows higher doses to be delivered without side effects that restrict dose levels in systemic delivery. Local delivery can be combined with controlled release to provide sustained high concentrations of drug in the immediate vicinity of affected tissue [1-3]. Local delivery is especially important in treating brain disorders, because most therapeutics administered intravenously do not cross the blood-brain barrier. Recent developments in treating brain gliomas, which are infiltrative tumors that present poor prognosis for patients, rely on local delivery methods. After resection of the tumor, malignant cells that have migrated from the tumor remain behind, surrounded otherwise by healthy tissue. These cells continue to grow, leading to the recurrence of the disease. CED is a local delivery technique in which therapeutics are infused directly into the brain interstitium through an implanted needle microcatheter [4, 5]. The infusion induces a convective flow of infusate through the interstitium. The infused drugs are subject to elimination via a variety of mechanisms. Therefore, the challenge in CED is to enhance penetration of infused therapeutics so that they reach migrating malignant cells before they are eliminated. Some of the most promising drugs for treating gliomas are large proteins and drugs packaged in nanoparticles, which, owing to their size, are especially difficult to move

CP1113, *8th International Symposium on Therapeutic Ultrasound,* edited by E. S. Ebbini
© 2009 American Institute of Physics 978-0-7354-0650-6/09/$25.00

through brain interstitium under the convective force of the infusion. Therefore, any method to enhance transport of infused drugs could benefit the outcome of the therapy.

The use of ultrasound to enhance drug delivery has evolved over several decades. Perhaps the most extensively studied example is the use of ultrasound to enhance transdermal drug delivery [6, 7]. Exposure of skin to ultrasound can increase the permeability of the stratum corneum, allowing transport across skin of some therapeutic compounds that would otherwise be excluded and enhancing transport rates of others. Although a variety of thermal and non-thermal mechanisms could be responsible for transport enhancement, acoustic cavitation and microstreaming [8, 9] may be the most important. At lower acoustic power, oscillations of endogenous microbubbles or microbubbles added to an infusate may induce similar microstreaming, even in the absence of cavitation.

We present results on the enhancement of Evans blue dye (EBD) transport into soft animal tissues using 1.58 MHz low spatial-average ultrasonic powers of 1.3 and 5.25 W in combination with an applied convective flow under conditions that simulate convection-enhanced drug delivery [10, 11].

METHODS

Sample preparation: Neurological-tissue-mimicking phantoms were prepared by filling 12 oz Solo Cups with a solution of 0.6 wt% agarose powder (MP Biomedicals, Solon, OH) [12]. The powder was dissolved in distilled water at 100° C for 5 min and then poured into the cups to a height of 1.5 cm. The cups were covered and allowed to cool and gel (about 20 min). Equine horse brain was harvested from the Cornell School of Veterinary Medicine immediately post-mortem and cut into 3 x 3 x 1.5 cm cortical slices. Experiments were conducted within 30 min of brain harvesting. Avian muscle tissue was purchased from a local supermarket and cut into 3 x 3 x 1.5 cm slices. A 0.25 wt% aqueous solution of Evans blue dye (MP Biomedicals, Solon, OH) was used to mimic a water-soluble drug. The EBD solution provided sufficient contrast to measure its extent of penetration into the phantom and tissue samples [10, 11, 13, 14].

Convection background and setup: In CED, an infusion into the brain establishes a radial flow outward from the needle tip. The average velocity of infusate in the tissue V_c decays as $1/r^2$, where r is the distance from the needle tip. For a volumetric infusion rate of 1 μL·min^{-1}, a typical value in rodent experiments, V_c ranges from 670 to 3.0×10^{-7} m·s^{-1}, from the needle tip to $r = 1.5$ cm [16, 17]. The pressure gradient associated with this flow can be calculated from Darcy's law, provided that the porosity Φ and hydraulic permeability κ of the tissue can be estimated. For brain tissue, avian muscle, and agarose brain phantom estimates are κ_{brain}=5.63 x 10^{-12}, κ_{muscle}=5.00 x 10^{-14}, $\kappa_{agarose}$=2.05 x 10^{-12} and Φ_{brain}=20%, Φ_{muscle}=1.6%, $\Phi_{agarose}$=90% [16-19]. To achieve values of V_c that are similar to those in CED, pressure gradients were applied across the equine brain, avian muscle and brain phantom samples in conjunction with topical application of EBD.

A convection chamber was constructed and used to apply pressure gradients of 1330 kPa·m^{-1} for the brain and phantom samples, and 6650 kPa·m^{-1} for the avian muscle samples. In this system, the average velocity flow due to the applied pressure gradient is unidirectional and constant throughout the sample. The sample was held in place at the bottom of a cylindrical chamber, which was filled with EBD solution to a height of 5 cm. The bottom of the chamber contained a hole that opened into a collection chamber. The tissue sample was placed on a screen that covered the hole. The pressure in the collection chamber was reduced to the appropriate value for each sample by drawing a vacuum (Model 2534B-01, Welch Inc., Niles, IL). The resulting values of V_c were estimated from the applied pressure difference across the sample, including the hydrostatic pressure from the liquid above the sample. For the specimens in this study we estimated V_c as 3.75×10^{-5}, 2.02×10^{-5} and 2.98×10^{-6} m·s^{-1} for the brain, muscle and phantom samples respectively.

Ultrasound setup and dosing: Ultrasound (US) energy was generated by a lead zirconate titanate (PZT-4), 1.58 MHz, 25.4 mm diameter piezoelectric ceramic with radius of curvature corresponding to 40 mm (EBL Products Inc., Hartford, CT). The transducer was driven at 1.58 MHz. US was applied at 100% duty cycle at the spatial-average power of 1.30 and 5.25 W in the sample's geometric center for durations of 1 to 4 min. The transducer was positioned with its focus at the sample-dye interface. To increase the sonicated volume of tissue, the transducer was translated periodically over a distance of 30 mm perpendicular to the sample's surface at 0.25 Hz. The transducer was driven by a custom-built portable system and calibrated using a force balance technique in which we measured the force that the ultrasound exerted on an acoustic absorbing object [20]. The temperatures of the sonicated samples were recorded with a calibrated thermocouple placed 1.5 cm from the focus (Model 52II, Fluke Inc. Everett, WA).

Data analysis: The experiment was run for the three tissue samples for 1, 2, 3 and 4 min with and without the applied pressure gradient and with and without exposure to ultrasound. For data analysis a 3 mm slice was taken from the geometric center of each sample. The intensity profile was measured as in our previous studies [10,11]. Area under the curve was calculated to quantify the amount of EBD uptake in each case.

RESULTS

The distance of EBD penetration into all samples increased in the following order: 1. No CED and no US, 2. CED and no US, 3. No CED and 1.3 W US, 4. No CED and 5.25 W US, 5. CED and 1.3 W US, 6. CED and 5.25 W US.

Ultrasound exposure led to increases in the sample temperature tabulated in table 1. For equine brain and brain phantom, temperature changes were similar among the samples. Temperature increases for avian muscle tissue were slightly larger. No tissue damage or changes in tissue morphology were observed in any sample.

Figures 1 and 2 show the EBD intensity as a function of distance into the sample for avian tissue after 4 min, brain tissue after 2 min and brain phantom after 1 min. The red curve shows the profile with no applied pressure gradient and no ultrasound; in this case EBD transport is purely diffusive. The green curve shows the profile with an applied pressure gradient but no ultrasound, which simulates CED. The blue curve shows the profile for tissue exposed to ultrasound with no applied pressure gradient.

The yellow curve shows the profile for tissue exposed to ultrasound with an applied pressure gradient, which simulates an ultrasound-enhanced CED. For both power levels the combined effect of ultrasound and an applied pressure gradient gave greatest EBD uptake in all tissues.

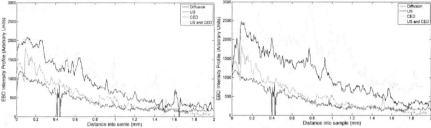

FIGURE 1. EBD profile of avian muscle tissue after sonication at 1.3 W (left) and 5.25 W (right) for 4 min. US combined with CED provided greatest EBD uptake enhancement of 240% (left) and 390% (right) as compared with diffusion alone.

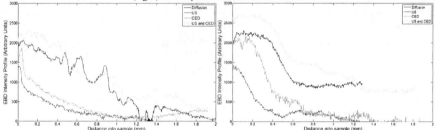

FIGURE 2. EBD profile of equine brain tissue (left) and brain-mimicking phantom (right) after 5.25 W sonication for 2 and 1 min, respectively. US combined with CED provided greatest EBD uptake enhancement of 560% (left) and 880% (right) compared with diffusion alone.

Figure 3 is a compilation of sectional EBD profile images used to produce figures 1 and 2. Moving from left to right across the columns in the image shows the enhancement of EBD penetration into the three samples.

As in our previous studies [10, 11], the EBD intensities at the tissue/dye interface (x=0 mm) are not identical in the four cases in each figure. This suggests the presence of a mass transfer resistance at the surface of the samples. Apparently, the application of ultrasound at 1.3 and 5.25 W decreases this mass transfer resistance at the interface and increases uptake into the sample.

TABLE 1. Percent enhancement of EBD uptake into tissue samples as compared with diffusion alone. The corresponding temperature changes in the samples during US application is also shown.

Sample and US Power	CED	US	CED and US	Temperature Change
Avian Muscle 1.3 W	130%	220%	240%	4 °C
Avian Muscle 5.25 W	130%	260%	390%	7 °C
Equine Brain 5.25 W	185%	450%	560%	1 °C
Brain Phantom 5.25 W	310%	590%	880%	2 °C

The shapes of the concentration profiles in figures 1 and 2 for cases with ultrasound suggest that ultrasound provides a mass transfer mechanism in addition to diffusion. The nearly flat profiles the EBD/sample interface (x=0) suggest a convection-dominated regime in this region. Further into the samples, the steeper concentration gradients that are found are consistent with mass transfer dominated by diffusion.

Temperature rise in the tissue samples from the absorption of ultrasound is a possible source of diffusion enhancement. According to the Stokes-Einstein relation, the diffusivity is directly proportional to temperature and inversely proportional to solvent viscosity. For a 4 and 7 °C increase in temperature, the diffusivity would increase by 11% and 16%, respectively, which is insufficient to explain the observed increases in EBD uptake, suggesting that enhanced diffusion due to tissue heating is not the dominant mechanism for enhanced EBD uptake.

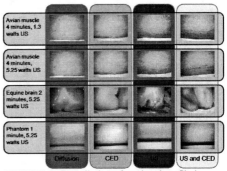

FIGURE 3. Compilation of sectional profile images to produce EBD profile curves in figures 1 and 2.

CONCLUSION

We studied effects of therapeutic 1.58 MHz focused ultrasound at 1.3 and 5.25 W spatial-average power levels in combination with convective flow on the uptake of Evans blue dye into avian muscle, equine brain and neurological-tissue-mimicking phantoms. Ultrasonic power levels were applied below tissue damage thresholds. Convection velocities were in the range of typical CED infusions in rodent brain. The study showed synergistic effects when ultrasound was combined with CED in all samples at both power levels. The results suggest that CED in combination with ultrasound may enhance the penetration of therapeutics in the brain and increase the concentration of infused drugs over the penetration distance, which may improve the outcome of CED therapy.

REFERENCES

1. C. Gueri et al., *Investigational New drugs*, **22**, 27-37 (2004).
2. J. Panyam and V. Labhasetwar, *Adv. Drug Del. Rev.,* **55**, 329-347 (2003).
3. M. Westphal et al., *Neuro-Oncology*, **5**, 79-88 (2003).
4. R. Bobo et al., *Proc. Nati. Acad. Sci.*, **91**, 2076-2080 (1994).
5. M. Vogelbaum, *J. of Neuro-Oncology*, **83**, 97-109 (2007).
6. S. Mitragotri, *Drug Discov Today*, **9**, 735-736 (2004).
7. I. Lavon and J. Kost, *Drug Discov. Today*, **9**, 670-676 (2004).
8. H. Guzman, D. Nguyen, A. McNamara, M. Prausnitz, *J. Pharm. Sci.*, **91**, 1693–1701 (2002).
9. K. Keyhani et al., *Pharm. Res.*, **18**, 1514–1520 (2001).
10. G. Lewis and W. Olbricht, *Proc. IEEE LISA 2007*, 67-70 (2007).
11. G. Lewis, W. Olbricht and G. Lewis Sr., *J. Acoust. Soc. Am.*, **122**, 3007 (2007).
12. Z. Chen et al., *J. Neurosurg.,* **101**, 314-322 (2004)
13. J. Woitzik and L. Schilling, *J Neurosurg.*, **106** ,872-880 (2007).
14 T Aoki, T Sumii, and et. al., *Journal of Stroke.* **33**, 2711 (2002).
15. P. Chan, R Fishman, J Caronna, and et.al., *Ann. Neurol.*, **13**, 625-32 (2006).
16. K. Neeves et al., *J. Controlled Release,* **111**, 252–262 (2006).
17. K. Neeves et al., *Brain* Research, **1180**, 121–132 (2007).
18. A. Datta, *Int. J. Food Properties*, **9**, 767–780 (2006).
19. F. Deumier, G. Trystram, A. Collignan and L. Guedider. *J. of Food Eng.*, **58**, 85–93 (2003).
20. S. Maruvada, G. R. Harris, and B. Herman , *J. Acoust. Soc. of Am.*, **121**, 1434-1439 (2007).

Qualitative and Quantitative Analysis of Molecular Delivery Through the Ultrasound-Induced Blood-Brain Barrier Opening in Mice

Shougang Wang[a], Babak Baseri[b], James J. Choi[b], Yao-Sheng Tung[b], Barclay Morrison[b], and Elisa E. Konofagou[a,b]

[a]Department of Radiology, Columbia University, New York, NY
[b]Department of Biomedical Engineering, Columbia University, New York, NY

Abstract. Recent studies have proven that focused ultrasound (FUS) in the presence of microbubbles can deliver large molecules across the blood-brain barrier (BBB) locally, transiently and non-invasively. In this study, the cellular effects, the size estimation of the opening and the amount delivered were inferred through qualitative and quantitative analysis of molecular delivery to the brain parenchyma in a murine model. The ultimate purpose was to build the foundation for future ultrasound-facilitated neurodegenerative disease treatment in humans. A bolus of microbubbles at 1 μl/g body weight concentration was intravenously injected. Pulsed FUS was applied to the left hippocampus through the intact skin and skull followed by intravenously administration of fluorescence-conjugated dextran at 3 kDa, 10 kDa and 70 kDa. The brain were either sectioned for fluorescence imaging or homogenized for quantitative analysis. The concentration of 3 kDa, 10 kDa and 70 kDa dextrans delivered to the left brain hemisphere was quantified to be 7.9±4.9 μg/g, 2.4±1.3 μg/g and 0.9±0.47μg/g of brain weight. Smooth muscle cells engulfing the arterioles exhibited higher fluorescence in the case of 70 kDa dextran, compared to the 3 kDa dextran, demonstrating that fluorescence imaging can help with the understanding of the type of mechanism of molecular uptake by different brain cells.

Keywords: blood brain barrier opening, dextran, fluorescence imaging, microbubble, ultrasound.
PACS: 87.50.Y−

INTRODUCTION

Drug delivery to the central nervous system is very difficult due to the blood brain barrier (BBB) [1]. The BBB is a specialized impermeability barrier of the cerebral capillaries that consists of endothelial cells, tight junction, basal lamina, pericytes and glial processes [2]. It selectively transfers some molecules between the blood and the brain parenchyma, protects the brain from harmful compounds and regulates its microenvironment [3]. On the other hand, this feature also limits the effectiveness of pharmacological agents by preventing their delivery to the brain region that needs treatment.

Recent studies have proven that focused ultrasound (FUS) in the presence of microbubbles can enable the delivery of large molecules across the blood-brain barrier (BBB) locally, transiently and non-invasively [5-7]. The feasibility of BBB opening in normal and transgenic AD mice monitored by MRI was also demonstrated [8]. In this technique, ultrasound was focused onto the brain region of interest at the presence of

CP1113, 8th International Symposium on Therapeutic Ultrasound, edited by E. S. Ebbini
© 2009 American Institute of Physics 978-0-7354-0650-6/09/$25.00

gas-filled microbubbles in the bloodstream. Upon sonication, either "inertial" or "non-inertial" cavitation was initiated, which caused the increased permeability of the BBB. This effect was demonstrated in rodents such as rabbits [9] and mice [10-11]. In this paper, the spatial distribution, the total amount of drugs delivered the cellular impact, and the physical size of the FUS-induced BBB opening was studied. with dextran at three molecular weights (3, 10, and 70 kDa) to qualitatively and quantitatively analyze the drug delivery efficiency of this technique and provide useful information for the future treatment of neurodegenerative diseases. In particular, the murine hippocampus was selected as our localized drug delivery target, because it is a subcortical structure that is most severely affected by Alzheimer's disease.

MATERIALS AND METHODS

All mice experiments were carried out in accordance with the Columbia University Institutional Animal Care and Use Committee guidelines and regulations. The anesthetized wild-type C57BL/6 mice were placed prone with its head immobilized by a stereotaxic apparatus. A single-element spherical segment FUS transducer was confocally aligned with a diagnostic transducer for sonication and imaging purposes. Ultrasound contrast agents (Definity®, Lantheus Medical Imaging, Inc, Billerica, MA) with a 1:20 dilution was injected into the tail vein at 1 μl/g body weight approximately 1 minutes prior to sonication. Pulsed FUS (pulse rate: 10 Hz, pulse duration: 20 ms, duty cycle: 20%) was then applied at a peak-negative pressure of 753 kPa in a series of two 30s sonication on the targeted hippocampus [6,7].

Fluorescent dextrans (Molecular Probes, Inc., Eugene, OR, USA), were prepared at at 20 mg/ml for Texas Red®-tagged of 3 kDa and 10 kDa and Alexa Fluor 647®-tagged of 10 kDa in phosphate buffered saline (PBS, 138 mM sodium chloride, 10 mM phosphate, pH 7.4) solution. Texas Red®-tagged of 70 kDa was prepared at 46.7 mg/ml to keep the mole concentration constant. The diameters of those dextrans were measured through a Nano-ZS zetasizer (Malvern Instruments, Ltd., Malvern, Worcestershire, UK). In this case, biotinylated rather than fluorescent-conjugated dextrans were used due to the less photon interference. Images were acquired using an inverted light and fluorescence microscope (IX-81; Olympus, Melville, NY, USA) with a filter set at excitation (ex.) 568±24 nm and emission (em.) 610±40 nm for Texas Red setting. For two color imaging, fluorescent tags were carefully selected so that the two dextrans were separable under different different filter set. A confocal fluorescence microscope (LSM 510 Meta, Carl Zeiss Inc., Thornwood, NY) was used with filters set at Texas Red and Cy5 (ex: 654±24nm, em:710±60nm). Fluorescence of Alex Fluor 647 was pseudo-colored in green for best contrast with Texas Red. All mice were perfused transcardially 20-min after the administration of dextrans according to the previously developed protocol [11]. Brain tissues were frozen sectioned into 300 μm slices in a horizontal orientation using a cryostat at -19 °C. It should be noted that for the dextran dose study, the mice were perfused with 60 ml PBS only. In a separate study, instead of sectioning, the brain was cut in half and homogenized. After centrifugation, the extracted dextrans were measured using a fluorometer (SpectraMAX M2, Molecular Devices, Sunnyvale, CA USA). The dextran diffusion was quantified using linear regression from seven separate administations of a priori known concentrations for each dextran size.

RESULTS AND DISCUSSION

The purpose of this study was to determine the drug load and distribution with respect to the drug's molecular weights in order to help elucidate the FUS-induced BBB opening's relevance for the treatment of neurodegenerative diseases. The deposition dose into the targeted hemisphere was 7.9±4.9 µg/g (n=5), 2.4±1.3 µg/g (m=4) and 0.9±0.45 µg/g (p=5) for the 3, 10 and 70 kDa dextrans, respectively (Table 1). The size distribution of the dextrans are also shown in Table 1. Dextrans with smaller molecular weight typically have smaller diameter, and,showed a greater dose into the targeted brain parenchyma through their largest diffusion area.

TABLE 1. The dosage of fluorescent dextrans at different molecular weights delivered to the mouse brain using ultrasound-induced blood-brain barrier opening.

# of mice	Dextran molecular weight (Da)[*]	Dextran in brain (µg/g brain weight)	Size (nm)
n=5	3,000	7.9±4.9	2.33±0.38
m=4	10,000	2.4±1.3	3.76±0.89
p=5	70,000	0.9±0.45	10.2±1.4

[*]All dextrans were Texas-Red® conjugated.

A separate set of experiments was performed to study the distribution of dextrans to the brain after BBB opening. Fluorescence images of 300-µm thick horizontal sections of the brain with a filter set for Texas Red (ex: 568±24 nm, em: 610±40 nm) are depicted in Fig. 1. The images show the left (targeted; (a), (c), and (e)) hippocampus and the right (control; (b), (d), (f)) hippocampus at molecular weights of 3, 10 and 70 kDa, respectively. The sonicated hippocampus showed significantly higher fluorescence compared to the control indicating successful trans-BBB delivery of dextrans. Smaller dextrans (i.e., 3 kDa in Fig. 1 (a)) showed more diffuse and larger areas of fluorescence that were more homogeneously distributed compared to those of the larger dextrans (i.e., 70 kDa in Fig. 1 (e)). At each molecular weight tested, fluorescence was observed along the major vessels throughout the hippocampus (Fig. 1(a), (c), and (e)). This may be attributed to the fact that those vessels have the largest microbubble concentration and, therefore, the most significant effect of ultrasound-microbubble interactions. There is a dense network of arterioles, capillaries and venules in the hippocampus. The fluorescence area in Fig. 1 (a),(c),(e) may thus be a combination of dextran leakage from adjacent BBB openings or diffusion from remote opening sites.

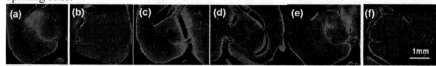

FIGURE 1. Horizontal fluorescence images of the mouse hippocampi. The (a, c, e) left hippocampus was sonicated while the (b, d, f) right hippocampus acted as the control. Following FUS-induced BBB opening, the mice were injected with Texas-Red® conjugated dextrans at distinct molecular weights: (a, b) 3 kDa, (c, d) 10 kDa, and (e, f) 70 kDa.

Figure 2 shows a series of magnified fluorescence images of 70 kDa dextran after BBB opening. The image of a complete horizontal section (Fig. 2(a)) depicts localized delivery of the dextran to the targeted left hippocampus. Figure 2(b) is the magnified region of interest (ROI) of the yellow box in Fig. 3(a). Figure 2(c) is the magnified ROI in the yellow box in Fig. 2(b). A structure with high fluorescence intensity around the vessel (pointed by white arrow) was shown in Fig. 2 (c). This structure is most similar to the smooth muscle cell (SMC) that sustains the vessel pressure [12]. Therefore, the endothelial and smooth muscle cells may both be affected by the ultrasound-microbubble interaction. However, SMC appear to have a stronger tendency to uptake the 70 kDa dextran by containing the 70 kDa diffusion.

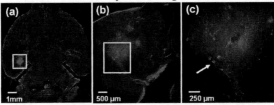

FIGURE 2. Horizontal luorescence images of the mouse brain. The left hippocampus was sonicated followed by intravenous injection of 70 kDa Texas-Red®-conjugated dextran. (a) Entire brain slice fluoresce image under 20X magnification, (b) Magnified region of the ROI (yellow box) in (a) under 40X magnification, (c) Magnified region of the ROI (yellow box) in (b) under 100X magnification. The white arrow indicates the localized high intensity region (a structure similar to smooth muscle cell).

To further study the distribution of dextran, and to minimize the effects of experimental variabilities, two dextrans at distinct molecular weights were simultaneously administered (i.e., 3 kDa and 10 kDa; 10 kDa and 70 kDa). Figure 3 (a) shows the fluorescence images of simultaneous injection of 3 kDa Texas-Red conjugated + 10 kDa Alex Fluor 647 conjugated dextran (mouse 1). Figure 5(b) shows the fluorescence images of 10 kDa Alex Fluor 647 conjugated dextran in combination with 70 kDa Texas-Red conjugated dextran (mouse 2). The images were obtained in a similar region within the sonicated left hippocampus with filter sets at TR and CY5. 3 kDa dextran showed consistently larger diffused area and distributed more evenly than the 10 kDa dextran in Fig. 3(a). Numerous focal fluorescent concentrations were observed along the vessel wall both in Fig. 3(a) and (b) for 10 kDa dextran (shown in bright green). Smooth muscle cell like structures were observed again in Fig. 3(b) (shown in red) at 70 kDa dextran.

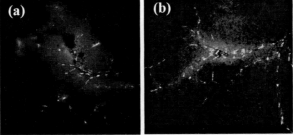

FIGURE 3. Confocal fluorescence imaging of the targeted hippocampus. (a) Fluorescence image with t dextrans at 3 kDa (Taxes-Red conjugated) and 10 kDa (Alex Fluor 647 conjugated), mouse 1. (b) Fluorescence image with dextrans at 10 kDa (Alex Fluor 647 conjugated) and 70 kDa (Texas-Red conjugated), mouse #2. Alex Fluor 647 was color coded with green for best contrast from Texas Red.

411

CONCLUSIONS

Localized ultrasound-induced BBB opening permits the delivery of dextran molecules selectively and non-invasively into the murine brain with molecular weights from 3 kDa to 70 kDa and physical sizes up to 10.2 nm. Large molecular weight dextrans (i.e., 70 kDa) exhibited a lower delivery dose and a smaller area of distribution compare to smaller dextrans (i.e., 3 kDa, 10 kDa). Smooth muscle cells seemed to have a more significant uptake of large dextrans, which may prevent larger molecules to diffuse further into the brain tissue. This study used dextrans as a model drug; however, the delivery dose and distribution of other molecules may be distinct from those of dextran.

ACKNOWLEDGMENTS

This study was supported in part by NSF CAREER 0644713, NIH R21 EY018505 and the Kinetic Foundation. We greatly appreciate Dr. Gordana Vunjak-Novakovic, Dr. Michael L. Shelanski, Dr. Karen Duff and Dr. Scott A. Small for their support. We also thank the Riverside Research Institute for providing the transducers. We appreciate Li Liu, Sujan Doshi and Abhiraj Modi, Jennifer Hui, Eugenia Kwon, Kristen Kim, Matt Herman, Melissa Simon of the Ultrasound and Elasticity Imaging Laboratory for their help.

REFERENCES

1. W.M. Pardridge, *Pharmaceutical research* **24**, 1733-1744(2007).
2. L. L. Rubin and J. M. Staddon, *Annu. Rev.Neurosci.,* **22**, 11-28(1999)
3. R. Ceccelli, V. Berezowski, S. Lundquist, M. Culot, M. Reftel, M.-P. Dehouck and L. Fenart, *Nature*, **6**, 650 (2007)
4. D. W. Laske, R. J. Youle, and E. H. Oldfield, *Nature, Medicine,* **3**, 1362-1368(1997)
5. K. Hynynen, N. McDannold, N. Vykhodtseva, and F.A. Jolesz, *Radiology*, **220**, 640-646(2001).
6. J. J. Choi, M. Pernot, S. Small, and E. E. Konofagou, *Ultrasound Med. Bio.*, **33**, 95-104(2007)
7. J. J. Choi, M. Pernot, T. Brown, S. Small and E. E. Konofagou *Phys. Med. Bio.*, **52**, 5509-5530 (2007)
8. J. J. Choi, S. Wang, S. Small and E. E. Konofagou, Ultrasound Imaging, 2008
9. L.H. Treat, N. McDannold, N. Vykhodtseva, Y. Zhang, K. Tam, and K. Hynynen, *International journal of cancer* **121**, 901-907(2007).
10. J. J. Choi, S. Wang, B. Morrison, and E.E. Konofagou, *IEEE Ultrasonics Symposium,* (2007),
11. S.B. Raymond, J. Skoch, K. Hynynen, and B.J. Bacskai, *J Cereb Blood Flow Metab* **27**, 393-403(2007).
12. S. Ugbes and T. Cban-Ling, *IOVS*, **45**, 2795-2806 (2004)

Sonodynamic Cytotoxicity In Controlled Cavitation Conditions

Jhony El MAALOUF[a,d], Arnaud SALVADOR[b,d], Laurent ALBERTI[c],
Sabrina Chesnais[a], Izella Saletes[a,d], Jean-Christophe Béra[a,d] and Jean-Louis MESTAS[a]

[a]INSERM, U556, Lyon, F-69003, France; Université de Lyon, France
[b]UMR 5180, Lyon; Université de Lyon, France
[c]INSERM, U590, F-69008, France; centre Léon Bérard France; Université Lyon 1, France
[d]Université Lyon 1, Lyon, F-69003, France

Abstract. *Sonodynamic cytotoxicity was always linked to the inertial cavitation phenomenon. In this work, sonodynamic effects with Photofrin® were evaluated in controlled cavitation conditions. Photofrin® potentiated significantly the cavitation cytotoxicity even for low setpoints where no inertial cavitation appeared. Moreover, the use of antioxidant histidine (10 mM) did not prevent the sonodynamic toxicity when inertial cavitation was preponderant. This was confirmed by mass spectrometry data showing no histidine transformation due to reactive oxygen species during sonodynamic experiments. The results show that sonodynamic mechanism would be principally mechanical, facilitated by the Photofrin® insertion in cellular cytoplasmic membranes.*

Keywords: Sonodynamic therapy, cavitation, hematoporphyrin, ultrasound, cavitation regulation, cytotoxicity, histidine, singlet oxygen.
PACS: 87.50.Y-, 43.35.Ei

INTRODUCTION

Different sonodynamic mechanisms were proposed in the literature based on the presence of the inertial ultrasonic cavitation phenomenon [1-5], but the exact mechanism is unknown. This phenomenon is characterized by the generation, motion and collapse of bubbles in medium irradiated with ultrasound. The bubble collapse creates sonoluminescence, local shockwaves and medium sonolysis generating medium derived free radicals. We have previously described the presence of a mechanical sonodynamic effect due to the membrane fragilization of cells by the photosensitizer insertion in cytoplasmic membranes. This study was completed here with a detection of the singlet oxygen generation, which represents the main toxic agent during light irradiation of photosensitizers in photodynamic therapy.

CP1113, 8th International Symposium on Therapeutic Ultrasound, edited by E. S. Ebbini
© 2009 American Institute of Physics 978-0-7354-0650-6/09/$25.00

MATERIALS AND METHODS

Cavitation device

The cavitation device previously described [6] consisted of the association of a flat transducer (LT01 EDAP) coupled with a home made hydrophone (cut-off frequency 10 MHz) submerged in degassed water bath (O_2 rate: 2.3 mg/L). Cells to be isonified were placed in RPMI medium in a 12 wells polystyrene plate (BD Biosciences) above the transducer with or without pretreatment with 20 µg/ml of Photofrin® for 30 minutes (fig 1). Cavitation control was based on a PXI module (National Instruments) composed of a sine wave generator card and an acquisition card which generated the signal to the transducer through an amplifier (Adece, 50 dB) and acquired the bubble activity signal from the hydrophone, respectively. The signal was then transferred to a computer where it was analyzed in the frequency range of 0.1 to 7.1 MHz. The ultrasonic setpoint used in this work, defined as CI, represents the mean of all the acoustic spectrum power density points in log scale.

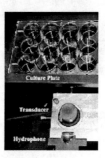

Figure 1. Experimental setup: general design

Mortality quantification

Mortality quantification was performed using the fluorescent Propidium Iodide (PI, Fluka Biochemika) which stained the dead cell DNA. Dead cell quantification was performed next using FACScan flow cytometer (Becton Dickinson).

Liquid chromatography-tandem mass spectrometry

The High Performance Liquid Chromatography (HPLC) device consisted of Agilent 1100 series pump and autosampler. As histidine is a very polar compound, Hydrophilic Interaction Chromatography (HILIC) was preferred. Histidine was chromatographied on a Zorbax SB-CN 3.5 µm (50 x 4.6 mm I.D.) from Agilent, operating at 800 μL/min. A gradient elution was performed using acetonitrile (A) and Water (B) Initial conditions: 5% B and linear increase in B to 90 % within 8 min. All separations were carried out at room temperature (22°C).

The HPLC device was coupled to a Sciex API 300 triple quadrupole mass spectrometer from MDS Sciex equipped with a TurboIonspray Source (TIS) operating in positive ion mode. Instrument control, data analysis and processing were performed using the associated Analyst 1.4.1 software. The mass spectrometer was initially calibrated using polypropylene glycol as standard (Applied Biosystems), setting the resolution, as peak width at half height, in the range 0.7±0.1 amu. The nebulizer (zero air) and the curtain gas flow (nitrogen) were set at 10 arbitrary units. The TIS source was operating at 400 ∘C, with the auxiliary gas flow (zero air) set at 8 L/min. The TIS voltage was set at 5500V. Dwell times were determined in order to define chromatographic peaks with about 30 points. Then, the dwell time was 100 ms. MS parameters were optimised using the autotune feature of the Analyst 1.4.1 software, by infusing histidine. Analysis were performed in single ion monitoring mode (m/z = 156.9). The orifice, ring and entrance voltage were set respectively at 6, 130 and 7.5 volts.

RESULTS AND DISCUSSION

Sonodynamic cytotoxicity was studied in regulated cavitation conditions [6]. A PF induced mortality gain was detected for all CI used. From the gain found, a relative mortality gain was defined showing high values at low CI in the absence of inertial cavitation phenomenon (fig 2). For low CI, the bubble oscillation and the induced microstreaming would be implicated in the sonodynamic mechanism. For high CI, microstreaming persists and other mechanical effects (such as shockwaves due to bubble collapse) could occur enhancing the mechanical effects.

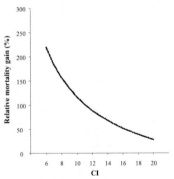

Figure 2. Relative mortality gain with CI [6]

Meanwhile, the bubble collapse induces sonoluminescence probably capable of activating PF and generating singlet oxygen [7] the essential actor in the photodynamic induced cytotoxicity. In order to detect the singlet oxygen generation, the anti-oxydant histidine, capable of reacting with different reactive oxygen species (ROS), notably singlet oxygen, was used. Cells incubated with PF were irradiated either with ultrasound or with light. Results did not show any histidine induced mortality decrease during the ultrasonic irradiations (CI = 14; 1 min), while mortality rates decreased of 49 +/- 7.5 % for the light irradiations (3000 Lux, 1 h). This shows indirectly that singlet oxygen was not involved in the sonodynamic mechanism in our conditions.

To confirm the previous result, the reaction of histidine with singlet oxygen and other ROS was studied. PF was irradiated either with light for 3000 Lux for 1h or with ultrasound for CI = 20 during 4 minutes in the presence of histidine in demineralized water. The quantification of intact histidine was then detected by mass spectrometer. Results showed that histidine concentration, given by the histidine specific spectrometer peak area (Fig 3), did not change with the ultrasonic irradiation while it decreased for 35 % for light irradiation. In accordance with our previous data [6], PF was not activated by ultrasonic cavitation and the sonodynamic mechanism is due to the cell sensibilization by PF insertion in cytoplasmic membranes,. This could be an interesting result for treatment with cavitation, since PF could be substituted with other compounds capable of membrane insertion without having the photosensitizers side effects (such as the prolonged skin sensitivity...).

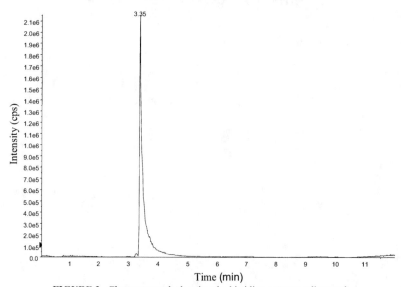

FIGURE 3. Chromatograph showing the histidine corresponding peak

ACKNOWLEDGMENTS

This work was supported by the "Association Française contre les Myopathies" AFM (grant # 9594) and the French national research agency "Agence Nationale de la Recherche" (grant ANR-06-BLAN-0405, Project Cavitherapus). The authors thank Adrien Mathias for his technical help.

REFERENCES

1. N. Yumita, R. Nishigaki, K. Umemura, and S. Umemura, *J. Jpn. Cancer Res.* 81, 304-308 (1990).
2. N. Yumita, K. Sasaki, S. Umemura and R. Nishigaki, *Jpn. J. Cancer Res.* 87, 310-316 (1996).
3. N. Yumita and R. Nishigaki, *Jpn. J. Cancer Res.* 84, 582-588 (1993).
4. K. Umemura, N. Yumita, R. Nishigaki and S. Umemura, *Cancer Lett.* 102, 151-157 (1996).
5. S. Umemura, N. Yumita, K. Umemura, R. Nishigaki, *Cancer Chemother. Pharmacol.* 43, 389-393 (1999).
6. J. El Maalouf, J. C. Béra, L. Alberti, D.Cathignol, J. L. Mestas, Ultrasonics, under press.
7. N. Yumita N, Q. S. Han, S. Umemura, , Anticancer Drugs. 18 (2007): 1149-56.

Characterization and Optimization of Trans-Blood-Brain Barrier Diffusion In Vivo

Elisa E. Konofagou[a,b], James Choi[a], Babak Baseri[a] and Ann Lee[a]

[a]Department of Biomedical Engineering, Columbia University, New York, NY
[b]Department of Radiology, Columbia University, New York, NY

Abstract. Current treatments of neurological and neurodegenerative diseases are limited due to the lack of a truly noninvasive, transient, and regionally selective brain drug delivery method. The brain is particularly difficult to deliver drugs to because of the blood-brain barrier (BBB). Over the past few years, we have been developing methods that combine Focused Ultrasound (FUS) and microbubbles in order to noninvasively, locally and transiently open the BBB so as to treat neurodegenerative diseases. In this paper, we will focus on the characterization of the type of molecular delivery that can be induced through the opened BBB. More specifically, we will characterize important properties of the BBB opening such as its reversibility and permeability using fluorescence and MR imaging techniques, respectively. Results on both wildtype and Alzheimer's model mice showed that the timeline of BBB opening is very similar between the presence and absence of amyloid plaques. The permeability change induced by BBB opening was found to increase by up to a 10-fold and to similar levels with those found in literature for glioma tumors.

Keywords: Alzheimer's; blood-brain barrier; brain drug delivery; focused ultrasound; HIFU; hippocampus; opening; permeability; dextran.
PACS: 43.80.Gx

INTRODUCTION

The BBB is a specialized substructure of the vascular system consisting of endothelial cells connected together by tight junctions. The luminal and abluminal membranes line the inner wall of the vessel and act as the permeability barrier. The combination of tight junctions and these two membranes characterizes the BBB as having low permeability to large and ionic substances. Certain molecules such as glucose and amino acids are exceptions, because they are actively transported. It has also been shown that lymphocytes can traverse the BBB by going through temporarily opened tight junctions of the endothelial walls. Several neurological disorders remain intractable to treatment by therapeutic agents because of the BBB, the brain's natural defense. By acting as a permeability barrier, the BBB impedes entry from blood to the brain of virtually all molecules with higher than around 400 Da of molecular weight [1]; thus, rendering many potent neurologically active substances and drugs ineffective simply because they cannot be delivered to where they are needed. As a result, traversing the BBB is the rate-limiting factor in brain drug delivery development [2]. The BBB opening has been demonstrated key in molecular delivery [3-9]. We have previously demonstrated the feasibility of BBB opening through intact skull and skin, i.e., without craniotomy or skin removal, and successful imaging of the BBB opening

CP1113, *8th International Symposium on Therapeutic Ultrasound*, edited by E. S. Ebbini
© 2009 American Institute of Physics 978-0-7354-0650-6/09/$25.00

in the area of the hippocampus at sub-millimeter imaging resolution using a 9.4T MR scanner in both wildtype [6, 7] and Alzheimer's mice [8,9]. This was the first time that a specific brain region (i.e., the hippocampus), which is typically affected in the case of neurodegenerative disease, such as Alzheimer's, was successfully and reproducibly targeted. In this paper, we will focus on the characterization regarding the reversibility, safety and permeability that is associated with the opened BBB. More specifically, we will characterize important properties of the BBB opening using histology and MR imaging techniques, respectively.

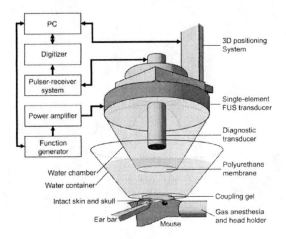

FIGURE 1. Schematic of the setup used in vivo

Methods

In vivo BBB opening in wildtype and Alzheimer's model (PS1-APP) mice (n=13) was achieved by systemically injecting microbubbles (Optison or Definity) and applying pulsed FUS (frequency: 1.525 MHz, peak-rarefactional pressure: 456 kPa) to the left hippocampus through the intact skin and skull. A sequence of MR T1-weighted images (9.4 T, Bruker Medical; Boston, MA) was obtained following intraperitoneal injection of gadolinium (596 Da; BBB impermeable) over 4 hours, both immediately after and 24 hours after the BBB opening. A relative increase in T1-weighted MR signal amplitude in the sonicated hippocampus as compared to the right (control) hippocampus confirmed trans-BBB diffusion. The permeability (Ki) of the BBB was quantified using a previously reported model [10] in order to measure the permeability changes of the BBB as a result of the FUS-induced opening. Immediately after sacrifice, H&E histology was also performed at the similar pressure amplitudes to determine any associated vascular or neuronal damage.

Results

Wildtype (Fig. 1(i)) and Alzheimer's model (Fig. 1(ii)) mice exhibited similar BBB opening properties after sonication indicating that the presence of amyloid plaques in mice does not affect the BBB properties, neither before nor after BBB opening. BBB opening was thus achieved at both reversible (Figs. 1 and 2) and safe levels. Histological studies indicated that, at the pressures used, red-blood cell extravasation (Fig. 3), but no discernible neuronal damage, may result in association with the BBB opening at the pressures used. Ki maps (Fig. 5) were obtained across the entire brain and were found highest at the BBB opening site equal to 7 μl/g-min using curve fitting methods on the MR signal amplitude variation after opening (Fig. 4).

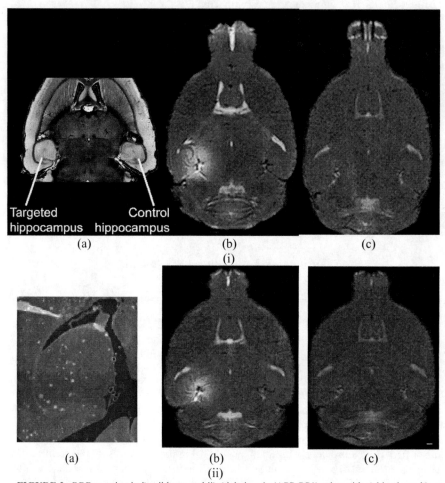

FIGURE 2. BBB opening in i) wildtype and ii) Alzheimer's (APP-PS1) mice with a) histology, b) BBB opening and c) BBB closure (i.e., recovery).

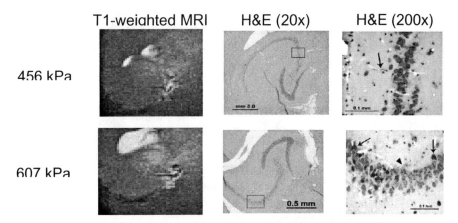

T1-weighted MRI   H&E (20x)   H&E (200x)

456 kPa

mm 3.0   8.1 mm

607 kPa

0.5 mm   8.1 mm

FIGURE 3. Safety window of BBB opening as detected on MR images: Increasing amounts of red blood cell extravasation were noted at higher pressure amplitudes.

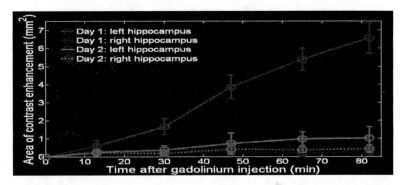

Day 1: left hippocampus
Day 1: right hippocampus
Day 2: left hippocampus
Day 2: right hippocampus

FIGURE 4. Variation of the T1-weighted MR amplitude after BBB opening in both sequential days over 90 min. The variation on Day 1 was used to calculate the permeability of the opened BBB.

MRI   Spatio-temporal   Permeability

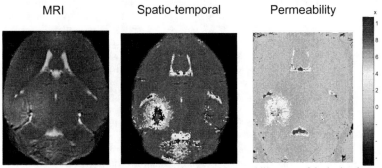

FIGURE 5. T1-weighted MR image, Spatiotemporal map and Permeability map of the brain after BBB opening on the left hippocampus.

Conclusions

FUS coupled with microbubbles opened the BBB sufficiently to allow passage of nanoparticles into the brain and permit subsequent regional increase of the blood-brain barrier permeability in the sonicated area with reversibility within 24 hours and associated minimal red blood cell extravasation as evidenced through histology.

ACKNOWLEDGMENTS

This study was supported by NSF CAREER 0644713, NIH R21 EY018505 and NIH R01 EB009041. The authors wish to thank Karen Duff, PhD, Department of Pathology for providing the APP-PS1 model, and Shougang Wang, PhD, Yao-Sheng Tung, MS, from the Ultrasound Elasticity Imaging Laboratory, Department of Biomedical Engineering at Columbia University, for their important input in the experiments.

REFERENCES

1. Pangalos MN et al. (2007) Drug development for CNS disorders: strategies for balancing risk and reducing attrition. *Nat Rev Drug Discov* 6(7):521-532.
2. Van Dam D & De Deyn PP (2006) Drug discovery in dementia: the role of rodent models. *Nat Rev Drug Discov* 5(11):956-970.
3. Kinoshita et al. (2006) Noninvasive localized delivery of Herceptin to the mouse brain by MRI-guided focused ultrasound-induced blood-brain barrier disruption. Proc Natl Acad Sci U S A 103(31):11719-11723.
4. Treat LH, et al. (2007) Targeted delivery of doxorubicin to the rat brain at therapeutic levels using MRI-guided focused ultrasound. International journal of cancer 121(4):901-907.
5. Sheikov N, *et al.* (2006) Brain arterioles show more active vesicular transport of blood-borne tracer molecules than capillaries and venules after focused ultrasound-evoked opening of the blood-brain barrier. *Ultrasound Med Biol* 32(9):1399-1409.
6. Choi JJ, et al. (2007) Spatio-temporal analysis of molecular delivery through the blood-brain barrier using focused ultrasound. (Translated from eng) Phys Med Biol 52(18):5509-5530 (in eng).
7. Choi JJ, et al.(2007) Noninvasive, transcranial and localized opening of the blood-brain barrier using focused ultrasound in mice. Ultrasound Med Biol 33(1):95-104.
8. Choi JJ, *et al.* (2008) Noninvasive and transient blood-brain barrier opening in the hippocampus of Alzheimer's double transgenic mice using pulsed Focused Ultrasound. (Translated from eng) *Ultrasonic Imaging* (in eng; in press).
9. Konofagou E.E. et al., Biomedical Applications of vibration and Acoustics in therapy, Bioeffects and modelling, Eds: A.Al-Jumaily and M. Fatemi, ASME Press, Chapter 3, pp. 63-80, 2008.
10. Jiang et al. (2005) Quantitative evaluation of BBB permeability after embolic stroke in rat using MRI. Journal of Cerebral Blood Flow and Metabolism. pp. 583-592.

Noninvasive Drug Delivery Using Ultrasound: Targeting Melanoma Using siRNA Against Mutant (V600E) B-Raf

Melissa A. Tran [a], Raghavendra Gowda [a], Eun-Joo Park [f], James Adair [d,g], Nadine Smith [d,f], Mark Kester [a,d] and Gavin P. Robertson [a,b,c,d,e]

Departments of Pharmacology[a], Pathology[b] and Dermatology[c], The Pennsylvania State University College of Medicine, Hershey, PA 17033
The Penn State Melanoma Therapeutics Program[d], The Foreman Foundation for Melanoma Research[e], Hershey, PA 17033.
Departments of Bioengineering[f], and Material Science and Engineering[g], Pennsylvania State University, University Park, PA, USA.

Abstract. Melanoma is the most deadly form of skin cancer. Currently early surgical removal is the best treatment option for melanoma patients with little hope of successful treatment of late stage melanoma. Clearly new treatment options must be explored. Topical administration of drugs provides the advantage of being able to apply large quantities of drug in close proximity to the tumor without the issue of systemic side effects. However, the natural barrier formed by the skin must first be overcome for topical treatment to become a viable option. With this in mind we have sought to use low-frequency ultrasound to transiently permeabilize the stratum corneum and successfully deliver liposomal siRNA to melanoma cells residing at the basement membrane. B-Raf is one of the most frequently activated genes in melanoma, making it an ideal candidate for targeting via siRNA. The novel liposomes used in this study load siRNA, protect if from the outside environment and lead to knockdown of target message. Combining ultrasound with liposomal siRNA we show that siRNA can be delivered into melanoma cells. Additionally, we show that siRNA to mutant B-Raf can effectively inhibit melanoma growth in reconstructs and in mice by 60% and 30% respectively. Therefore, ultrasound with liposomal siRNA is a potentially valuable treatment option for melanoma patients.

Keywords: melanoma, ultrasound, B-Raf, liposomes, siRNA.
PACS: 87.50.yt

INTRODUCTION

Melanoma is a cancer of melanocytes, which are pigmented skin cells residing at the epidermal-dermal junction [1]. While early stage melanomas can be treated effectively by surgical removal, there are no effective topical agents that prevent the development and spread of melanocytic lesions [2]. The skin consists of an outer epidermal and inner dermal region, which are protected by a surface keratinized layer called the stratum corneum [3, 4]. The keratinized layer prevents most topically applied agents from reaching early melanocytic lesions developing at the epidermal-dermal junction or from reaching cutaneous metastases, which are locally invasive lesions in the skin dermis [5]. Therefore, topical agents targeting early lesions or

CP1113, *8th International Symposium on Therapeutic Ultrasound*, edited by E. S. Ebbini
© 2009 American Institute of Physics 978-0-7354-0650-6/09/$25.00

cutaneous metastases hold significant potential to decrease melanoma incidence and mortality rates. Furthermore, localized application of topical therapies could enable high concentrations of agents to be administered directly to skin lesions, limiting toxicity caused by systemic administration [3, 6, 7]. Thus, effective topical inhibitory agents need to be developed as well as delivery approaches established for skin penetration.

The purpose of this study is to develop a unique liposomal-ultrasound mediated approach for delivering siRNA into melanocytic lesions present in skin, which inhibits early melanocytic lesion development, as well as, that of cutaneous metastases. Topical delivery of novel siRNA containing cationic liposomes following low-frequency ultrasound can decrease early melanocytic lesion development or spread of metastases in skin.

MATERIALS AND METHODS

Initially, liposomal-siRNA complex was topically applied to the skin; however, the complex only penetrated the upper layers of the stratum corneum. This occurs because skin forms a natural barrier preventing uptake of agents, including lipids [3, 5]. Therefore, a strategy was developed to permeabilize the skin to enable topically administered liposomes containing siRNA to reach skin melanocytic lesions. This involved a combination approach using ultrasound followed by topical administration of siRNA-liposomal complex to skin. A lightweight cymbal array was used for ultrasonic treatment prior to administration of the siRNA-liposomal complex (Fig. 1(a)). Using calibrated miniature omnidirectional reference hydrophone (TC4013, RESON, Inc., Goleta, CA), the profile of acoustic intensity has been determined (Fig. 1(b)). In order to permeabilize the skin, the array was operated at the special-peak temporal-peak intensity (I_{sptp}) of 50.1 ± 0.8 mW/cm^2.

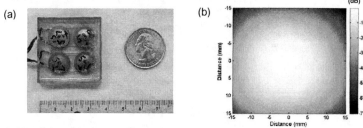

Figure 1. (a) A lightweight, low-profile cymbal array for ultrasonic treatment to permeabilize skin. (b) The profile of acoustic intensity for the 2x2 cymbal array used in this study.

Skin reconstructs were treated with ultrasound by removing media and submerging skin reconstructs in PBS. Ultrasound was administered for 20 minutes at 20 kHz and a duty cycle of 20% [8]. Liposomal-siRNA complex was then topically applied at a concentration of 1 μM and allowed to soak into the skin. For damage studies, ghost liposome was applied after ultrasound treatment. Hematoxylin and eosin (H&E) stained paraffin embedded cross sections were examined for skin damage using microscopy. For uptake studies skin reconstructs were treated with Alexa Fluor 546 containing liposomes (1 µM) or ghost liposomes and harvested one hour after treatment. Uptake was analyzed using stereo fluorescence microscopy. Laboratory generated skin reconstructs were treated on alternate days starting on day 10 up to day 20 and on day 21, skin was harvested. Skin reconstructs from all experiments were fixed in 4% paraformaldehyde at 4°C overnight. After fixation skin was stored in 0.5 M EDTA pH 8.0 (Fisher Scientific, Waltham, MA). To quantify differences between treatment groups following nucleofection or ultrasound treatment + siRNA-liposomal complex, 4-6 images of each reconstruct were taken. Total area occupied by GFP-tagged tumor nodules in each image was analyzed. Average area was then calculated for each piece of skin and for each treatment group.

In order to investigate the siRNA-liposomal complex treatment for tumors in mice, 1×10^6 UACC 903-GFP cells were injected subcutaneously into the right flank of nude mice. After 24 hours, mice were treated by ultrasound for 15 minutes followed by topical addition of liposomal-siRNA (siMutB-Raf or siScrambled) complex (25 µg) on alternate days up to day 23. Aquaflex Gel Pads (Parker Laboratories, Inc., Fairfield, NJ) were used as an ultrasound standoff. Ultrasound was administered for 15 minutes at a frequency of 20 kHz and a duty cycle of 20% [8]. Liposomal siRNA was administered to the ultrasound treated area overlying the tumor and allowed to soak into the skin.

RESULTS

From the comparison of untreated skin to ultrasound treated skin, the array configuration did not cause significant damage to the skin at the settings used for this study. Next, penetration of skin by the siRNA-liposomal complex following ultrasound treatment was examined using stereo fluorescence microscopy. Top down views of the skin reconstructs show uptake of liposomal siRNA by both keratinocytes and GFP tagged UACC 903-GFP melanoma cells (Fig. 2 (a)). Compared to treatment with control ghost liposomes, cross sections of skin treated with liposomes containing siRNA (red) showed presence of the complex in melanoma cells located in both the epidermis and at the epidermal-dermal junction (Fig. 2 (b)). From the comparison,

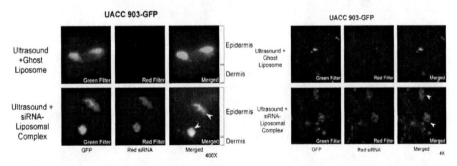

Figure 2. (a) Top down view of skin reconstructs treated with ultrasound and siRNA-liposomal complex (400×). (b) Cross sections of skin treated with ultrasound followed by siRNA-liposomal complex treatment (4×).

ultrasound treatment of skin prior to topical application with a siRNA-liposomal complex enables delivery of siRNA to melanocytic lesion cells located within skin.

To determine whether ultrasound followed by topical treatment of liposomal-siRNA complex could decrease skin lesion development in animals, 1×10^6 GFP-tagged UACC 903 were subcutaneously injected into the flanks of nude mice. Twenty-four hours later and on every alternate day thereafter, mice under anesthesia were treated with ultrasound for 15 minutes at the tumor site followed by topical application of liposomal-siRNA complex (Fig. 3 (a)).

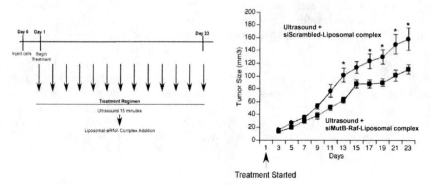

Figure 3. (a) Schematic showing treatment regime. (b) Melanocytic tumor development in animal skin treated with ultrasound and liposomal-siRNA complex.

Along with measurement of developing tumors (Fig. 3(b)), mice were also weighed on alternate days. A statistically significant ~30-40% reduction in tumor size compared to mice treated with the control ultrasound + siScrambled-liposomal complex was observed starting at day 13 and on days 17, 19, 21 and 23. Ultrasound followed by topical treatment of liposomal-siRNA complex targeting [V600E]B-Raf in melanocytic lesions significantly decreased cutaneous tumor development in animals.

DISCUSSION

Novel therapeutic regimens must be developed for treating early melanocytic lesions and cutaneous metastases since aside from surgical excision few treatment options are available (2). Current therapeutic approaches are frequently limited by toxicities associated with systemic administration and various off target effects (3). These issues would be decreased for topical and localized treatment regimes, which could permit high concentrations of agents to be used with less associated systemic toxicity [3, 6].

Application of liposomes topically to skin, including those containing tretinoin, have been shown to deliver drugs primarily to cells in the upper layers of the epidermis [5]. This requires development of strategies for delivery to melanocytic lesions in epidermis, at the epidermal-dermal junction or in the dermis [3, 5]. In this study, low-frequency ultrasound using the lightweight cymbal array was used to successfully permeabilize the skin enabling delivery of the siRNA-liposomal complex into melanoma cells residing at the dermal-epidermal junction of skin reconstructs validating this method as a feasible way to deliver siRNA.

In conclusion, a unique liposomal-ultrasound mediated approach for delivering siRNA into melanocytic lesions present in skin has been developed. The novel cationic liposome effectively encapsulates siRNA that specifically targets mutant ^{V600E}B-Raf present in melanocytic lesions, protects the siRNA from degradation and facilitates its entry into cells. Following non-damaging low-frequency ultrasound of skin the siRNA-liposomal formulation penetrates epidermal and dermal layers leading to a 1-2 fold decrease in early lesion or cutaneous metastasis development by causing a 4-5 fold decrease in cellular proliferative potential. Thus, topical delivery of novel siRNA containing cationic liposomes following low-frequency ultrasound can decrease early melanocytic lesion development or spread of metastases in skin.

ACKNOWLEDGMENTS

This study was supported by NIH/National Cancer Institute grant 1-RO3-CA128033-01, American Cancer Society grant RSG-04-053-01-GMC, The Foreman Foundation for Melanoma Research, State of Pennsylvania Non-formulary Tobacco Settlement Funds, and Department of Defense Technologies for Metabolic Monitoring grant W81XWH-05-1-0617.

REFERENCES

1. Satyamoorthy K, Herlyn M. Cellular and molecular biology of human melanoma. Cancer Biol Ther 2002;1:14-7.
2. Garbe C, Eigentler TK. Diagnosis and treatment of cutaneous melanoma: state of the art 2006. Melanoma Res 2007;17:117-27.
3. El Maghraby GM, Williams AC, Barry BW. Can drug-bearing liposomes penetrate intact skin? J Pharm Pharmacol 2006;58:415-29.
4. Lee SH, Jeong SK, Ahn SK. An update of the defensive barrier function of skin. Yonsei Med J 2006;47:293-306.
5. Ting WW, Vest CD, Sontheimer RD. Review of traditional and novel modalities that enhance the permeability of local therapeutics across the stratum corneum. Int J Dermatol 2004;43:538-47.
6. Radny P, Caroli UM, Bauer J, et al. Phase II trial of intralesional therapy with interleukin-2 in soft-tissue melanoma metastases. Br J Cancer 2003;89:1620-6.
7. Lavon I, Kost J. Ultrasound and transdermal drug delivery. Drug Discov Today 2004;9:670-6.
8. Smith NB, Lee S, Shung KK. Ultrasound-mediated transdermal in vivo transport of insulin with low-profile cymbal arrays. Ultrasound Med Biol 2003;29:1205-10.

Ultrasound Delivery of an Anti-Aβ Therapeutic Agent to the Brain in a Mouse Model of Alzheimer's Disease

Jessica F. Jordão[a,b,c], Carlos A. Ayala-Grosso[b,f], Rajiv Chopra[a,d], JoAnne McLaurin[c,e], Isabelle Aubert[b,c] and Kullervo Hynynen[a,d]

[a]Imaging Research and [b]Neuroscience, Sunnybrook Research Institute, Toronto, ON, Canada; [c]Dept of Laboratory Medicine and Pathobiology, [d]Dept of Medical Biophysics, and [e]Centre for Research in Neurodegenerative Diseases at the University of Toronto, Toronto ON, Canada; [f]Unidad de Biología Molecular, Facultad de Farmacia, Universidad Central de Venezuela, Caracas, Venezuela

Abstract. Plaques composed of amyloid-beta (Aβ) peptides represent a pathological hallmark in the brain of patients with Alzheimer's disease. Aβ oligomers are considered cytotoxic and several therapeutic approaches focus on reducing Aβ load in the brain of Alzheimer's patients. The efficacy of most anti-Aβ agents is significantly limited because they do not cross the blood-brain-barrier. Innovative technologies capable of enhancing the permeability of the blood-brain barrier, thereby allowing entry of therapeutic agents into the brain, show great promise in circumventing this problem. The application of low-intensity focused ultrasound in the presence of an ultrasound contrast agent causes localized and transient permeability of the blood-brain barrier. We demonstrate the value of this technology for the delivery of anti-Aβ antibodies to the brain of TgCRND8 mice, a mouse model of Alzheimer's disease exhibiting Aβ plaques. BAM-10, an anti-Aβ antibody, was injected into the tail vein simultaneously with exposure to MRI-guided, low-intensity focused ultrasound (FUS) to one hemisphere of TgCNRD8 mice. Four hours after treatment, antibodies were detected at significant amounts only in the brain of mice receiving FUS in addition to BAM-10. This data provides a proof-of-concept that FUS allows anti-Aβ therapeutics to efficiently enter the brain and target Aβ plaques. Four days following a single treatment with BAM-10 and MRI-guided FUS, a significant decrease in the number of Aβ plaques on the side of the treated hemisphere was observed in TgCRND8 mice. In conclusion low-intensity, focused ultrasound is effective in delivering Aβ antibodies to the brain. This technology has the potential to enhance current anti-Aβ treatments by allowing increased exposure of amyloid plaques to treatment agents.

Keywords: Focused ultrasound; microbubbles; antibody; Alzheimer's disease; transgenic mouse model; drug delivery; immunotherapy
PACS: 87.14em, 87.15.rs, 87.19xr, 87.19um

INTRODUCTION

Alzheimer's disease (AD) is characterized by neuronal loss, paired helical filaments and senile plaques composed of amyloid-beta (Aβ) peptides. Due to evidence that Aβ is neurotoxic[1], recent therapies have focused on using anti-Aβ antibodies to bind and clear Aβ. However, only 0.1-1% of systemically administered antibodies cross the BBB[2], making targeting of Aβ within the brain inefficient. Magnetic resonance image-guided focused ultrasound (MRIgFUS) in combination with microbubbles has the potential to increase the delivery of anti-Aβ antibodies to the brain in a non-invasive, transient and localized manner [3].

The present study has two main objectives. First, we aimed to demonstrate that low-intensity MRIgFUS in combination with microbubbles can be used to deliver BAM-10, an anti-Aβ antibody, to the brain of TgCRND8 mice. Second, we evaluated the efficacy of BAM-10 delivered by MRIgFUS to clear Aβ plaques in TgCRND8 mice. TgCRND8 mice have a double mutation in the human amyloid precursor protein gene, which results in significant Aβ plaque load at 4 months of age, as observed in the current study.

Our data indicate that MRIgFUS delivers BAM-10 to the brain and that this treatment significantly reduces the number of Aβ plaques in TgCRND8 mice.

METHODS AND RESULTS

Delivery of anti-Aβ antibody via MRIgFUS

To demonstrate the delivery of the anti-Aβ antibody BAM-10 to the brain of 4 month-old TgCRND8 mice, we used 3T MRI scans to position 4 foci (1.5 mm apart) along the right hemisphere. A spherically-focused transducer with a diameter of 10 cm, focal length of 78 mm and a resonant frequency of 0.558 MHz was used for sonication (pressure amplitude of 0.3MPa for 2 min; 10ms bursts; PRF=1Hz). Definity microbubbles (80 μl/kg), MRI contrast agent, gadolinium (0.2 mg/kg) and biotinylated anti-Aβ antibody BAM-10 (40 μg), were administered via tail vein injection simultaneously with low-intensity FUS application After sonication, MRI was used to confirm disruption of the blood-brain barrier (**Figure 1**).

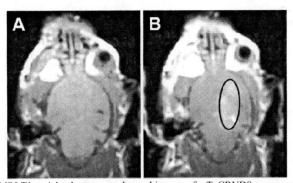

FIGURE 1. 3T MRI T1-weighted contrast enhanced images of a TgCRND8 mouse prior to sonication (**A**) and post-treatment (**B**). BBB disruption (**outlined**) was achieved using simultaneous sonication and systemic administration of microbubbles. BBB disruption is visualized by the leakage of gadolinium into the brain (A, B: 256x256, TE/TR=10.4/500.0, FOV=4cm, Slice 1mm, ETL=4, 3NEX).

TgCRND8 mice treated with MRIgFUS and biotynylated-BAM-10 were sacrificed 4 hr post-treatment. Following brain perfusion with fixative, coronal sections were cut (40 μm) and processed with strepavidin-horseradish peroxidase and 3,3'-diaminobenzidine (DAB). We found that the biotinylated BAM-10 antibody delivered in the bloodstream crossed the BBB and entered the right hemisphere where ultrasound was applied (**Figure 2A**). In **Figure 2B**, the same anti-Aβ antibody was applied directly on an adjacent brain section to illustrate that Aβ-plaques are present on both sides of the brain in TgCRND8 mice. In **Figure 2C**, a negative control (not injected with antibody nor treated with ultrasound) is shown. Similar images for negative controls were observed for mice receiving BAM-10 with no MRIgFUS, reinforcing the finding that BAM-10 enters the brain efficiently only with the use of MRIgFUS at 4 hr post-BAM-10 injection.

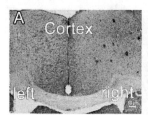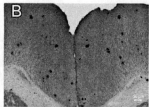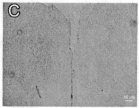

FIGURE 2. Biotinylated-BAM-10 antibody enters the brain and binds to Aβ plaques in TgCRND8 mice following MRIgFUS treatment. After systemic injection of biotinylated anti-Aβ antibody, biotinylated-BAM-10 was detected only in the MRIgFUS targeted (right) hemisphere (**A**). Biotinylated-BAM-10 directly applied on brain sections reveals Aβ plaques in both hemispheres of TgCRND8 mice (**B**). Negative controls including those from untreated brains without antibody and/or without ultrasound (**C**).

MRIg FUS Delivery of an Anti-Aβ Antibody Reduces Plaque Load

The efficacy of the anti-Aβ treatment with MRIgFUS (parameters previously stated) to reduce plaque load in TgCRND8 mice was evaluated using stereological approaches to generate unbiased estimates of plaque number (optical fractionator probe) and size (nucleator probe) within the region of the brain where the BBB was disrupted. Measurements from post-treatment MRI scans (**Figure 1B**) were used to define the inclusion zones in which Aβ plaques were counted and measured. Plaque number and size were counted separately in both hemispheres of TgCNRD8 mice for all groups 4 days post-treatment: treated with ultrasound delivered antibody (USAb), antibody alone (Ab), ultrasound alone (US) and untreated (UT).

MRIgFUS-delivered antibody treatment resulted in a significant reduction in plaque number on the treated side of the brain (right) compared to the untreated side (left) (USAb group, **Figure 3A, 3B**).

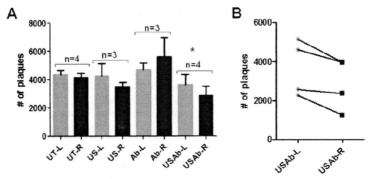

FIGURE 3. MRIgFUS delivery of BAM-10 antibody in TgCRND8 mice significantly reduced the number of plaques on the right treated side (USAb-R) compared to the left untreated side (USAb-L) (*$p<0.05$, paired t-test ; mean $\pm$ SEM, n is indicated above each pair of columns) (**A**). Intra-animal comparison of the right and left hemisphere for the USAb group shows that plaque count on the right US-targeted side of the brain is consistently lower than plaque count on the contralateral left side (**B**).

Qualitative observations of Aβ plaques in all treatment groups indicated a range of plaque sizes and appearance among TgCRND8 mice, independent of treatment. The mean plaque size was not statistically different between groups or between the right and left hemisphere within each group (**Figure 4**).

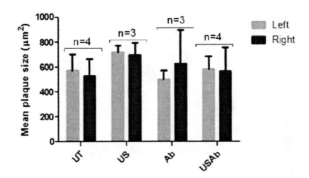

FIGURE 4. Plaque mean size is not statistically different between treatment groups, or within treatment groups comparing the right treated side to the left untreated side of the brain (mean $\pm$ SEM shown above, n is indicated above each pair of columns).

CONCLUSION

We demonstrated that MRIgFUS allows the localized delivery of systemically administered anti-Aβ antibody to the brain of TgCRND8 mice, a mouse model of AD. The amount of anti-Aβ antibody delivered to the brain by MRIgFUS was sufficient to significantly decrease the number of plaques in the targeted hemisphere of the brain, within a short-time frame of 4 days. These results provide a proof-of-concept that MRIgFUS delivery of therapeutic agents to the brain is feasible and effective, as demonstrated here by the delivery anti-Aβ antibodies to the brain causing a decrease in the number of plaques observed.

ACKNOWLEDGMENTS

We would like to thank Ping Wu, Dr. Laura Curiel and Yue-Xi Huang for their technical assistance during MRIgFUS experiments, as well as Shawna Rideout-Gros, Ying-Qi Weng and Mary Hill for their help with TgCRND8 mice. This study was supported by grants from NIH (KH), CIHR (JM), and Sunnybrook Research Institute (IA).

REFERENCES

1. Selkoe DJ. *JAMA.* **283**:1615-17 (2000).
2. Nitsch RM and Hock C. *Neurotherapeutics.* **5**:415-20 (2008).
3. Hynynen K, *et al. Radiology* **220**, 640-6 (2001).

Ultrasound Gene Transfer into Fibroblast Cells using Microbubbles

Yoji Nakamura[1], Kota Hirayama[2], Kiyoshi Yoshinaka[1],
Yuichi Tei[1], Shu Takagi[2] and Yoichiro Matsumoto[2]

1 Department of Bioengineering, School of Engineering, The University of Tokyo
7-3-1 Hongo, Bunkyo-ku, Tokyo 113-8656 JAPAN
2 Department of Mechanical Engineering, The University of Tokyo,
7-3-1 Hongo, Bunkyo-ku, Tokyo 113-8656 JAPAN

Abstract. Ultrasound is widely applied in the medical field and offers the strong advantages of non-invasiveness and high-selectivity. Gene transfer using ultrasound, which is called sonoporation, is one application. Ultrasound has the potential to deliver therapeutic materials such as genes, drugs or proteins into cells. Microbubbles are known to be able to improve delivery efficiency. This is attributed to therapeutic materials passing through the cell membrane after permeability is increased by destruction or oscillation of microbubbles. The present study tried to deliver the GFP plasmids into fibroblast cells. Cells were cultured in 6-well culture plates and exposed to ultrasound (frequency, 2.1 MHz; wave pattern, duty cycle 10%; intensity, 0-26 W/cm^2; time, 0-200 s) transmitted through medium containing microbubbles (Levovist® (void fraction, 8×10^{-5}) or Sonazoid® (void fraction, 0-24×10^{-4})) and GFP plasmids at a concentration of 15 μg/mL. Density of microbubbles after ultrasound irradiation was measured. When ultrasound intensity was increased with Levovist® 8×10^{-4}, transfection efficiency increased, cell viability decreased and microbubbles disappeared. With Sonazoid®, transfection efficiency and cell viability were basically unchanged and microbubbles decreased, but did not disappear. Transfection efficiency also improved with increased ultrasound irradiation time or microbubble density. Microbubble destruction appeared to have the main effect on gene transfection under Levovist® and microbubble oscillation had the main effect under Sonazoid®.

INTRODUCTION

Progress in medical technology over recent years has required not only the treatment of disease, but also the amelioration of physical and mental distress in patients. Various noninvasive treatments have thus been proposed. Attenuation and permeability of ultrasound *in vivo* are known to be suitable, and ultrasound is currently applied in medical fields as diverse as imaging, noninvasive treatment of tumors [1, 2] and lithotripsy [3]. Ultrasound also has the potential to deliver therapeutic materials such as genes, drugs or proteins into cells. This method is called sonoporation. Moreover, microbubble contrast agents have been shown to enhance the efficiency of sonoporation [4, 5]. However, the mechanisms underlying sonoporation remain unclear and efficiency is still insufficient. The present study attempted to deliver GFP plasmids into fibroblast cells. We investigated the number of transfected cells, cell viability and the density of microbubbles under several experimental conditions (ultrasound intensity, ultrasound exposure time, and concentration of microbubble).

CP1113, *8th International Symposium on Therapeutic Ultrasound*, edited by E. S. Ebbini
© 2009 American Institute of Physics 978-0-7354-0650-6/09/$25.00

EXPERIMENTAL SETUP AND CONDITIONS

Figure 1 shows the experimental apparatus. Cultured cells on 6-well culture plates were exposed to 2.1-MHz ultrasound (duty cycle, 10% (40/360); exposure time, 100 s; intensity, 0~32 W/cm^2) transmitted through media containing GFP plasmids (concentration, 15 μg/mL) and microbubbles (Levovist® or Sonazoid®; void fraction, 0-24 ×10^{-4}[-]).NIH3T3 fibroblast cells were selected as target cells, the GFP plasmid as the gene, and Levovist® and Sonazoid® as microbubble contrast agents. When GFP plasmid is transfected into the cell, the cell appears green under fluorescence microscopy. Figure 2 shows fluorescence images using Levovist® and Sonazoid® as microbubble contrast agents.

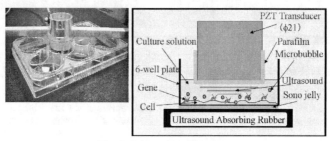

Figure 1: Experimental apparatus

Table 1: Experimental Conditions

Ultrasound	**Frequency**	**2.1 MHz**
	Wave profile	**Burst 40/360 (on/off)**
	Exposure time (s)	10, 20, 30, 50, 100, 200
	Intensity (W/cm^2)	1.3, 5.4, 12.0, 16.3, 20.8, 26.3
Microbubbles	Levovist®	**10% (v/v)** **(void fraction, 8 ×10^{-5})**
	Sonazoid®	0–30% (v/v) **(void fraction, 0-24 ×10^{-4})**
Cell	**Fibroblast cells**	**NIH3T3**
Gene	**GFP plasmid**	**15 μg/ml**

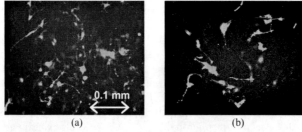

(a) (b)

Figure 2: Fluorescence images of cells according to ultrasound intensity. Microbubbles: (a) Levovist® (b) Sonazoid® at a void fraction of 8 ×10^{-4}[-]; ultrasound intensity, 16.3 W/cm^2; ultrasound exposure time, 100 s; GFP density, 15 μg/ml).

RESULTS AND DISCUSSIONS

Figures 3 and 4 show how numbers or rates of transfected cells, cell viability and density of microbubbles vary with ultrasound intensity.

When using Levovist®, numbers of transfected cells increased with stronger ultrasound intensity. When ultrasound intensity increased from 12.0 W/cm² to 16.3 W/cm², the number of transfected cells decreased. Taking the decreased cell viability into consideration, a threshold exists beyond which damage to cells exceeds effectiveness of transfection. From the measurement of the density of microbubbles, we know that dissolution of microbubbles occurs under any ultrasound intensity. We can thus consider that the dissolution of microbubbles mainly affects transfection [5].

When using Sonazoid®, rates of cell transfection and cell viability displayed only minor changes, but density of microbubbles decreased. Other main factors thus appear to affect transfection, such as microbubble oscillation [5].

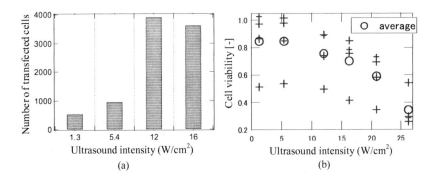

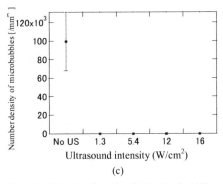

Figure 3: a) Number of transfected cells, b) cell viability and c) density of microbubbles according to ultrasound intensity Ultrasound intensity: 1.3, 5.4, 12.0, 16.3 and 26.3 W/cm². Microbubbles: Levovist® at void fraction 8 ×10⁻⁴ [-], ultrasound exposure time, 100 s; GFP density, 15 μg/ml.

435

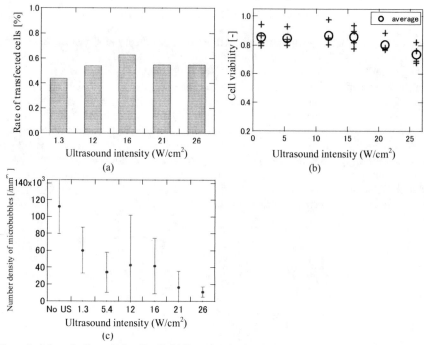

(a)

(b)

(c)

Figure 4. a) Rate of cell transfection, b) cell viability and c) density of microbubbles according to ultrasound intensity. Ultrasound intensity: 1.3, 5.4, 12.0, 16.3 and 26.3 W/cm². Microbubbles: Sonazoid® at void fraction of 8 ×10⁻⁴ [-]; ultrasound exposure time, 100 s; GFP density, 15 μg/ml.

Figure 5 shows the number of transfected cells according to ultrasound exposure time under an ultrasound intensity of 5.4 W/cm² using Sonazoid®. We can see that the number of transfected cells increases with longer exposure time. The result of exposure for 100 s does not differ widely from that for 200s. Microbubbles may thus have disappeared, reducing increased transfection.

Figure 6 shows the number of transfected cells according to the concentration of microbubbles under an ultrasound intensity of 5.4 W/cm² using Sonazoid®. We can see that the number of transfected cells also increases with higher microbubble concentrations.

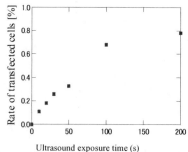

Ultrasound exposure time (s)

Figure 5: Number of transfected cells according to ultrasound exposure time (ultrasound exposure times: 0, 10, 20, 30, 50, 100 or 200 s. Ultrasound intensity, 5.4 W/cm². Microbubbles: Sonazoid® at void fraction of 8 ×10⁻⁴ [-]; GFP density, 15 μg/ml.

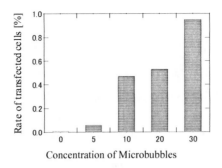

Concentration of Microbubbles

Figure 6: Number of transfected cells according to concentration of microbubbles (concentration of microbubbles: 0%, 5%, 10%, 20% or 30% (void fraction: 0, 4×10^{-4}, 8×10^{-4}, 16×10^{-4} or 24×10^{-4}[-]. Ultrasound intensity, 5.4 W/cm^2. Microbubbles: Sonazoid® at void fraction of 8×10^{-4} [-]. Ultrasound exposure time, 100 s; GFP density, 15 µg/ml.

CONCLUSIONS

This study experimented with the delivery of GFP plasmids into fibroblast cells using ultrasound and microbubbles, reaching the following conclusions:

[1] When using Levovist®, the number of transfected cells is increased with stronger ultrasound intensity, but cell viability decreases. Microbubbles disappear because of the ultrasound irradiation at any intensity.

[2] When using Sonazoid®, rate of transfected cells and cell viability is unchanged when ultrasound intensity is changed. In addition, microbubbles decrease after ultrasound irradiation.

[3] With longer ultrasound exposure, the rate of transfected cells increases.

[4] With higher concentration of microbubbles, the rate of transfected cells increases.

ACKNOWLEDGMENTS

This work was partially supported by a grant for Center for NanoBio Integration (CNBI) and Scientific Research (A)18206020, from the Ministry of Education, Culture, Sports, Science and Technology of Japan.

REFERENCES

1. Kawashima H. Ichihara M. et al., Oscillation of a vapor/gas bubble with heat and mass transport, 2000, Transactions of JSME, B, vol. 67, pp. 2234-2242.
2. Yoshizawa S., Ph. D. thesis, The University of Tokyo, 2006.
3. Holt R. G. and Roy R. A., Measurements of bubble-enhanced heating from focused, MHz-frequency ultrasound in a tissue-mimicking material, 2001, Ultrasound Med. Biol., vol. 27, pp. 1399-1412.
4. Umemura S., Kawabata K., et al., In vivo acceleration of ultrasonic tissue heating by microbubble agent, 2005, IEEE Trans. UFFC, vol. 52, pp. 1690-1698.
5. Wamel A., et al., Vibrating microbubbles poking individual cells: Drug transfer into cells via sonoporation, 2006, J. Control. Release, vol. 112, pp. 149-155.

MRI-Controlled Rapidly Scanned Focused Ultrasound Hyperthermia for Temperature Sensitive Localized Drug Delivery

Robert Staruch[a], Jeff Wachsmuth[b], Rajiv Chopra[a,b] & Kullervo Hynynen[a,b]

[a]*Department of Medical Biophysics, University of Toronto*
[b]*Imaging Research, Sunnybrook Health Sciences Centre*
2075 Bayview Avenue, Toronto, Ontario, Canada M4N 3M5

Abstract. Temperature sensitive drug delivery systems have been limited by a lack of versatile, noninvasive methods for applying uniform non-ablative heating. The objective of this study was to characterize and demonstrate an MRI-controlled scanned focused ultrasound system capable of maintaining temporally and spatially uniform target temperatures *ex vivo*. Degassed turkey breast was heated in a clinical 3T MRI using a single-element focused transducer rapidly scanned along a circular trajectory by an MRI-compatible transducer positioning system. Spatial temperature distribution was measured every 5s using the proton resonance frequency shift. Temperature at the center of the scan trajectory was used as input for proportional-integral control of applied acoustic power. Uniform temperature elevation of 10°C was maintained for several minutes in a 5 mm target diameter using controller gain values identified by numerical simulations. Simultaneous scanning and imaging caused a correctable periodic drift in baseline phase. Temporally and spatially uniform MRI-controlled scanned focused ultrasound hyperthermia was demonstrated *ex vivo* with a simple feedback control system.

Keywords: Focused ultrasound, hyperthermia, MRI, thermometry, control, drug delivery.
PACS: 87.50.yk, 87.50.yt, 87.61.-c.

INTRODUCTION

The development of temperature-sensitive drug delivery systems has been limited by the lack of versatile, noninvasive methods for applying uniform non-ablative heating. MRI-guided scanned focused ultrasound is a noninvasive modality capable of controlling temperature distributions deep within tissue, but few groups have demonstrated systems capable of applying uniform, mild heating over a clinically relevant volume of tissue for a sustained period of time [1,2].

In order to study the use of focused ultrasound hyperthermia as a means of enhancing drug delivery and triggering temperature-sensitive drug release, we are developing a small animal scanned focused ultrasound system designed to achieve temperature elevations of 5-10°C in tumors measuring 1.0-2.0 cm in diameter. This study describes the system characterization and *ex vivo* testing of single-point temperature control using a new MRI-compatible transducer positioning system for preclinical scanned focused ultrasound experiments.

CP1113, *8th International Symposium on Therapeutic Ultrasound*, edited by E. S. Ebbini
© 2009 American Institute of Physics 978-0-7354-0650-6/09/$25.00

METHODS

Controlled heating was performed in degassed turkey breast in a clinical 3T MRI using a single-element focused ultrasound transducer (2.787 MHz, 5 cm aperture, 10 cm radius) scanned through circular trajectories of 0-10 mm diameter by a motorized MRI-compatible positioning system. Acoustic coupling was provided by a degassed water-filled flexible plastic sleeve clamped both to the outer edge of the transducer fixture and to the inner edge of an aperture in the experiment stage above (Figure 1).

Temperature maps were computed by the proton resonance frequency (PRF) shift method [3] from phase images acquired every 5 seconds using a spoiled gradient-echo sequence (FSPGR, TE: 10 ms, TR: 38.6 ms, 30° flip angle, 128 x 128, 10-14 cm FOV, 3 mm slice, PRF temperature coefficient α = -0.0097 ppm/°C). A custom 64 mm receive coil was fitted around the water sleeve, directly under the sonicated tissue.

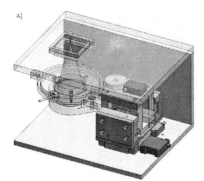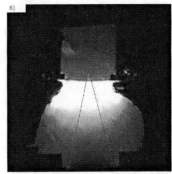

FIGURE 1. A) Schematic of small animal MRI-compatible scanned focused ultrasound system showing acoustic field sonicating up through the top plate of the apparatus. B) Axial image showing transducer position with respect to ex vivo sample and the ultrasound focus.

The mean temperature in a 3 x 3 pixel region of interest at the center of the circular scan trajectory was used as input for proportional-integral control of applied acoustic power. Proportional and integral gain values for uniform temperature profiles were identified in simulations based on the Pennes bioheat transfer equation [4].

RESULTS

A periodic baseline phase drift was observed during simultaneous transducer scanning and MR imaging that corresponded to temperature fluctuations of up to ±5°C. Figure 2 shows the mean ± SD temperatures calculated from a coronal imaging slice through the ultrasound focus in a sample of degassed turkey breast, within an ROI encompassing the scanning area, with no acoustic power applied. In this example, a circular path was scanned in the coronal plane with radius 2.5 mm and period 4 seconds, starting from before imaging began until 4 minutes 20 seconds later, at which point the device held its final position and temperature fluctuations decreased from ±3 to ±0.5°C.

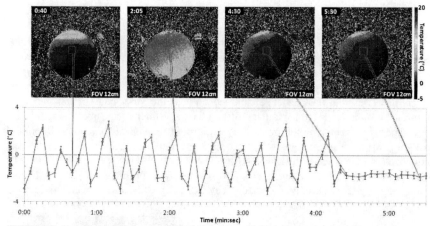

FIGURE 2. Periodic baseline temperature drift in coronal MR thermometry caused by simultaneous scanning (2.5 mm radius, 4 s period) and imaging. Circular scanning ceased at time 4:20.

To identify whether the source of this phase drift was caused by susceptibility changes due to positioning system motion, transducer motion, or water motion, the standard deviation of the baseline temperature was measured during scanning in three sets of experiments: scanning with the positioner alone, the positioner with FUS transducer, and the positioner with FUS transducer and water sleeve. Figure 3 shows the baseline temperature drift for scanning radii of 0, 1, 2.5 and 5 mm at scan rates of 3 and 6 mm/s. Identical imaging parameters were used in all cases (128x128 matrix, 12 cm FOV, 5 second acquisition time).

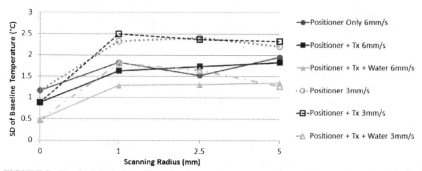

FIGURE 3. Standard deviation of baseline temperatures vs. scanning radius, speed, and positioning system setup. Standard deviation increases with increasing speed, decreases when loaded with water.

A proportional-integral controller was used to dynamically update output power based on the error between the current temperature and the temperature goal, as well as the integral temperature error over all previous update periods. Using a proportional gain of 0.040 and integral gain of 0.001, which worked well in simulation for a scan radius of 2.5 mm and period of 5 seconds, the time series shown in Figure 4 was achieved when heating turkey breast.

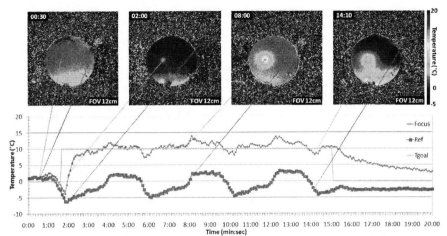

FIGURE 4. Single-point temperature control of scanned heating in degassed turkey breast. Focal point temperatures are maintained near 10°C despite periodic variations in baseline phase.

The temperature profile in Figure 5 demonstrates the spatial uniformity of scanned heating across the meat sample in the experiment shown above. Mean temperatures ± SD from 3:00 to 15:00 are shown. Solid lines denote the 5 mm scan diameter of the focus, while the dashed lines show the full-width at half-maximum of the heating profile, which was estimated to be 13 mm.

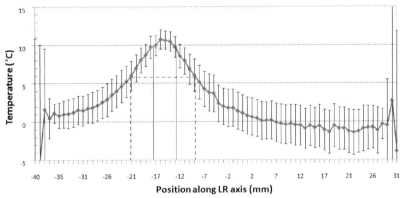

FIGURE 5. Temperature mean ± SD through the focus from time 3:00 to time 15:00 for the scanned heating experiment shown in Figure 4. The 5 mm scan diameter and 13 mm FWHM are shown.

DISCUSSION

Figure 3 suggests that temperature variation does not increase with scanning radius, and increased scanning speeds result in larger errors. The volume of water appears to improve temperature measurements, but this is likely due to improved SNR with improved impedance matching for the custom-tuned receive coil.

Correction of the artifacts shown in Figure 2 by subtracting the reference phase of a single mineral oil phantom proved unsuccessful as drift artifacts varied across the imaging plane. Interpolation between multiple reference phantoms, or the application of atlas correction schemes designed for periodic motion artifacts [2] should prove to reduce the error to levels acceptable for temperature control applications.

In these preliminary experiments with a prototype positioning system, scanning speed was limited to less than 10 mm/s by errors caused by positional drift seen only during simultaneous scanning and imaging. These were later determined to be caused by vibrations of the MR bed induced by the imaging gradients of the 3T MRI.

As shown in Figures 4 and 5, despite periodic phase drift of ±4°C, good temporal and spatial control of temperature was achieved by scanning a 1 mm ultrasound focus along a 5 mm diameter circular trajectory, with power updated every 5 seconds by a single-point proportional-integral controller taking MR temperature measurement as input. To extend these results to *in vivo* MR-guided scanned FUS hyperthermia in small animals, multi-point control [1,5] will be applied to account for anticipated temporal and spatial inhomogeneities in tissue perfusion and absorption.

CONCLUSION

Temporally and spatially uniform hyperthermia using MR-guided scanned focused ultrasound was demonstrated *ex vivo* using a new MRI-compatible transducer positioning system and a basic single-point feedback controller. Simultaneous scanning and temperature imaging resulted in a periodic drift in the baseline phase that increased with increasing speed and decreased with increased image SNR. Future work to reduce phase artifacts by improving the susceptibility profile of the positioning system is warranted, as is the exploration of correction schemes for any remaining scanning-induced periodic phase drift, and evaluation of scanned heating produced by this and other temperature control algorithms *in vivo*.

ACKNOWLEDGMENTS

Funding provided in part by an NSERC Alexander Graham Bell Canada Graduate Scholarship. Hardware and software support for the MR-compatible positioning system were provided by Anthony Chau and Sushil Kumar.

REFERENCES

1. N. B. Smith *et al*, "Control system for an MRI compatible intracavitary ultrasound array for thermal treatment of prostate disease," *Int. J. Hyperthermia* 17(3), 271-282 (2001).
2. B. D. de Senneville *et al*, "Real-time adaptive methods for treatment of mobile organs by MRI-controlled high-intensity focused ultrasound," *MRM* 57, 319-330 (2007).
3. Y. Ishihara *et al*, "A precise and fast temperature mapping using water proton chemical shift," *MRM* 34, 814-823 (1995).
4. H. H. Pennes, "Analysis of tissue and arterial blood temperatures in the resting human forearm," *J. Appl. Physiol.* 1(2), 93-122 (1948).
5. E. Hutchinson, "The feasibility of MRI feedback control for intracavitary phased array hyperthermia treatments," *Int. J. Hyperthermia.* 14(1), 39-56 (1998).

Impact of Focused Ultrasound-enhanced Drug Delivery on Survival in Rats with Glioma

Lisa Hsu Treat[a,b], Yongzhi Zhang[b], Nathan McDannold[b], and Kullervo Hynynen[c]

[a]Harvard-MIT Division of Health Sciences and Technology, 77 Massachusetts Avenue, E25-518, Cambridge, Massachusetts 02139, USA
[b]Department of Radiology, Harvard Medical School and Brigham and Women's Hospital 221 Longwood Avenue, EBRC 521, Boston, Massachusetts 02115, USA
[c]Department of Imaging Research, Sunnybrook Health Sciences Centre, 2075 Bayview Avenue, Room S6 65b, Toronto, Ontario M4N 3M5, Canada

Abstract. Malignancies of the brain remain difficult to treat with chemotherapy because the selective permeability of the blood-brain barrier (BBB) blocks many potent agents from reaching their target. Previous studies have illustrated the feasibility of drug and antibody delivery across the BBB using MRI-guided focused ultrasound. In this study, we investigated the impact of focused ultrasound-enhanced delivery of doxorubicin on survival in rats with aggressive glioma. Sprague-Dawley rats were implanted with 9L gliosarcoma cells in the brain. Eight days after implantation, each rat received one of the following: (1) no treatment (control), (2) a single treatment with microbubble-enhanced MRI-guided focused ultrasound (FUS only), (3) a single treatment with i.v. liposomal doxorubicin (DOX only), or (4) a single treatment with microbubble-enhanced MRI-guided focused ultrasound and concurrent i.v. injections of liposomal doxorubicin (FUS+DOX). The survival time from implantation to death or euthanasia was recorded. We observed a modest but significant increase in median survival time in rats treated with combined MRI-guided focused ultrasound chemotherapy, compared to chemotherapy alone ($p < 0.001$). There was no significant improvement in survival between those who received stand-alone chemotherapy and those who did not receive any treatment ($p > 0.10$). Our study demonstrates for the first time a therapeutic benefit achieved with ultrasound-enhanced drug delivery across the blood-brain barrier. This confirmation of efficacy in an *in vivo* tumor model indicates that targeted drug delivery using MRI-guided focused ultrasound has the potential to have a major impact on the treatment of patients with brain tumors and other neurological disorders.

Keywords: ultrasound, blood-brain barrier, glioma, doxorubicin, drug delivery, survival
PACS: 43.80.Sh, 87.50.yt, 87.61.Tg

INTRODUCTION

The BBB remains a formidable obstacle in the treatment of patients with brain malignancies. Its restrictive permeability prohibits the passage of many therapeutic agents from systemic circulation into brain parenchyma[1,2] or prevents their accumulation at sufficient concentrations.[3] The high spatial resolution and noninvasive nature of ultrasound-induced BBB disruption make it an advantageous technique for targeted drug delivery to the brain. The feasibility of trans-BBB delivery by focused ultrasound has been well established for numerous agents.[4-8] Furthermore, BBB

CP1113, 8th International Symposium on Therapeutic Ultrasound, edited by E. S. Ebbini
© 2009 American Institute of Physics 978-0-7354-0650-6/09/$25.00

disruption by MRI-guided focused ultrasound and concurrent i.v. administration of doxorubicin has been demonstrated to achieve therapeutic drug levels in localized areas of the brain.[7] In this study, we investigated the impact of focused ultrasound-enhanced delivery of doxorubicin across the BBB on survival in rats with aggressive glioma.

MATERIALS AND METHODS

Male Sprague-Dawley rats (~200 g) were anesthetized and the hair covering the top of the head removed. Each rat was implanted with $(0.5 - 1) \times 10^5$ 9L gliosarcoma cells at a depth of 3.5 mm from the dorsal surface of the brain through a burr hole drilled 2 mm lateral to the bregma. Eight days after implantation, each rat received one of the following: (1) no treatment (control), (2) a single treatment with microbubble-enhanced MRI-guided focused ultrasound (FUS only), (3) a single treatment with i.v. liposomal doxorubicin (DOX only), or (4) a single treatment with microbubble-enhanced MRI-guided focused ultrasound and concurrent i.v. injections of liposomal doxorubicin (FUS+DOX).

For groups 2 and 4, the rat was laid on the MR table in a standard 3-Tesla scanner so that its skull was acoustically coupled with degassed water and exposed to pulsed ultrasound from a single-element focused transducer (diameter = 10 cm; radius of curvature = 8 cm; frequency = 1.7 MHz) mounted on a positioning device (Fig. 1). T2-weighted and contrast-enhanced T1-weighted (Magnevist, 0.25 mL/kg) MR images of the brain were obtained to determine the size and location of the tumor. Sonications were pulsed (burst length 10 ms, pulse repetition frequency 1 Hz, duration 60–120 s) at 1-mm spacing targeted in and around the tumor. At the start of each sonication, a bolus of microbubble-based ultrasound contrast agent (Definity, 0.01-0.02 mg/kg) was injected simultaneously into the catheterized tail vein, and flushed with 0.2 mL normal saline. Post-treatment contrast-enhanced T1-weighted MR images were obtained to confirm targeting of ultrasound-induced BBB disruption.

For groups 3 and 4, liposomal doxorubicin (Doxil, 5.67 mg/kg) was injected into the catheterized tail vein at regular intervals following the sonication schedule, each injection followed by 0.2 mL normal saline to flush the catheter. Additional T2-weighted images of the brain were acquired weekly to track tumor growth. Rats were survived up to 55 days after implantation; their date of death was recorded.

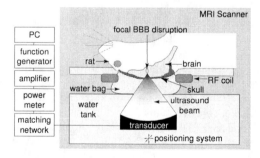

FIGURE 1. Experimental set-up of MRI-guided focused ultrasound for targeted drug delivery.

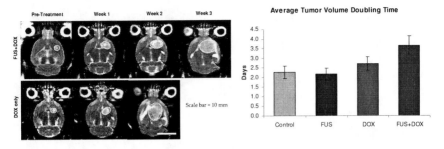

FIGURE 2. *Left*: Weekly T2-weighted MR images of the brain in a rat treated with FUS+DOX (top) and with DOX only (bottom); *Right*: Average tumor volume doubling time by treatment group.

RESULTS

Delayed Tumor Growth in Rats Treated with FUS+DOX

Figure 2 (left panel) shows an example of T2-weighted MR images of the brain of a rat treated with FUS+DOX (top row) and of one treated with DOX only (bottom row). On a week-by-week basis, the rat treated with FUS+DOX seemed to exhibit a tumor growth pattern comparable to that of the rat treated with DOX only until two weeks after treatment, when noticeable differences in the growth patterns emerged. While the tumor in the DOX-only-treated rat continued to grow exponentially ($R^2 = 0.999$) even after treatment, tumor growth in the FUS+DOX-treated rat was visibly delayed, allowing the ultrasound-enhanced treated rat to survive longer.

Exponential growth time constants for each rat were calculated from least-squares regression analyses. Animals in treated with FUS+DOX exhibited an average tumor volume doubling time ($T\_1/2 \pm$ SD) of 3.7 ± 0.5 days, whereas those treated with DOX only had a doubling time $T\_1/2 = 2.7 \pm 0.4$ days. Animals who received FUS only or no treatment exhibited similar tumor growth rates as the latter group with $T\_1/2 = 2.2 \pm 0.3$ days and $T\_1/2 = 2.3 \pm 0.3$ days, respectively. These results confirmed that rats treated with FUS+DOX had longer average tumor volume doubling times than any other group (Fig. 2, right panel).

Improved Survival in Rats Treated with FUS+DOX

Figure 3 shows the Kaplan-Meier estimates of survival in rats which received (1) no treatment (black solid line), (2) FUS only (blue dotted line), (3) DOX only (red dashed line), or (4) FUS+DOX (purple dotted-dashed line). The median survival times for each group were 26, 25, 29, and 33 days, respectively. Thus, rats which received a single treatment of FUS+DOX had a 14-32% greater median survival time than those which did not. Using the Log-Rank test to compare survival curves, we found that the FUS+DOX treatment yielded significantly different survival results than the DOX only treatment ($X^2 = 11.97$, $p < 0.001$). There was no significant difference in survival between animals treated with FUS only and untreated controls.

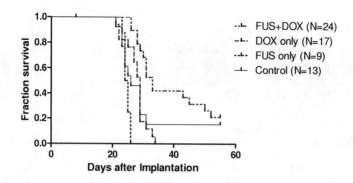

FIGURE 3. Kaplan-Meier survival estimate.

DISCUSSION

While doxorubicin is highly effective against many extracranial cancers, it has been ineffective against malignancies within the brain because it does not readily cross the intact BBB.[3] We have previously demonstrated that it is possible to achieve therapeutic levels of doxorubicin in localized areas of the brain by using MRI-guided focused ultrasound to induce transient BBB disruption in rats.[7] In this study, we have shown that targeted delivery of doxorubicin by ultrasound-induced BBB disruption significantly slows disease progression and improves survival in rats with aggressive glioma. Follow-up MRI confirmed that rats who received the combined treatment experienced slower tumor growth with increased tumor volume doubling times. In addition, rats who received ultrasound-enhanced chemotherapy showed a modest but highly significant increase in median survival time, as well as an increase in the proportion of long-term survivors, compared to those who received stand-alone chemotherapy. Neither ultrasound nor intravenous chemotherapy was sufficient on its own to achieve the improved survival benefit observed when the two treatments were combined. It is likely that the therapeutic benefit of the ultrasound-enhanced treatment resulted primarily from the increased penetration of doxorubicin across the BBB and its accumulation in and around the tumor, thus improving the antitumoral efficacy of the systemic agent.

The enhanced therapeutic efficacy of the combined treatment is attributable to the augmented penetration of doxorubicin through the ultrasound-induced BBB disruption. The interaction of low-power focused ultrasound with intravascular microbubbles is thought induce mechanical stresses on the brain microvascular endothelial wall, which can be exploited to induce focal and transient BBB opening.[9] Immunoelectron microscopy studies indicate that passage through the BBB after treatment with microbubble-enhanced ultrasound occurs via both paracellular and transcellular routes, including (1) open endothelial cell tight junctions (TJ), (2) enhanced active vesicular transport, (3) endothelial cell fenestration and channel formation, and (4) free passage through injured endothelium.[10-12]

CONCLUSIONS

Ultrasound-mediated drug delivery is a novel technique which enables the passage of diagnostic and therapeutic agents across the blood-brain barrier in a noninvasive and localized manner. In this study, ultrasound-enhanced delivery of doxorubicin across the blood-brain barrier is shown to improve survival and slow disease progression in a rodent model of aggressive glioma. This study provides the first *in vivo* demonstration of the therapeutic benefit of this technique, which has the potential to have a major impact on the treatment of patients with malignancies of the central nervous system and other neurological disorders.

ACKNOWLEDGMENTS

This research was supported by NIH grants #R01EB003268 and #U41RR019703. LHT was supported by graduate research fellowships from the MIT Whitaker Health Sciences Fund and from the Harvard-MIT Division of Health Sciences and Technology. Cell cultures (9L GL) were kindly provided by the University of California–San Francisco/Neurosurgery Tissue Bank.

REFERENCES

1. W. M. Pardridge, *Neuron* **36**, 555-558 (2002).
2. S. Banerjee and M. A. Bhat, *Annu. Rev. Neurosci.* **30**, 235-258 (2007).
3. H. von Holst, E. Knochenhauer, H. Blomgren, V. P. Collins, L.Ehn, M. Lindquist, *et al.*, *Acta Neurochir. (Wein)* **104**, 13-16 (1990).
4. M. Kinoshita and K. Hynynen, *Biochem. Biophys. Res.* **335**, 393-399 (2005).
5. M. Kinoshita, N. McDannold, F. A. Jolesz and K. Hynynen, *Biochem. Biophys. Res.* **340**, 1085-1090 (2006).
6. M. Kinoshita, N. McDannold, F. A. Jolesz and K. Hynynen, *Proc. Nat. Acad. Sci. USA* **103**, 11719-11723 (2006).
7. L. H. Treat, N. McDannold, N. Vykhodtseva, Y. Zhang, K. Tam and K. Hynynen, *Int. J. Cancer* **121**, 901-907 (2007).
8. S. B. Raymond, L. H. Treat, J. D. Dewey, N. J. McDannold, K. Hynynen and B. J. Bacskai, *PLoS ONE* **3**, e2175 (2008).
9. K. Hynynen, N. McDannold, N. Vykhodtseva and F. A. Jolesz, *Radiology* **220**, 640-646 (2001).
10. N. Sheikov, N. McDannold, N. Vykhodtseva F. A. Jolesz and K. Hynynen, *Ultrasound Med. Biol.* **30**, 979-989 (2004).
11. N. Sheikov, N. McDannold, F. A. Jolesz, Y. Zhang, K. Tam and K. Hynynen, *Ultrasound Med. Biol.* **32**, 1399-1409 (2006).
12. N. Sheikov, N. McDannold, S. Sharma and K. Hynynen, *Ultrasound Med. Biol.* **34**, 1093-1104 (2008).

Long, T., 246
Lu, X., 30

M

Mahonen, A., 35
Maier, F., 372
Maleke, C., 236
Marsac, L., 18
Martin, E., 397
Maruvada, S., 286, 291
Mast, T. D., 43, 73
Matsumoto, Y., 48, 362, 433
McDannold, N., 443
McGough, R. J., 210
McLaurin, J., 428
Melodelima, D., 101, 139, 144, 175
Merouche, S., 347
Mestas, J.-L., 413
Miller, E. L., 96
Miller, N. R., 175
Milonas, N., 367
Miyata, T., 362
Montaldo, G., 8
Moonen, C. T. W., 159, 228, 231
Morel, A., 397
Moros, E. G., 387
Morrison, B., 25, 408
Mougenot, C., 159, 228, 231, 296
Mukundan, S., 342
Muratore, R., 25
Murillo-Rincon, A., 347
Murray, T. W., 270

N

Nakamura, Y., 433
Nam, K.-H., 124
Nandlall, S. D., 205
Nau, W. H., 318
N'Djin, W. A., 101, 139, 144, 175
Novák, P., 387

O

Ohto, M., 81, 86
Olbricht, W., 403

Olkku, A., 35
Ota, R., 362
Owen, N. R., 347

P

Padilla, F., 185
Park, E.-J., 423
Parker, D., 170, 215
Parmentier, H., 101, 139
Partanen, A., 159, 281, 296
Pauly, K. B., 149
Payne, A., 170, 215
Pernot, M., 8, 18
Petrusca, L., 332
Pichardo, S., 352
Pua, E. C., 30

Q

Qin, J., 337
Quesson, B., 159, 228, 231

R

Raju, B. I., 200
Rapoport, N., 124
Rauschenberg, J., 372
Raymond, J., 96
Rieke, V., 149, 223, 318, 392
Rivoire, M., 101, 139, 144
Roberts, W. W., 129
Robertson, G. P., 423
Roell, S., 215
Roemer, R., 170, 215
Roland, J., 215
Roy, R. A., 270

S

Sakamoto, A., 81, 86
Saletes, I., 53, 413
Salgaonkar, V. A., 73
Salomir, R., 332
Salvador, A., 413
Sankin, G., 337